THE CLINICIAN'S GUIDE TO
Inflammatory
Bowel Disease

THE CLINICIAN'S GUIDE TO
Inflammatory Bowel Disease

Gary R. Lichtenstein, MD

Professor of Medicine
Director, Center for Inflammatory Bowel Disease
Hospital of the University of Pennsylvania
University of Pennsylvania School of Medicine
Department of Medicine
Division of Gastroenterology
Philadelphia, Pennsylvania

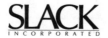

An innovative information, education and management company
6900 Grove Road • Thorofare, NJ 08086

Care has been taken to ensure that drug selection, dosages, and treatments are in accordance with currently accepted/recommended practice. Due to continuing research, changes in government policy and regulations, and various effects of drug reactions and interactions, it is recommended that the reader review all materials and literature provided for each drug use, especially those that are new or not frequently used.

The work SLACK Incorporated publishes is peer reviewed. Prior to publication, recognized leaders in the field, educators, and clinicians provide important feedback on the concept and content that we publish. We welcome feedback on this work.

The clinician's guide to inflammatory bowel disease / edited by Gary R. Lichtenstein.

    p. ; cm.

Includes bibliographical references and index.

ISBN 1-55642-554-6 (alk. paper)

1. Inflammatory bowel diseases--Handbooks, manuals, etc.

[DNLM: 1. Inflammatory Bowel Diseases--Handbooks. WI 39 C641 2003]

I. Lichtenstein, Gary R., 1958-

RC862.I53 C556 2003

616.3'44--dc21

                        2002015488

Printed in the United States of America.

Published by: SLACK Incorporated
                       6900 Grove Road
                       Thorofare, NJ 08086 USA
                       Telephone: 856-848-1000
                       Fax: 856-853-5991
                       www.slackbooks.com

CONTENTS

ACKNOWLEDGMENTS

I am grateful for the wonderful job my fellow contributors have provided. They have done detailed, critical, and well thought-out uniformly superb reviews. I am appreciative that they were able to contribute to this important educational endeavor during their already busy schedules. My sincere gratitude is also expressed to the staff at SLACK Incorporated for their outstanding editorial assistance and guidance with this handbook. Lastly, I am most appreciative and extend my thanks to my family, colleagues, patients, and those who have supported my research in the field and have enabled me to care for patients and extend the boundary of my knowledge to uncover new material for patients with inflammatory bowel disease.

POTENTIAL CONFLICT OF INTEREST DECLARATION	
Centocor, Inc.	Consultant, Research, Speakers Bureau
Celltech, Inc.	Research
Inkine, Inc.	Research
Intesco Corp.	Research
Astra-Zenecca, Inc.	Speakers Bureau, Consultant
Solvay Pharmaceuticals	Speakers Bureau, Consultant
Faro Pharmaceuticals	Speaker's Bureau
Celgene Corp.	Research
Otsuka, Corp.	Research
Abbott Corp.	Research
Proctor and Gamble	Speaker's Bureau, Consultant
Smith Kline Beecham Corp.	Consultant
Protein Design Labs	Consultant, Research
Shire Pharmaceuticals	Consultant, Speakers Bureau
Salix Pharmaceuticals	Consultant, Speaker's Bureau, Research
Protomed Scientific	Research, Consultant
ISIS Corporation	Research
Genetics Institute	Research
Axcan Corp.	Speakers Bureau, Consultant

About the Contributors

Jean-Paul Achkar, MD
Department of Gastroenterology
The Cleveland Clinic Foundation
Cleveland, Ohio

Mohammed Al Haddad, MD
Department of Gastroenterology
The Cleveland Clinic Foundation
Cleveland, Ohio

Robert N. Baldassano, MD
Division of Gastroenterology and Nutrition
Children's Hospital of Philadelphia
Philadelphia, Pennsylvania

L. Arturo Batres, MD
Division of Gastroenterology and Nutrition
Children's Hospital of the King's Daughters
Norfolk, Virginia

Alain Bitton, MD, FRCPC
McGill University Health Centre
Royal Victoria Hospital Site
Division of Gastroenterology
Montreal, Quebec

David Black, MD
McGill University Health Centre
Royal Victoria Hospital Site
Division of Gastroenterology
Montreal, Quebec

Brian Brauer, MD
Washington University School of Medicine
St. Louis, Missouri

Alan L. Buchman, MD, MSPH
Norwestern University Medical School
Division of Gastroenterology and Hepatology
Chicago, Illinois

Russell D. Cohen, MD
Department of Medicine, Section of Gastroenterology
The University of Chicago Medical Center
Chicago, Illinois

Francis A. Farraye, MD, MSc
Section of Gastroenterology
Boston University School of Medicine
Boston Medical Center
Boston, Massachusetts

Brian G. Feagan, MD
Robarts Clinical Trials
London, Ontario

David G. Forcione, MD
Harvard Medical School
Gastrointestinal Unit
Massachusetts General Hospital
Boston, Massachusetts

Lawrence S. Friedman, MD
Harvard Medical School
Gastrointestinal Unit
Massachusetts General Hospital
Boston, Massachusetts

Peter D. Han, MD
Department of Medicine, Section of Gastroenterology
The University of Chicago Medical Center
Chicago, Illinois

Jeffry A. Katz, MD
Department of Gastroenterology
Case Western Reserve University School of Medicine
University Hospitals of Cleveland
Cleveland, Ohio

Walter A. Koltun, MD
Peter and Marshia Carlino Professor of Inflammatory Bowel Disease
Chief, Section of Colon and Rectal Surgery
Penn State Milton S. Hershey Medical Center
Hershey, Pennsylvania

Asher Kornbluth, MD
The Henry D. Janowitcz Division of Gastroenterology
The Mount Sinai Medical Center
New York, New York

Joshua R. Korzenik, MD
Washington University School of Medicine
St. Louis, Missouri

Bret A. Lashner, MD
Center for Inflammatory Bowel Disease
Department of Gastroenterology
The Cleveland Clinic Foundation
Cleveland, Ohio

Thomas Lee, MD
Norwestern University Medical School
Division of Gastroenterology and Hepatology
Chicago, Illinois

Peter Legnani, MD
The Henry D. Janowitcz Division of Gastroenterology
The Mount Sinai Medical Center
New York, New York

Norman Marcon, MD
The Centre for Therapeutic Endoscopy and Endoscopic Oncology
St. Michael's Hospital
Toronto, Ontario

Jaime Oviedo, MD
Section of Gastroenterology
Boston University School of Medicine
Boston Medical Center
Boston, Massachusetts

Lisa S. Poritz, MD
Section of Colon and Rectal Surgery
Penn State Milton S. Hershey Medical Center
Hershey, Pennsylvania

James S. Scolapio, MD
Mayo Clinic
Division of Gastroenterology and Hepatology
Jacksonville, Florida

Enrico Souto, MD
The Centre for Therapeutic Endoscopy and Endoscopic Oncology
St. Michael's Hospital
Toronto, Ontario

Radhika Srinivasan, MD
University of Pennsylvania School of Medicine
Presbyterian Medical Center
Philadelphia, Pennsylvania

Chinyu Su, MD
University of Pennsylvania School of Medicine
Presbyterian Medical Center
Philadelphia, Pennsylvania

Richmond Sy, MD
St. Joseph's Hospital
London, Ontario

PREFACE

It is an exciting time for gastroenterologists caring for patients with inflammatory bowel disease (IBD). IBD constitutes multisystem disorders of uncertain origin. Since Drs. Crohn, Ginzburg, and Opppenheimer were credited with the initial description of Crohn's disease in 1932 in the *Journal of the American Medical Association,* and Drs. Wilks and Moxon were credited with the original description of ulcerative colitis in 1875, a significant amount of information has been learned about these disorders. Both disorders are found worldwide and they spare no socioeconomic group. These disorders are effectively treated with many different medications; however, approximately 25% of patients with ulcerative colitis will undergo surgery, and over half the patients with Crohn's disease will follow similar suit despite our best efforts to do so.

In the development of this handbook, entitled *The Clinician's Guide to Inflammatory Bowel Disease,* a highly talented and internationally renown group of sophisticated physician-scientists has been assimilated to present an up-to-date guide of the current status of selected topics in IBD. This handbook, which is intended to be a user-friendly manual, has a primary clinical focus for the clinician—whether he or she is a gastroenterologist, medical student, fellow, resident, specialist, internist, or family practitioner. The articles in this book focus on many of the advances established in various areas of IBD, highlighting many sophisticated topics. These issues will not only inform physicians of the recent progress that has been made in these specific areas, but they will also prepare the physician for the future.

The varied subjects covered in this book encompass a broad scope, however, not every aspect of IBD is focused upon. Rather, those clinically important areas that have undergone recent changes or discoveries will be addressed.

Gary R. Lichtenstein, MD

chapter 1

Epidemiology of Inflammatory Bowel Disease

Brian G. Feagan, MD and Richmond Sy, MD

Although the term *inflammatory bowel disease (IBD)* describes a wide range of inflammatory states, it generally refers to ulcerative colitis and Crohn's disease. Methodologically rigorous studies, which evaluate the epidemiology of these disorders, are relatively rare. Furthermore, much of the available literature is limited by referral bias and inadequate case definition. The latter issue is particularly relevant since the current concept that Crohn's disease and ulcerative colitis are unique entities has been challenged by recent genetic discoveries. Nevertheless, our current phenotypic-based classification is clinically useful and provides a valuable framework for research. Ultimately, a more sophisticated classification scheme will evolve that will further assist epidemiological studies.

DESCRIPTIVE EPIDEMIOLOGY

INCIDENCE AND PREVALENCE RATES

For the most part, ulcerative colitis and Crohn's disease are diseases of young people. However, the distribution of the age of onset is bimodal with the greatest incidence in adolescents and young adults and a second, smaller peak between the fifth and eighth decades. Although some studies suggest a difference in gender ratio (a small female preponderance for Crohn's disease and a male preponderance for ulcerative colitis), this finding has not been consistent. Moreover, in those studies that identified such a difference the absolute magnitude of the variance was small. Overall, the evidence suggests that ulcerative colitis and Crohn's disease affect males and females equally.

In recent studies the incidence (ie, the number of new cases per annum) of Crohn's disease and ulcerative colitis is approximately 4 to 7/100,000 and 7 to 15/100,000, respectively. A striking observation is that the incidence of Crohn's disease increased three to six fold in the interval between 1960 and 1980. Although improved diagnostic testing and increased awareness of the disease by clinicians may partially explain this phenomenon, it seems highly likely that a real increase in incidence has occurred. No satisfactory explanation has been accepted for this "epidemic;" however, the data strongly suggest an underlying environmental cause. In more recent years this increase in incidence has stabilized. In comparison, during the same period of observation, a relatively stable incidence has been observed for ulcerative colitis.

Prevalence refers to the number of individuals with a given condition residing in a specific jurisdiction at a specific time. Current estimates of the prevalence of Crohn's disease and ulcerative colitis are 100 to 200/100,000 and 150 to 250/100,000, respectively. It is noteworthy that the prevalence of IBD varies considerably by geographic location with the highest rates originating in Northern Europe and Canada.

MORTALITY AND MORBIDITY

Mortality

A modest increase in mortality is present in most population-based studies. In a typical study, performed in Sweden, the observed survival rate following 15 years of disease was 93.7% (95% confidence interval [CI] 91.8% to 95.7%) of that expected for the general population for patients with Crohn's disease and 94.2% (95% CI 92.4% to 96.1%) for those with ulcerative colitis. Patients with pancolitis are at increased risk, especially during the first attack of the disease. Accordingly, the standardized mortality ratio is increased the first year following a diagnosis of ulcerative colitis.

Morbidity

Very few large-scale studies have evaluated the burden of these diseases. Because IBD develops early in life, a large socioeconomic effect might be anticipated. Several studies have documented increased rates of chronic disability and unemployment. Because surgery is frequently required to treat either disease related complications or patients who become refractory to medical management, the rate of hospitalization is also increased.

RISK FACTORS AND IBD

Identification of risk factors is an important goal for epidemiologists because better understanding of pathological mechanisms may result in new concepts of causation or treatment. The most popular model of pathogenesis speculates that these disorders are the consequence of an interaction existing between environmental and genetic factors. Accordingly, genetically susceptible individuals who encounter specific environmental triggers develop an abnormal immune response that leads to chronic inflammation and tissue damage. Several risk factors are well established in IBD while others remain tenuous.

ENVIRONMENTAL RISK FACTORS

Cigarette Smoking

The intriguing relationship between smoking and IBD was first identified in the early 1980s. Since then numerous studies have demonstrated a consistent finding—Crohn's disease is positively associated with cigarette smoking, while a negative association exits between smoking and ulcerative colitis.

In various studies the relative risk of developing Crohn's disease among current smokers and ex-smokers has been estimated to be 1.2 to 3.9 and 0.8 to 3.2, respectively. Similarly, patients with Crohn's disease in remission who are ex-smokers or nonsmokers have a lower risk of developing a disease exacerbation than those who continue to smoke. For example, in a Canadian study the annual risk of relapse was 53% in smokers compared with 30% in nonsmokers and 35% in ex-smokers. These findings have been confirmed by other investigators. In a European cohort study weight loss and diarrhea were more prominent in smokers than nonsmokers, suggesting that the harmful effects of smoking may selectively influence specific symptoms. A multivariate analysis found smoking status to be the only definable predictor of surgical recurrence (hazard ratio 2.0). Thus, although data from randomized trials of smoking cessation are lacking, the results of observational studies strongly indicate that smoking may worsen the clinical course of Crohn's disease and increase the risk of disease development in individuals at risk. Given this information, notwithstanding the other harmful effects of smoking, gastroenterologists should strongly advocate smoking cessation for patients with Crohn's disease and their first-degree relatives.

Remarkably, smoking is inversely associated with the risk of developing ulcerative colitis. Caulkins and colleagues who performed a meta-analysis of epidemiological studies estimated that the risk of developing ulcerative colitis among smokers is only 40% that of nonsmokers. The risk also was greater for ex-smokers compared with those who have never smoked. Limited evidence also indicates that smoking may ameliorate disease severity; a lower rate of hospitalization in smokers compared to nonsmokers has been reported.

As a result of these observations, mechanistic studies have examined the potential effects of smoking on immune function and intestinal permeability.

Although some plausible biologic effects have been demonstrated, these findings do not adequately explain the epidemiological observations. Randomized controlled trials have evaluated the efficacy of the nicotine patch in patients with active colitis. In one trial, 49% of patients assigned to receive nicotine entered remission, as compared with 24% of patients who received a placebo. However, no anti-inflammatory effect was demonstrated on colonic biopsies. Moreover, a second trial failed to demonstrate a benefit of nicotine as a maintenance therapy. Although some experts have suggested that patients with refractory symptoms might be encouraged to smoke, in our opinion it is inappropriate to advocate this practice.

Oral Contraceptives

The relationship between oral contraceptive use and IBD is controversial. Smoking may be a confounding factor because oral contraceptive use is more common among smokers. Nevertheless, the previously described rise in the incidence of Crohn's disease closely parallels the increased use of oral contraceptives. A case control study found an increased risk of both Crohn's and ulcerative colitis in women who reported use of oral contraceptives within 6 months of disease onset (relative risk [RR] 2.0, 95% CI 1.2 to 3.3 for ulcerative colitis and an RR of 2.6, 95% CI 1.8 to 14.3 for Crohn's disease). The relative risk decreased on discontinuation of oral contraceptive use after 4 years to 1.2 (95% CI 0.5 to 2.6) for Crohn's disease. Another study found a positive interaction with smoking; the odds ratio for developing the disease in women who had both risk factors was estimated to be 2.64 (95% CI 1.22 to 5.75). Data regarding oral contraceptive use and ulcerative colitis are less clear. In one study a positive association was demonstrated with a relative risk of 2.5. In contrast, multiple studies have not identified any association between oral contraceptive use and IBD. These contradictory findings may be due to differences in estrogen formulation since most oral contraceptives in current use have a much lower concentration of estrogen than those previously available. At the present time insufficient evidence exists to recommend discontinuation of oral contraceptives in patients with IBD.

Geography

IBD is more common in northern latitudes. Accordingly, the United States, Canada, the United Kingdom, and the Scandinavian countries have the highest reported incidence of the disease. In contrast, countries such as South Africa, Australia, and southern Europe have low incidence rates. IBD is rare in Asia and South America. A European study found an 80% increase in the incidence of Crohn's disease and a 40% increase in the risk of ulcerative colitis in the north of Europe in comparison to the south. This difference was not explained by differences in smoking. Although the basis for this observation remains unknown, differences in exposure to sunlight, experience with infectious agents, and physical activity have been suggested as potential explanations. It is noteworthy that the north-south gradient is not likely explainable on the basis of genetic differences. Perhaps the gradient is unstable; some southern countries now report incidence rates that are similar to their northern neighbors.

Limited evidence exists that indicates IBD is more common in urban centers. IBD may also be more common in people with high socioeconomic status. Although risk factors such as exposure to pollutants or toxins, increased indoor activity, and infectious agents have also been suggested, the potential interactions among place of residence, lifestyle, socioeconomic class, and environmental exposure are complex.

Diet

The concept of a dietary etiology is attractive to patients. Nevertheless, multiple studies have consistently been unable to identify any dietary factor that increases the risk of IBD. The possible roles of refined sugars, fish, fruits, vegetables, margarine, and coffee have been evaluated. Although some studies have demonstrated an increased consumption of carbohydrates among patients, it is plausible that this finding is a consequence of the disease rather than a causal factor.

Nonsteroidal Anti-Inflammatory Drugs

The potential causative role of nonsteroidal anti-inflammatory drugs (NSAIDs) is controversial. Much of the available literature regarding the subject consists of case reports. The possibility that NSAIDs might make IBD worse is plausible biologically. Animals treated with indomethacin develop colitis and patients with rheumatoid arthritis have been shown to develop ulceration of the small bowel with chronic administration. However, strong scientific evidence that shows NSAIDs either cause IBD or consistently cause worsening of existing disease is lacking.

Mycobacteria

The search for a bacterial agent has continued since the first description of these diseases. Most of this activity has focused on Crohn's disease in which *Mycobacterium avium* subspecies paratuberculosis is the leading candidate. This organism causes Johne's disease, an IBD of ruminants. *M. paratuberculosis* is widely dispersed in the environment, and people are exposed through consumption of contaminated food, milk, and water. However, epidemiological data are inconsistent with a causal role for this organism since spouses of patients with Crohn's disease are not at increased risk. Moreover, immunological and genetic testing have not shown evidence of persistent infection. Finally, randomized controlled trials of antimycobacterial therapy have failed to show a benefit on the course of the disease.

Measles Virus

Crohn's disease has pathological features that are consistent with a focal granulomatous vasculitis similar to that found in some viral infections. Subsequent to a report that identified paramyxovirus-like particles from vascular endothelial cells in the colon of patients with Crohn's disease multiple investigations focused on measles virus as a potential cause of the disease. However, these studies did not consistently identify measles virus genetic material or evidence of a host immune response to this pathogen.

Appendectomy

An inverse relationship has been shown between appendectomy and the development of ulcerative colitis. A Belgian cohort study found that patients who underwent appendectomy for a perforated appendix before the age of 20 had a marked reduction in the risk of developing ulcerative colitis (hazard ratio 0.58, 95% CI 0.38 to 0.87). Interestingly, those patients who underwent an appendectomy for reasons other than appendicitis had the same risk of developing ulcerative colitis as the control population (adjusted hazard ratio of 1.06, 95% CI 0.74 to 1.52). It is possible that the protective effects of appendectomy may be the result of functional changes in the immune system that occur following this surgery.

GENETIC RISK FACTORS

Several lines of evidence support the role of genetic factors in the etiology of IBD. Identification of disease specific genes is complex because these diseases do not follow a simple mendelian pattern of inheritance. Moreover, a considerable degree of overlap probably exists among clinical phenotypes. Despite these difficulties, considerable progress has been made in this area over the past decade.

Familial Aggregation

Five percent to 10% of patients have a first-degree relative with IBD. In a European study, the risk of developing Crohn's disease was increased 35 times in first-degree relatives whereas the risk of developing ulcerative colitis was increased 15 fold. In a study of Ashkenazi Jews, the lifetime risk of developing IBD among first-degree relatives was 8.9% in offspring, 8.8% in siblings, and 3.5% for parents. Usually, concordance is observed; relatives of people with Crohn's disease tend to develop Crohn's rather than ulcerative colitis. Several studies have not documented any increase in disease incidence among spouses of patients with IBD, which confirms that genetic rather than environmental factors are responsible for the previously described observations.

Twin studies also provide strong evidence for the importance of genetic factors. In a Danish study, 5 out of 10 monozygotic twin pairs were concordant for Crohn's disease whereas none of 27 dizygotic twins were concordant. For ulcerative colitis, three of 21 monozygotic pairs were concordant while two of 44 dizygotic twins were concordant. Another study from Scotland demonstrated a 50% concordance rate for monozygotic twins in Crohn's disease compared with a 3% rate in dizygotic twins and 2% in other siblings. These data suggest that genetic factors are more important in Crohn's disease rather than ulcerative colitis.

Race/Ethnicity

Assessment of the influence of race on IBD is difficult because the issue is both sensitive and hard to quantify. Measurement of the effects of race may also be confounded by cultural factors such as eating habits and health practices.

Nonetheless, the increased incidence of IBD in Ashkenazi Jews is well documented. In this population the incidence of Crohn's disease is increased three to eight fold whereas ulcerative colitis is two to four times as common.

Gene Identification

The application of linkage disequilibrium studies in multiplex families has yielded the first of what will undoubtedly be many outstanding discoveries. Two groups of investigators independently identified a Crohn's disease susceptibility gene in 2001. The NOD2 gene, located on chromosome 16, codes for a protein that is analogous to plant disease resistance gene products. Normally, the wild type protein activates nuclear factor NF-kappaβ making it responsive to bacterial lipopolysaccharides. It is speculated that patients with this defect respond inappropriately to endogenous gut bacteria and thus develop chronic intestinal inflammation. Although further phenotypic and genotypic characterization of patients has only just begun, it has already been demonstrated that mutations in NOD confer a greater likelihood of developing ileal and right colonic disease. Although patients with defects in NOD2 are in a minority, this finding demonstrates the potential for genetic discoveries to change our approach to phenotypic classification.

With respect to ulcerative colitis considerable evidence exists for an association between HLA class II haplotypes and increased risk of the disease. Specifically, multiple studies have shown an association with HLA DR 2. Since the products of HLA class II genes are essential to immune regulation, it is easy to speculate how genetic variability might increase susceptibility to ulcerative colitis.

FUTURE DIRECTIONS

The identification of specific gene associations will greatly enhance future epidemiological studies. If the current theory of pathogenesis is correct, both environmental and genetic factors must contribute to disease development. In the future, prospective cohort studies performed in individuals at increased genetic risk must be performed to clarify the potential role of putative environmental factors. Assessment of gene-environment interactions has become the next frontier in the quest to determine the cause of IBD.

BIBLIOGRAPHY

Andersson RE, Olaison G, Tysk C, Ekbom A. Appendectomy and protection against ulcerative colitis. *New Engl J Med.* 2001;344(11):808-814.

Andres PG, Friedman LS. Epidemiology and the natural course of inflammatory bowel disease. *Gastro Clin N Am.* 1999;28(2):255-281.

Binder V. Genetic epidemiology in inflammatory bowel disease. *Dig Dis.* 1998;16(6):351-355.

Boyko EJ, Perera DR, Koepsell TD, Keane EM, Inui TS. Effects of cigarette smoking on the clinical course of ulcerative colitis. *Scand J Gastroenterol.* 1988;23(9):1147-1152.

Boyko EJ, Theis MK, Vaughan TL, Nicol-Blades B. Increased risk of inflammatory bowel disease associated with oral contraceptive use. *Am J Epidemiol.* 1994;140(3):268-278.

Calkins BM. A meta-analysis of the role of smoking in inflammatory bowel disease. *Dig Dis Sci.* 1989;34(12):1841-1854.

Chamberlain W, Graham DY, Hulten K, et al. Review article: mycobacterium avium subsp. Paratuberculosis as one cause of Crohn's disease. *Aliment Pharmacol Ther.* 2001;15(3):337-346.

Cosnes J, Beaugerie L, Carbonnel F, Gendre JP. Smoking cessation and the course of Crohn's disease: an intervention study. *Gastroenterology.* 2001;120(5):1093-1099.

Ekbom A, Helmick CG, Zack M, Holmberg L, Adami HO. Survival and causes of death in patients with inflammatory bowel disease: a population-based study. *Gastroenterology.* 1992;103(3):954-960.

Orholm M, Binder V, Sorensen TI, Rasmussen LP, Kyvik KO. Concordance of inflammatory bowel disease among Danish twins. Results of a nationwide survey. *Scan J Gastroenterol.* 2000;35(10):1075-1081.

Persson PG, Bernell O, Leijonmarck CE, Farahmand BY, Hellers G, Ahlbom A. Survival and cause-specific mortality in inflammatory bowel disease: a population-based cohort study. *Gastroenterology.* 1996;110(5):1339-1345.

Pullan RD, Rhodes J, Ganesh S, et al. Transdermal nicotine for active ulcerative colitis. *N Engl J Med.* 1994;330(12):811-815.

Rubin DT, Hanauer SB. Smoking and inflammatory bowel disease. *Eur J Gastroenterol Hepatol.* 2000;12(8):855-862.

Russel MG, Stockbrugger RW. Epidemiology of inflammatory bowel disease: an update. *Scan J Gastroenterol.* 1996;31:417-427.

Russel MG, Volovics A, Schoon EJ, et al. Inflammatory bowel disease: is there any relation between smoking status and disease presentation? European Collaborative IBD Study Group. *Inflamm Bowel Dis.* 1998;4(3):182-186.

Shivananda S, Lennard-Jones J, Logan R, et al. Incidence of inflammatory bowel disease across Europe: is there a difference between north and south? Results of the European Collaborative Study on Inflammatory Bowel Disease (EC-IBD). *Gut.* 1996;39(5):690-697.

Thomas GAO, Rhodes J, Mani V. Transdermal nicotine as maintenance therapy for ulcerative colitis. *New Engl J Med.* 1995;332:998.

Timmer A, Sutherland LR, Martin F. Oral contraceptive use and smoking are risk factors for relapse in Crohn's disease. The Canadian Mesalamine for Remission of Crohn's Disease Study Group. *Gastroenterology.* 1998;114(6):1143-1150.

Vessey M, Jewell D, Smith A, Yeates D, McPherson K. Chronic inflammatory bowel disease, cigarette smoking, and use of oral contraceptives: findings in a large cohort study of women of childbearing age. *Br Med J (Clin Res Ed).* 1986;292(6528):1101-1103.

chapter 2

Imaging in Inflammatory Bowel Disease

Enrico Souto, MD and Norman E. Marcon, MD

INTRODUCTION

Inflammatory bowel disease (IBD) is an idiopathic, chronic intestinal condition with diverse clinical presentations and courses. Imaging techniques are crucial for the disease management, helping to establish the correct diagnosis, determine severity and extent of disease, as well as monitor response to therapy.[1] Radiologic and endoscopic techniques are complementary[2] and should be both considered, at any stage of the disease, for a more complete evaluation of the patient's condition. Both techniques are sensitive and safe, but a clear understanding of their diagnostic yield and associated complications is essential for their optimal use in the different situations that one faces when caring for a patient with IBD.

Endoscopy is the most sensitive means for evaluating mucosal changes and is especially useful in patients with a mild disease. Moreover, endoscopy can provide important histologic information. It is the only procedure available for colorectal neoplasia surveillance in IBD. In selected cases, therapeutic endoscopic procedures, such as stricture dilation,[3-5] stent placement,[6] and bleeding control techniques, can also be safely performed with a great impact in the patient's management.

Endoscopic techniques are limited for defining IBD involvement of the colon, terminal ileum, and upper gastrointestinal (GI) tract. However, novel techniques, such as wireless capsule diagnostic endoscopy,[7] are under investigation that promises accurate assessment of the extent of small bowel disease in Crohn's disease (CD).

GI radiology, although less invasive and expensive, has been replaced by endoscopy in most of its indications, but it still has a definitive role in some aspects of IBD. Its major applications in IBD are for the evaluation of complicating strictures, fistulas, and masses or whenever endoscopy is contraindicated (eg, toxic megacolon or suspicious free bowel perforation). It is also pivotal in the assessment of the small bowel, where endoscopic evaluation has always been limited (as discussed above).

DIAGNOSING INFLAMMATORY BOWEL DISEASE

The initial IBD diagnosis can be a challenge,[1] as a variety of conditions share the same clinical presentations (Table 2-1). Infectious and ischemic colitis are on the top of the long list of differential diagnosis and can be difficult conditions to rule out. As no specific finding or serologic marker has yet been shown to be pathognomonic of IBD, its diagnosis is in most part one of exclusion and can usually only be firmly defined after a close follow-up of the patient's condition and response to therapy.

Mucosal artifacts induced by colonic cleansing agents can occasionally pose a diagnostic dilemma. Sodium phosphate oral lavage, for example, was shown to induce aphthoid-like lesions in a normal colon, similar to the ones seen in CD,[8] and for that reason it should be avoided as a colonoscopy preparation solution in patients suspected of having IBD.

The first step in a diagnostic evaluation of a patient suspected of having IBD is to confirm the presence of mucosal inflammation and determine the pattern and extent of disease involvement. Particular types of mucosal abnormality and disease distribution are usually more accurate in defining a specific IBD diagnosis than a histopathologic examination of mucosal biopsy.

Endoscopy is the procedure of choice for this initial evaluation. It has great accuracy in defining mucosal abnormalities and can precisely establish the limits of disease involvement in the colon when combined with histopathologic information.

Endoscopy is also helpful in differentiating types of IBD.[9,10] For example, no other imaging technique can demonstrate the violaceous hue of ischemic mucosal injury, a tip-off that neither corticosteroids nor antibiotics are required.

In most patients with colitis, a full colonoscopy (including a terminal ileum examination) with colonic preparation can be safely performed. However, a limited colonoscopy without colonic preparation is usually preferred in patients with severe colitis. Multiple mucosal biopsies should be obtained during the procedure. Another option for extremely sick colitis patients is the use

Table 2-1

DIFFERENTIAL DIAGNOSIS OF INFLAMMATORY BOWEL DISEASE

- Infectious colitis
- Ischemic colitis
- Pseudomembranous and drug-induced colitis
- Microscopic colitis
- Radiation colopathy
- Malignancy (eg, lymphoma)
- Diversion colitis
- Diverticulitis
- Behçet's syndrome
- Graft-versus-host disease

of a very small scope (6 mm outer diameter) for assessment of the rectum and sigmoid. This technique virtually eliminates the risk of perforation and gives an accurate impression of disease severity with more patient comfort. Proximal extent is then determined radiologically, using supine flat plate or computed tomography (CT), looking for mucosal edema.

The definition of the specific type of IBD has great impact on the patient's management and prognosis but can be equally challenging, as ulcerative colitis and Crohn's colitis can present with overlapping features. *Indeterminate colitis* is the term used when this distinction cannot be made and occurs in 5% to 10% of IBD patients.

ULCERATIVE COLITIS

In ulcerative colitis (UC), the inflammatory response is directed exclusively to the colon and is limited to the mucosa and submucosa. The colon is usually involved in a circumferential, contiguous pattern, and the disease starts at the rectum in 95% of cases. Rectum sparing should raise the possibility of a different diagnosis or a previous local treatment, such as the use of suppositories or retention enema. The disease distribution in UC is extremely helpful in differentiating it from CD.

The disease presentation varies accordingly with the distribution, severity, and duration of the inflammatory response. The disease can be limited to the rectum or involve the whole colon. At early stages, loss of vascular pattern and congestion will dominate the picture. As mucosal congestion becomes more prominent, edema and friability occur. The edematous mucosa acquires a sandpaper-like appearance and bleeding occurs in response to minor trauma. In more severe cases, disruption of the colonic mucosa develops and can progress from superficial erosions to large, deep ulcerations that can eventually coalesce to form areas of completely destroyed mucosa. In these denuded areas, isolated, congested mucosal remnants can acquire the appearance of a mucosal bridge or form polyp-like projections, known as *pseudopolyps* or *inflammatory polyps*. Pseudopolyps follow disease distribution and can be found throughout the colon, although they are relatively uncommon in the rectum.[11] Occasionally, they can be associated with chronic bleeding or be large enough to cause obstructive symptoms. Usually, pseudopolyps do not pose any clinical significance, other than causing differential diagnostic dilemmas with adenomatous and malignant polyps in patients with long-standing disease during surveillance.

In patients with severe colitis, toxic damage to neural plexus and muscularis propria may lead to neuromuscular dysfunction. This can result in progressive colonic dilation associated with signs of severe systemic compromise, a condition known as *toxic megacolon*. This ominous condition, although more frequently associated with UC, can also occur in CD.

In 10% to 20% of patients with UC who present with pancolitis the terminal ileum can be involved with mild inflammation, with similar characteristics as in the colon (backwash ileitis). Macroscopically, the usual findings consist of erythema, abnormal vascular pattern, and superficial erosions in the distal 5 cm of the terminal ileum. They are almost always associated with a dilated, patulous ileocecal valve. Although terminal ileum involvement in UC is never symptomatic, the recognition of backwash ileitis can be of clinical significance, as there is data demonstrating that it causes an increased risk of colorectal cancer.[12] The reason for the association is not clear.

Finally, at advanced stages, there is colonic shortening with loss of haustral folds that is caused by muscularis mucosa thickening and submucosal fibrosis. This gives the colon a "pipe" appearance on endoscopy and barium enema.

ENDOSCOPY

Lower Flexible GI Endoscopy
(Colonoscopy and Flexible Sigmoidoscopy)

The management of IBD, and particularly of UC, has been strongly influenced by the development of a thinner endoscope with better image resolution that permits a more thorough mucosal evaluation with a better safety and comfort profile. Different types of endoscopes can be selected according to the patient's clinical condition. Usually any full-length colonoscope (165 cm), whether regular (12 mm) or pediatric (10 mm), is appropriate for a complete evaluation of the colon and terminal ileum. A pediatric colonoscope is particularly useful in patients suspected of having strictures. When the disease is very active, the use of a regular or pediatric gastroscope (because of their smaller diameter and increased flexibility) almost completely eliminates the risk of colonic perforation, while providing quick distal colonic examination. When a very tight, distal stricture is present, a transnasal-type (6 mm) endoscope can be used. This ultra-thin scope can be advanced through tight strictures with minimal trauma, so the stricture itself and the adjacent colon can be observed appropriately and biopsied. This technique is also useful for guidewire placement through a stricture, so a balloon dilation can be safely performed. When a colonoscopy is predicted to be technically challenging, the use of fluoroscopy may be of great help in selected cases.

Currently, a complete colonoscopic exam with cecum visualization can be safely and successfully performed in at least 98% of nonobstructed cases.[13] The use of colonic cleansing agents for an optimal colonoscopic examination is the main limitation for the procedure in patients with severe symptoms. These agents, such as a polyethylene glycol based-solution, can contribute to further metabolic and electrolyte imbalances in patients with already severely compromised general clinical status, and can precipitate the development of toxic megacolon. Although disease severity is a relative contraindication to endoscopy, patients with severe symptoms can still have a limited examination (the extent of the examination is determined by the degree of difficult and severity of disease) without a colonic cleansing, but enabling examination of rectum and sigmoid.

The most common indications for colonoscopy in UC are listed in Table 2-2. Colonoscopy is pivotal for the establishment of disease diagnosis, the determination of the disease extent and activity, and to monitor a response to therapy. As UC characteristically involves the rectum, extending proximally and circumferentially, for the initial diagnosis or for the evaluation of a recent flare up a limited examination of the rectum and sigmoid is usually sufficient. UC can involve the whole colon or only part of it, usually with an abrupt demarcation of diseased mucosa from normal mucosa and formed stool. The determination of disease distribution has a great impact for patient management and prognosis, and can be outlined by a full colonoscopy with an optimal colonic cleansing that is usually performed after the disease activity is under control. A careful inspection of the mucosa with an appropriate biopsy is then performed. Colonic biopsies should be obtained from the involved and adjacent normal-appearing mucosa, as the disease activity may not be apparent macroscopically.[14] The terminal ileum should be examined in patients with pancolitis. As discussed above, the presence of backwash ileitis may be significant in determining the patient's risk of colorectal cancer. On the other hand, the finding of severe terminal ileum ulceration associated with strictures will point the diagnosis toward CD instead of UC.

Endoscopically, a normal colonic mucosa is salmon-pink, smooth, and has a delicate visible network of finely branching vessels. In UC, diffuse erythema and vascular congestion represent the earliest findings. The delicate vascular network is replaced by irregular, engorged, and tortuous vessels. As the disease progresses, edema and friability develop; the mucosa acquires a granular, sandpaper appearance. Bleeding easily occurs with the touch of the scope. Ulcers and yellowish exudate develop and become progressively more prominent in a gross correlation with the patient's clinical condition. Spasm and loss of normal distensibility can also be observed, especially in the rectum.

Table 2-2

INDICATIONS FOR LOWER ENDOSCOPY IN INFLAMMATORY BOWEL DISEASE

- Early diagnosis
- Disease extension and activity
- Perioperative evaluation
- Postoperative follow-up
- Monitor therapy
- Stricture management
- Cancer screening

As the healing process continues, an improvement of the mucosal friability and vascular pattern associated with scar and pseudopolyp formation, as well as the presence of solid stools, can be observed. Pseudopolyps can be numerous and involve the whole colon. They usually have an uniform appearance and whenever one differs from the surroundings, it should be sampled histologically to rule out another possible diagnosis. Although pseudopolyps are rarely symptomatic they can spontaneously bleed and present as new onset of hematochezia, which can be confused with flare up of UC in a patient with quiescent disease. Rarely, giant pseudopolyps cause obstructive symptoms. They can be removed with a snare when symptomatic.

Endoscopic Ultrasound

The role of endoscopic ultrasound (EUS) for the evaluation of UC is yet to be clearly defined, but it is likely to be minor. For example, it may be helpful in distinguishing UC from CD by demonstrating the depth of mucosal involvement. Additionally, an ultrasound probe may be of potential use in characterizing colonic strictures and staging superficial carcinomas. However, EUS has a definitive indication in unusual patients with both UC and perianal disease (see further discussion of perianal disease in CD in this chapter).

Chromoendoscopy and Magnifying Colonoscope

Novel techniques using chromoendoscopy and magnifying colonoscopes have been studied in at attempt to increase the sensitivity and specificity of colorectal cancer surveillance in UC. For example, the use of 0.4% indigo carmine spray (with magnification to observe pit pattern) can help the targeting and mapping of suspicious dysplastic or neoplastic areas for biopsy. This technique is not standardized yet and its usefulness in the IBD patient is still under investigation.

RADIOLOGY

Abdominal Radiography Without Contrast

Flat and upright abdominal x-ray without contrast is still extremely valuable in the evaluation of patients with UC. Hospitalized patients with severe colitis should have daily abdominal x-rays to rule out impending toxic megacolon or bowel perforation. If an intestinal obstruction is suspected, an abdominal x-ray will also help to determine the location and completeness of the obstruction. Additionally, in a patient with severe bloody diarrhea we routinely obtain an abdominal radiography after a limited flexible sigmoidoscopy. The air carefully inflated in the colon during the procedure will work as a contrast agent that highlights mucosal edema and distribution of solid stool on the flat abdominal radiography and gives a very accurate estimate of extent of disease. When there is solid stool, the mucosa is usually normal.

Barium Studies

Barium enema can be performed as a single barium or double contrast (barium-air contrast) exam. Double contrast exam assesses colonic distensibility and better defines the mucosa details, so it is preferred. However, the use of barium interferes with an endoscopic examination, sometimes for days, until all barium is eliminated. For that reason, in situations in which an endoscopic examination is considered for the immediate management of patient's condition (eg, severe bleeding) a barium enema should be deferred at least until after an endoscopic evaluation is completed.

Barium enemas require more expertise to interpret than endoscopy. It has limited sensitivity in recognizing the early stages of UC and accurately defining the extent of the disease. When erythema and/or abnormal mucosal vascular pattern are the sole abnormalities, the barium enema is usually normal. Gabrielsson et al showed that barium enemas underestimate the extent of colonic involvement in two-thirds of cases as compared to colonoscopy.[15] Similarly, when compared to histopathologic results, barium enema does not correlate well with disease activity. For this reason, it should not be used to monitor response to therapy.[2,14]

Fine mucosal granularity represents the earliest abnormalities seen in the barium enema of a patient with UC. As the disease evolves, this granularity becomes progressively coarse and eventually nodular. Thumbprinting, caused by mucosal edema, can also be observed. Limited distensibility of an involved segment is also a very sensitive radiologic finding. As the disease progresses, the mucosa and the haustral folds become thickened and superficial ulcerations are seen. Polyps can be found and although they usually represent pseudopolyps, a differential diagnosis with adenomatous and malignant polyps should be considered.

In 10% to 20% of patients with pancolitis, backwash ileitis can be detected. Typically, in backwash ileitis the ileal-cecum valve is patulous and deformed, and the barium can easily reflux into the terminal ileum (which appears dilated with irregular mucosa, although without deep ulcerations or strictures).

Finally, in chronic, longstanding colitis, fibrosis develops in the muscularis propria and results in a shortened, narrowed, and straightened colon with loss of the haustral folds. In the rectum, this muscularis propria fibrosis typically leads to an increased distance from the sacrum to the barium-filled lumen that can be appreciated on lateral radiographies.

Although barium enemas represent a safe imaging technique, it should be avoided in patients with moderate to severe symptoms of colitis due to the risk of precipitating toxic megacolon.

Computed Tomography

CT techniques have become easily accessible and cheap—to the point that it would not be a surprise if in the near future it completely substituted conventional radiography.

Abdominal CT is usually indicated for the evaluation of UC patients with severe symptoms, complicated strictures, or intra-abdominal mass lesions. Although CT findings are usually not specific in patients with severe symptoms of colitis (eg, inhomogeneous wall density with mural thickening), it can be of great help in determining disease extension when a colonoscopic evaluation is contraindicated. In patients with a stricture, it helps characterize the nature of the stricture by determining the pattern of wall thickness and the presence of regional or distant lymphadenopathy or metastasis. CT is also of great assistance in determining the nature of intra-abdominal mass lesions, specifically for the differentiation of inflammatory versus malignant lesions.

Virtual CT colonoscopy may in the future substitute for endoscopic evaluation, but at this current stage of its development it does not have a defined role in the evaluation of IBD patients.

Magnetic Resonance Imaging

Magnetic resonance cholangiopancreatography (MRCP) is a noninvasive and sensitive technique usually indicated for the evaluation of a nonjaundice patient with UC suspected of having associated primary sclerosing cholangitis (PSC) (see discussion on page 22 regarding PSC).

CROHN'S DISEASE

CD and UC harbor many overlapping features. However, it is characteristic of CD that the transmural and segmental inflammation pattern have the potential to involve any part of the GI tract, including the perianal area. Also, when compared to classical UC, it has a higher tendency to be complicated by fistulas, abscesses, and strictures, as well as a lower propensity to develop associated colorectal malignancy.

The most common patterns of disease distribution are ileocolitis (40% to 55%), ileitis (30% to 40%), and colitis (15% to 25%). The small bowel, particularly the terminal ileum, is the most commonly affected segment. The disease is typically discontinuous, with affected segments interspersed with uninvolved ones. Additionally, the rectum is frequently spared in Crohn's colitis.

A unique pattern of mucosal involvement is also seen in CD. At an early stage, aphthous ulcers are typically seen on the background of normal mucosa. As the disease progresses, these superficial ulcerations enlarge and coalesce to become long and linear. They can also deepen throughout the bowel wall, eventually to possibly be complicated with fistula and abscess formation. Longitudinal and transverse linear ulcerations can circumscribe islands of nonulcerated mucosa, which then acquires a cobblestone appearance. Transmural inflammation can also lead to the formation of large inflammatory masses of intestine loops matted together. Finally, in areas with transmural circumferential inflammation, the healing process of scar formation leads to stricture development.

Granulomas are the histopathologic hallmark of CD, although they are only present in 10% to 25% of biopsy specimens. They are more commonly seen in the early stages of the disease[16] and can be found throughout the GI tract—even in macroscopically uninvolved areas. For example, in random rectal biopsies granulomas and microgranulomas were shown to be present in 6% and 14% of cases, respectively.[17] Granulomas can also be found in random biopsy of the upper GI tract[18] and, for that reason, gastroscopy with biopsy has been advocated in all patients with colitis when the differentiation between UC and CD is not clear.

The small bowel involvement poses an additional challenge for the imaging evaluation of CD. Imaging the small bowel is not an easy task. The majority of the small bowel is not accessible to an endoscopic examination. As the terminal ileum is involved for the majority of patients with CD, colonoscopy with terminal ileum examination is of great diagnostic value. However, different types of imaging studies should be combined for a full small bowel evaluation.

ENDOSCOPY

The most common endoscopic findings consist of superficial (93%) and deep erosions (74%).[19] Aphthous ulcers in the background of normal mucosa are the typical early endoscopic findings in CD, although they are present in only 10% of cases. Aphthous ulcers are small, discrete, and surrounded by an erythematous halo. As the disease progresses, aphthous ulcers increase in number and coalesce to form large, stellate, or linear ulcers.

Although the severity of the endoscopic findings weakly correlates with the clinical activity in CD,[20,21] these findings are of no value in guiding continuation of therapy after clinical remission.[22]

Oesophagogastroduodenoscopy

Oesophagogastroduodenoscopy (OGD) is the imaging modality of choice in patients with CD and upper GI tract symptoms. CD involvement of the upper GI tract is a difficult diagnosis to establish, as associated symptoms and the endoscopic findings are often nonspecific. An abnormal OGD was found in 56% of consecutive IBD patients in a prospective study.[18] Although multiple additional factors for development of upper GI disease were present, such as steroid use and the presence of *Helicobacter pylori*, granulomas were seen in 26% of patients. Furthermore, 11% of patients with normal esophagogastro-duodenoscopy (EGD) had granulomas found on the protocol biopsy. For that reason, a staging EGD might well be indicated in the initial evaluation of patients with CD when the differential diagnosis with UC is not clear.

Colonoscopy

As in UC, colonoscopy has been pivotal in the diagnosis and management of Crohn's colitis. Whenever a patient's condition permits, a full colonoscopy with special attention to the terminal ileum can be performed. The use of a pediatric rather than a regular, "adult size" colonoscope can be better tolerated in CD patients complicated with strictures. Colonoscopy is the most effective procedure in differentiating CD from UC. The most striking findings that characterize Crohn's colitis include the presence of aphthous ulcerations; uninvolved, skip segments; and terminal ileum ulcerations.

Enteroscopy

In the vast majority of Crohn's patients, the duodenum and terminal ileum can be readily assessed endoscopically, but the small bowel is mostly inaccessible to conventional endoscopy. Push and intraoperative enteroscopy have been traditionally used for the endoscopic imaging of the small bowel. Push enteroscopy consists of either using a 160-cm pediatric colonoscope or a very flexible 200-cm enteroscope, which permits an extended examination to the midjejunum. The use of a long, flexible, enteroscope usually requires the use of an overtube to bypass the stomach and prevents gastric looping. The procedure can be easily and safely performed, although the use of an overtube increases the risk and adds discomfort to the patient. On the other hand, a pediatric colonoscope avoids the use of an overtube and the extent of the examination is usually only 20 cm shorter than when using enteroscopes. Therefore, we prefer to use the pediatric colonoscope for the evaluation of proximal small bowel lesions.

Alternatively, the use of an enteroscope (200 to 240 cm) with a sigmoid overtube for the examination of lesions in the distal ileum instead of a regular colonoscope may allow passage of 50 to 80 cm of the terminal ileum.

Intraoperative enteroscopy is another option for visualizing the extent of CD. The surgeon makes a small enteric incision, and the enteroscope is introduced and advanced in both directions. By telescoping the intestines over the endoscope, the whole length of the small bowel can be evaluated by this technique. Occasionally, more than one enteric incision is necessary for small bowel evaluation in its full extension. Intraoperative enteroscopy can be done either by a conventional laparotomy or, more recently, by laparoscopic-assisted guidance. However, although it is more sensitive than barium studies in determining small bowel involvement, the additional findings obtained by intraoperative enteroscopy do not predict postoperative recurrence of CD.[23] For all these reasons, intraoperative enteroscopy for the surgical management of CD is seldom indicated.

The Given wireless capsule enteroscopy (Given Imaging Limited, Yoqneam, Israel) is a novel technique of great potential for the evaluation of CD with nonobstructive small bowel involvement. Trials are currently under evaluation, and it remains a possibility that this technique will bring new insights in the management of CD.

Endoscopic Ultrasound

As in UC, more studies are needed to define the role of endoscopic US in CD. As discussed below, EUS can be helpful in the management of perianal disease and may have a role in better defining the nature of complicating strictures.

RADIOLOGY

Barium Studies

Barium studies of small bowel can be performed by the small bowel follow-through (SBFT) or enteroclysis techniques. The fundamental difference between these two procedures is that enteroclysis involves the insertion of a nasoduodenal tube that is then injected with methylcellulose and barium solution. Small bowel lesions are better defined by enteroclysis because of the resulting higher pressure and concentration that the barium is infused into the small bowel. However, in one study, Bernstein et al showed that enteroclysis does not add diagnostic benefits to SBFT in CD.[24] For that reason, and because of the discomfort of a nasoduodenal tube placement, SBFT is our procedure of choice.

In CD, the earliest finding in barium contrast studies is the presence of aphthous ulcers, represented by small, discrete collections of barium surrounded by radiolucent halos of inflammation and infiltration with intervening normal mucosa. As the disease progresses, these aphthous ulcerations increase in number, enlarge, deepen, and coalesce to form linear, serpiginous, or stellate ulcerations. A cobblestone appearance of the mucosa, caused by longitudinal and transverse ulceration with normal intervening mucosa, can be observed at this stage. Deep ulcerations may be complicated by the development of fistulas and abscesses. Transmural inflammation can also progress to fibrosis and, when circumferential, it can form strictures. Fistulas and strictures represent the best indications for barium studies, which are superior in sensitivity and specificity to endoscopy in their recognition. Occasionally, when the stricture involves a long area of circumferential fibrosis and narrowing, a long segment of luminal narrowing acquires the appearance of a string (ie, the string sign). Transmural inflammation also leads to significant thickening of bowel wall, which is observed as wide gaps between the barium-filled lumen of the small bowel loops.

Computed Tomography

Abdominal CT is usually indicated in the evaluation and management of complicating abscesses and fluid collections as discussed below. Abdominal CT can also be helpful in differentiating CD from UC. Findings that suggest CD over UC include mucous thickening of the small bowel, isolated right colon involvement, mesenteric fat stranding, and intra-abdominal abscesses.

Magnetic Resonance Imaging

MRI enteroclysis has been used, and although sensitive and specific, it adds expenses without diagnostic advantages over conventional barium studies for the evaluation of the small bowel.[25] High-spatial resolution MRI is accurate in detecting anal fistulas and providing important preoperative information.[26]

DIAGNOSING COMPLICATIONS OF IBD

BENIGN STRICTURES

Benign strictures frequently complicate the clinical course of patients with IBD, specifically in cases of CD. Most of these strictures result from circumferential fibrosis in a short segment of the bowel and are involved by a resulting inflammatory process. The reversibility of the obstructive symptoms associated with a particular stricture will be related directly to the amount of potential reversible inflammation.

Barium studies and endoscopy give complementary information in the assessment of stricture. Radiology studies define their location and full extension, while endoscopic biopsies help determine their nature.

Patients with CD who present with stricture will have their clinical course marked by a tendency for stricture recurrence, especially postoperatively at the anastomotic site. Small bowel strictures occur more frequently than the colonic ones and are usually located in the distal ileum. These strictures have a very low malignancy potential and usually do not require surveillance biopsies. They can be single or multiple and involve a few inches up to large small bowel segments.

Unfortunately, the Given capsule enteroscopy, as currently constructed, is contraindicated in patients with suspected small bowel stricture because of the potential for entrapment at the stricture site. This can result in worsening of the obstructive symptoms and perhaps necessitating laparotomy.

Balloon dilation of strictures at the very distal terminal ileum or at the duodenum/proximal jejunum sites can be safely performed and give significant and immediate relief of patient's obstructive symptoms.[3] However, the results of balloon dilation are usually temporary.[4,27]

Radiologic studies are the cornerstone of the diagnosis of small bowel stricture. An SBFT can usually define the location, extension, and severity of a stricture and is pivotal in the preoperative evaluation of patients with obstructive symptoms associated with benign strictures.

Colonic strictures occur in both UC and CD and, in marked contrast to the small bowel, have a strong association with malignancy. They require an aggressive malignancy surveillance plan, and surgery should be considered when a satisfactory histologic sampling of part of the stricture is not possible.

As part of the initial evaluation of colonic strictures, an abdominal CT should be obtained. Special attention should be directed to the wall thickness and the presence of lymphadenopathy or metastases.

As in the small bowel, treatment of colonic strictures with balloon dilation is usually only temporarily efficient, but extremely helpful, specifically in patients that are considered poor surgical candidates. Dilations are more effective in fibrotic, chronic strictures with minimal inflammation. When associated with active inflammation, steroid injection can be useful.[28]

Experience with using stents in IBD patients is limited. The available colonic stents are metallic, uncovered, and permanent. These stents always induce a severe granulation reaction that, over time, can obstruct the stent and interfere with its removal. The use of expandable, plastic, or degradable stents may overcome most of the complications of permanent stents and be of great potential for IBD patients with benign stricture, but published experience is scant.

FISTULA

Fistulas occasionally complicate the clinical course of patients with CD. They are usually between small bowel loops (enteroenteric) and often associated with worsening diarrhea and weight loss. Barium studies can precisely define the fistula location. It can also estimate the severity of the fistula by determining its flow volume and the amount of bowel bypassed. Endoscopy has no role for the diagnostic assessment of fistula, and no endoscopic therapies (such as clipping or glue-like compounds injection aimed to seal off the fistula) have shown any benefit.

MASSIVE GASTROINTESTINAL BLEEDING

Massive bleeding in IBD is uncommon. It is more common in CD than UC.[29] When it does occur, the approach taken is similar to that in patients with GI bleeding without IBD, which includes bowel prep, endoscopy, and possible intervention for isolated lesion (although the presence of an endoscopically treatable lesion is uncommon).

TOXIC MEGACOLON

Toxic megacolon is one of the most feared complications of IBD. It can happen in both UC and CD, although it is more commonly associated with UC. Clinical diagnosis is best confirmed by a plain abdominal radiography that demonstrates a transverse colon with a diameter of more than 6.0 cm and shows either loss of haustration or intramucosal air. Colonoscopy and barium studies are absolutely contraindicated in this situation. Daily plain abdominal radiography is indicated to follow-up the patient's condition and rule out the development of complicating intestinal perforation.

POLYPS

Polyps are common in IBD. Most often they are inflammatory polyps. Patients with long-standing colitis of severe activity are the ones who usually develop multiple pseudopolyps and, at same time, are at the greatest risk of developing colorectal neoplasia. It is not an unusual scenario to face a patient with several polyps throughout the colon that leads to difficulties in determining which polyps are neoplastic, requiring removal. Our approach is to perform a full colonoscopy and biopsy polyps that are more than 1 cm, have spontaneous surface bleeding, irregular surface configuration, or which clearly differ from the other surrounding polyps.

PERIANAL DISEASE

Patients with CD are especially prone to the development of complicating perianal disease. Fistulas and abscesses involving the perianal and perineum are usually associated with pain and/or continuous discharge. As their management is usually surgical, a precise imaging definition is mandatory. Schwartz et al demonstrated an MRI accuracy of 86% in detecting perianal fistula in CD, similar to EUS and EUA (exam under anesthesia). This accuracy was increased to 100% when two of these diagnostic procedures were combined.[30]

PRIMARY SCLEROSING CHOLANGITIS

Primary sclerosing cholangitis (PSC) is a cholestatic disease in which a nonsuppurative, chronic inflammation involves the biliary tree. There is a strong correlation between PSC and IBD. Patients with PSC will have a concomitant or future diagnosis of IBD in 65% of cases, while patients with IBD will have associated PSC in 5% of cases.

All patients with IBD, as part of their initial evaluation, should have liver function test (LFT) determination. An abnormal LFT should always raise the possibility of PSC, although drug-related hepatotoxicity, virus hepatitis, autoimmune hepatitis (AIH), and primary biliary cirrhosis (PBC) should also be considered. In PSC, the typical LFT profile is of cholestasis, with a more significant rise in serum alkaline phosphatase than alanine aminotransferase (ALT) or aspartate aminotransferase (AST).

In early stages, abdominal US and CT can be normal. However, as the disease progresses, signs of biliary dilatation or cirrhosis can develop. MRCP, percutaneous transhepatic cholangiography (PTC), and endoscopic retrograde cholangiopancreatography (ERCP) are the best diagnostic tools available for the evaluation of the biliary tree. MRCP is the least invasive and has shown great sensitivity and specificity for PSC diagnosis.[31,32] It is best indicated when a therapeutic procedure, such as biliary stenting or brushing, is not contemplated.

ERCP and PTC are the gold standards for PSC diagnosis. Both have the advantage of providing the possibility of a therapeutic approach as biliary stricture brushing and stenting. ERCP is less invasive and can be easily performed even in patients without significant biliary dilatation. PTC is more invasive and requires a certain degree of biliary dilatation. When biliary drainage is indicated, a temporary external bag is necessary. Therefore, our approach is to initially use ERCP and refer the patient for a PTC if ERCP is unsuccessful.

SCREENING FOR CANCER

Patients with chronic colitis, especially UC, have an increased risk of developing colorectal malignancy.[33,34] This risk increases with the duration and extent of the disease. Patients with pancolitis and long-term disease activity are at the highest risk.[35] It is estimated that after 10 years of active pancolitis the risk of developing colorectal malignancy is increased about 1% per year. Additionally, recent studies have linked the presence of backwash ileitis with the development of this neoplasia.[12]

In patients with chronic colitis, colorectal cancer usually arises in a flat dysplasia or dysplasia-associated lesion or mass (DALM). This is in contrast to patients with sporadic or familial forms of this malignancy that arise in an adenomatous polyp. Early stages of colitis associated cancer may be very difficult to identify macroscopically,[36] and radiology usually fails to detect these early small flat lesions. On the other hand, clinical studies of colonoscopic surveillance indicate that colon cancers can be detected early and that mortality may therefore be improved. The sensitivity of random colonic biopsies is directly proportional to the number of histologic samples obtained. Itzkowitz[33] has shown that the most cost effective approach is to obtain four mucosal biopsies of each colonic segment, to a typical total of 33 biopsies. We specifically separate the biopsies of each segment in different labeled bottles before submitting them to pathology.

Patients with subtotal colectomy with a retained rectum are still at high risk of developing rectal cancer, so surveillance must be continued indefinitely.

The usual endoscopic surveillance is done using standard white light endoscopes, and biopsies are obtained randomly or are targeted to visually abnormal areas. Currently, there is interest in technology that could augment white light endoscopy in order to improve the accuracy and efficiency of directed biopsies. One of these novel technologies is chromoendoscopy with magnification. Jaramillo[37] suggests that this might improve the detection of flat adenomas in UC. Another novel but experimental technology utilizes fluorescence imaging with blue light illumination to detect autofluorescence or the fluorescence from intrinsic protoporphyrin IX. This results in the administration of the precursor agent 5-aminolevulinic acid (ALA). For a dysplastic area, tissue fluorescence is seen brick red and normal tissue images in blue green. While these technologies have great potential to aid in mapping dysplastic areas, there are major limitations due to costs and inflammation-related false positive findings.

CONCLUSION

IBD is a complex disease with several different manifestations. Management of the disease needs to be carefully tailored for each clinical situation. Imaging studies supply a snapshot of the patient's clinical condition and allow appropriate management decisions to be made. Radiologic and endoscopic imaging complement each other.

New technologies, such as wireless capsule endoscopy, will improve the diagnosis of small bowel disease. Screening for colorectal malignancy may be improved with novel photo diagnostic devices. However, until the culprit agent(s) is identified and specific therapy is developed, our management continues to be imperfect.

REFERENCES

1. Bernstein CN. On making the diagnosis of ulcerative colitis. *Am J Gastroenterol.* 1997;92(8):1247-1252.

2. Dijkstra J, Reeders JW, Tytgat GN. Idiopathic inflammatory bowel disease: endoscopic-radiologic correlation. *Radiology.* 1995;197(2):369-375.

3. Breysem Y, Janssens JF, Coremans G, Vantrappen G, Hendricks G, Rutgeerts P. Endoscopic balloon dilation of colonic and ileocolonic Crohn's strictures: long-term results. *Gastrointest Endosc.* 1992;38(2):142-147.

4. Blomberg B. Endoscopic balloon-dilatation of strictures due to inflammatory bowel disease. *Bildgebung.* 1992;59(Suppl 1):12.

5. Kelly SM, Hunter JO. Endoscopic balloon dilatation of duodenal strictures in Crohn's disease. *Postgrad Med J.* 1995;71(840):623-624.

6. Matsuhashi N, Nakajima A, Suzuki A, Yazaki Y, Takazoe M. Long-term outcome of non-surgical strictureplasty using metallic stents for intestinal strictures in Crohn's disease. *Gastrointest Endosc.* 2000;51(3):343-345.

7. Appleyard M, Glukhovsky A, Swain P. Wireless-capsule diagnostic endoscopy for recurrent small-bowel bleeding. *N Engl J Med.* 2001;344(3):232-233.

8. Zwas FR, Cirillo NW, el-Serag HB, Eisen RN. Colonic mucosal abnormalities associated with oral sodium phosphate solution. *Gastrointest Endosc.* 1996;43(5):463-466.

9. Patel Y, Pettigrew NM, Grahame GR, Bernstein CN. The diagnostic yield of lower endoscopy plus biopsy in nonbloody diarrhea. *Gastrointest Endosc.* 1997;46(4):338-343.

10. Mantzaris GJ, Hatzis A, Archavlis E, et al. The role of colonoscopy in the differential diagnosis of acute, severe hemorrhagic colitis. *Endoscopy.* 1995;27(9):645-653.

11. de Dombal FT, Watts JM, Watkinson G, Goligher JC. Local complications of ulcerative colitis. Stricture, pseudopolyps and cancer of the colon and rectum. *American Journal of Proctology.* 1967;18(3):198-201.

12. Heuschen UA, Hinz U, Allemeyer EH, et al. Backwash ileitis is strongly associated with colorectal carcinoma in ulcerative colitis. *Gastroenterology.* 2001;120(4):841-847.

13. Alemayehu G, Jarnerot G. Colonoscopy during an attack of severe ulcerative colitis is a safe procedure and of great value in clinical decision making. *Am J Gastroenterol.* 1991;86(2):187-190.

14. Mitros FA. The biopsy in evaluating patients with inflammatory bowel disease. *Med Clin N Am.* 1980;64(6):1037-1057.

15. Gabrielsson N, Granqvist S, Sundelin P, Thorgeirsson T. Extent of inflammatory lesions in ulcerative colitis assessed by radiology, colonoscopy, and endoscopic biopsies. *Gastrointestinal Radiology.* 1979;4(4):395-400.

16. Potzi R, Walgram M, Lochs H, Holzner H, Gangl A. Diagnostic significance of endoscopic biopsy in Crohn's disease. *Endoscopy.* 1989;21(2):60-62.

17. Fochios SE, Korelitz BI. The role of sigmoidoscopy and rectal biopsy in diagnosis and management of inflammatory bowel disease: personal experience. *Am J Gastroenterol.* 1988;83(2):114-119.

18. Alcantara M, Rodriguez R, Potenciano JL, Carrobles JL, Munoz C, Gomez R. Endoscopic and bioptic findings in the upper gastrointestinal tract in patients with Crohn's disease. *Endoscopy.* 1993;25(4):282-286.

19. Modigliani R, Mary JY, Simon JF, et al. Clinical, biological, and endoscopic picture of attacks of Crohn's disease. Evolution on prednisolone. Groupe d'Etudes Therapeutiques des Affections Inflammatoires Digestives. *Gastroenterology.* 1990;98(4):811-818.

20. Mary JY, Modigliani R. Development and validation of an endoscopic index of the severity for Crohn's disease: a prospective multicentre study. Groupe d'Etudes Therapeutiques des Affections Inflammatoires du Tube Digestif (GETAID). *Gut.* 1989;30(7):983-989.

21. Cellier C, Sahmoud T, Froguel E, et al. Correlations between clinical activity, endoscopic severity, and biological parameters in colonic or ileocolonic Crohn's disease. A prospective multicentre study of 121 cases. The Groupe d'Etudes Therapeutiques des Affections Inflammatoires Digestives. *Gut.* 1994; 35(2):231-235.

22. Landi B, Anh TN, Cortot A, et al. Endoscopic monitoring of Crohn's disease treatment: a prospective, randomized clinical trial. The Groupe d'Etudes Therapeutiques des Affections Inflammatoires Digestives. *Gastroenterology.* 1992;102(5):1647-1653.

23. Perez-Cuadrado E, Macenlle R, Iglesias J, Fabra R, Lamas D. Usefulness of oral video push enteroscopy in Crohn's disease. *Endoscopy.* 1997;29(8):745-747.

24. Bernstein CN, Boult IF, Greenberg HM, van der Putten W, Duffy G, Grahame GR. A prospective randomized comparison between small bowel enteroclysis and small bowel follow-through in Crohn's disease. *Gastroenterology.* 1997;113(2):390-398.

25. Umschaden HW, Szolar D, Gasser J, Umschaden M, Haselbach H. Small-bowel disease: comparison of MRI enteroclysis images with conventional enteroclysis and surgical findings. *Radiology.* 2000;215(3):717-725.

26. Beets-Tan RG, Beets GL, van der Hoop AG, et al. Preoperative MR imaging of anal fistulas: does it really help the surgeon? *Radiology.* 2001;218(1):75-84.

27. Blomberg B, Rolny P, Jarnerot G. Endoscopic treatment of anastomotic strictures in Crohn's disease. *Endoscopy.* 1991;23(4):195-198.

28. Ramboer C, Verhamme M, Dhondt E, Huys S, Van Eygen K, Vermeire L. Endoscopic treatment of stenosis in recurrent Crohn's disease with balloon dilation combined with local corticosteroid injection. *Gastrointest Endosc.* 1995;42(3):252-255.

29. Pardi DS, Loftus EV Jr, Tremaine WJ, et al. Acute major gastrointestinal hemorrhage in inflammatory bowel disease. *Gastrointest Endosc.* 1999;49(2):153-157.

30. Schwartz DA, Wiersema MJ, Dudiak KM, et al. A comparison of endoscopic ultrasound, magnetic resonance imaging, and exam under anesthesia for evaluation of Crohn's perianal fistulas. *Gastroenterology.* 2001;121(5):1064-1072.

31. Angulo P, Pearce DH, Johnson CD, et al. Magnetic resonance cholangiography in patients with biliary disease: its role in primary sclerosing cholangitis. *J Hepatol.* 2000;33(4):520-527.

32. Vitellas KM, Enns RA, Keogan MT, et al. Comparison of MR cholangiopancreatographic techniques with contrast-enhanced cholangiography in the evaluation of sclerosing cholangitis. *American Journal of Roentgenology.* 2002;178(2):3273-34.

33. Itzkowitz SH. Inflammatory bowel disease and cancer. *Gastroenterol Clin North Am.* 1997;26(1):129-139.

34. Eaden JA, Mayberry JF. Colorectal cancer complicating ulcerative colitis: a review. *Am J Gastroenterol.* 2000;95(10):2710-2719.

35. Eaden JA, Abrams KR, Mayberry JF. The risk of colorectal cancer in ulcerative colitis: a meta-analysis. *Gut.* 2001;48(4):526-535.

36. Lynch DA, Lobo AJ, Sobala GM, Dixon MF, Axon AT. Failure of colonoscopic surveillance in ulcerative colitis. *Gut.* 1993;34(8):1075-1080.

37. Jaramillo E, Watanabe M, Befrits R, Ponce de Leon E, Rubio C, Slezak P. Small, flat colorectal neoplasias in long-standing ulcerative colitis detected by high-resolution electronic video endoscopy. *Gastrointest Endosc.* 1996;44(1):15-22.

chapter 3

Clinical Features, Course, and Laboratory Findings in Ulcerative Colitis

Peter Legnani, MD and Asher Kornbluth, MD

A. Assessment of Disease Severity

1. Truelove and Witts Classification of Severity[1]

    a. This classification divides patients into mild, moderate, or severe disease based upon diarrheal symptoms, vital signs, and simple laboratory values (Table 3-1).

    b. This index is simple, quick, and easily applied and rapidly identifies the sickest patients with ulcerative colitis.

2. Ulcerative Colitis Disease Activity Index

    a. The ulcerative colitis disease activity index (UCDAI) was designed to provide an objective basis for assessment of drug efficacy.

    b. Four variables are measured: stool frequency, amount of blood in the stool, endoscopic appearance of colonic mucosa, and physician's assessment of disease activity. Each variable is given a numerical value ranging from 0 (normal) to 3 (most severe), with a value of 12 indicating most severe disease (Table 3-2).

    c. A potential strength of this index is the incorporation of endoscopic appearance into determination of disease severity.

    d. A positive response to therapy is usually defined as a reduction in the UCDAI score by 2 or more points. A complete response to therapy is a reduction of the UCDAI score by less than 3 points.

Table 3-1

TRUELOVE AND WITTS' CLASSIFICATION OF SEVERITY[1]

Mild
- Diarrhea: fewer than four bowel movements per day, with only small amounts of blood
- No fever
- No tachycardia
- Erythrocyte sedimentation rate (ESR) <30 mm/hr

Severe
- Diarrhea: six or more bowel movements daily, with blood
- Fever: mean evening temperature >37.5°C or a temperature of >37.5°C on at least 2 of 4 days at any time of the day
- Tachycardia: mean pulse >90/min
- Anemia: Hemoglobin <7.5 g/dL compared to normal, allowing for recent transfusions
- ESR: > 30 mm/hr

Moderate
- Activity between mild and severe

Table 3-2

ULCERATIVE COLITIS DISEASE ACTIVITY INDEX

Stool Frequency
- 0 = Normal
- 1 = One to two stools/day above normal amount
- 2 = Three to four stools/day above normal amount
- 3 = >Four stools/day above normal amount

Rectal Bleeding
- 0 = None
- 1 = Streaks of blood
- 2 = Obvious blood
- 3 = Mostly blood

continued on next page

> ### *Table 3-2 continued*
>
> ## ULCERATIVE COLITIS DISEASE ACTIVITY INDEX
>
> ### Mucosal Appearance
> - 0 = Normal
> - 1 = Mild friability
> - 2 = Moderate friability
> - 3 = Exudation of mucosa, spontaneous bleeding
>
> ### Physicians Rating of Disease Activity
> - 0 = Normal
> - 1 = Mild
> - 2 = Moderate
> - 3 = Severe
>
> Maximum score = 12
>
> Adapted from Sutherland LR, Martin F, Greer S, et al. 5-aminosalicylic acid enema in the treatment of distal ulcerative colitis, proctosigmoiditis, and proctitis. *Gastroenterology.* 1987;92:1894.

    e. There are multiple derivations of this index incorporating histologic severity and the patient's self-evaluation of wellness.

  3. Lichtiger Score

    a. As with the UCDAI, this score is designed to allow assessment of drug efficacy and is often utilized in drug trials in patients with severe colitis.

    b. This score incorporates the patient's subjective pain, self-assessment of general well-being, and findings on physical exam.

    c. This score also recognizes that antidiarrheal therapy can alter the number of bowel movements and assigns an additional point for its use.

    d. The maximum score is 21 and a clinical response has been defined as a score of <10 for 2 consecutive days (Table 3-3).

B. Ulcerative Proctitis

  1. Symptoms

    a. *Diarrhea* is usually frequent in number and small in volume. The patient's definition of diarrhea varies widely. Ask the patient to quantify daily number, time of day, relation to meals, consistency, and whether nocturnal stools are present.

Table 3-3

LICHTIGER SCORE

Symptom   Score

- Diarrhea (# Daily Stools)
  - 0 to 2 0
  - 3 to 4 1
  - 5 to 6 2
  - 7 to 9 3
  - 10 or more 4

- Nocturnal Diarrhea
  - No 0
  - Yes 1

- Visible Blood in Stool (% Bowel Movements)
  - 0 0
  - <50% 1
  - 50% or more 2
  - 100% 3

- Fecal Incontinence
  - No 0
  - Yes 1

- Abdominal Pain or Cramping
  - None 0
  - Mild 1
  - Moderate 2
  - Severe 3

- General Well-Being
  - Perfect 0
  - Very good 1
  - Good 2
  - Average 3
  - Poor 4
  - Terrible 5

- Abdominal Tenderness
  - None 0
  - Mild and localized 1
  - Mild to moderate and diffuse 2
  - Severe 3

continued on next page

Table 3-3 continued

LICHTIGER SCORE

Symptom   Score

- Need for Antidiarrheals
  - No 0
  - Yes 1

Maximum score = 21
Score <10 denotes clinical response

Adapted from Lichtiger S, Present DH, Kornbluth A, et al. Cyclosporine in severe ulcerative colitis refractory to steroid therapy. *N Engl J Med.* 1994;330:1841.

b. *Bleeding* is visibly present at some time in almost all patients. By definition, ulcerative colitis is a mucosal ulcerating process with the consequence of mucosal blood loss. Although diarrheal stools are not always bloody, the absence of any history of bloody stools makes the diagnosis of ulcerative colitis suspect. Patients may describe the stools as grossly bloody, streaked or mixed with blood, or as passage of only blood. The typical patient description of a local anal problem such as a hemorrhoid or fissure will usually suggest these diagnoses.

c. *Tenesmus* is best described as "dry heaves of the rectum." Patients describe the sensation of a full rectum, rectal pressure, and the desire to defecate, but without satisfaction. Some patients may describe this as constipation, which in some cases may be the only symptom of proctitis besides bleeding.

d. *Urgency* is often the most troubling symptom of all to patients and sometimes leads to the much-dreaded incontinence. Patients will plot their daily activities with the constant awareness of where the next bathroom is located.

e. *Pain* may be located in the left lower quadrant or described as an aching, tugging back pain. Severe pain should suggest the possibility of a fissure or a complicated hemorrhoid.

2. Physical Examination

a. Systemic or constitutional findings are uncommon: pallor may reflect anemia, which is far less common than in patients with more extensive colitis (see the discussion that follows). Tachycardia may reflect anemia or dehydration. Fever is uncommon.

     b. There may be tenderness in the left lower quadrant or in the infraumbilical region.

     c. Rectal exam will reveal evidence of bleeding.

     d. Extraintestinal manifestations are far less common than in patients with more extensive colitis (see below).

3. Laboratory Features

     a. *Anemia* is usually mild and due to iron deficiency when present.

     b. *Erythrocyte sedimentation rate (ESR)* may be elevated and correlate with the severity of disease activity. However, a significant number of patients may have severe flares, while the ESR remains normal or barely elevated. Similarly, thrombocytosis may be present as a nonspecific acute phase reactant.

4. Clinical Course

     a. At the time of diagnosis of ulcerative colitis, approximately 30% to 50% of patients will have the disease confined to the rectum (ie, proctitis). The incidence in more recent series tends to be toward the higher end of this range, probably due to the more widespread use of sigmoidoscopy.

     b. A minority of patients (less than 15%) will have severe disease (see disease activity indexes under section A) at their initial presentation.

     c. Up to half of all patients will develop more extensive inflammatory disease documented by endoscopy when followed for over 10 years. However, less than 10% will have extension of the disease proximal to the splenic flexure (disease involvement proximal to the splenic flexure is termed *extensive colitis*).

     d. Proctitis is generally characterized by mild disease with infrequent relapses. However, up to one-fifth of patients will have continuous symptoms requiring prolonged therapy with immunomodulators.

     e. Surgery (proctocolectomy) is ultimately required in 15% of patients, usually for refractory disease.

C. Ulcerative Colitis

1. Definitions of Anatomic Extent

     a. Proctitis or proctosigmoiditis—limited to the rectum of rectosigmoid, respectively.

     b. Left-sided disease—extends proximal to sigmoid but not extending proximal to the splenic flexure.

     c. Extensive disease—extends proximal to the splenic flexure but does not involve the entire colon.

     d. Pancolitis—involves the entire colon.

2. Symptoms

     a. All symptoms described above in ulcerative proctitis occur in patients with more extensive colitis as well and vary in intensity based upon the severity of the flare.

b. Constitutional findings of fatigue, malaise, fever, and weight loss are more common and are generally correlated with the severity of the attack.

c. Note that the classic Truelove and Witts criteria for disease severity (see Table 3-1) utilized the number of daily bowel movements and presence of bleeding as the only symptoms in their score, while the Lichtiger score also included symptoms of nocturnal movements, abdominal pain, overall patient sense of well-being, and need for antidiarrheals.

d. The development of constitutional toxicity in the absence of a megacolon is no less cause for concern than in patients developing colonic dilation; patients with toxic colitis may proceed to perforation without intervening dilatation.

e. Patients may present with symptoms of extraintestinal manifestations (see below) that are comparable in severity and, in some cases, even overshadow the distress caused by the bowel symptoms.

3. Physical Examination

a. The anatomic extent of colitis may be suggested by the distribution of tenderness on abdominal exam, which may be generally characterized as mild, moderate, or severe. All "normal" findings on abdominal exam should be interpreted with caution in the patient on steroids because these may mask even severe findings. Distension is indicative of colonic dilation and possible megacolon, while guarding and peritoneal signs are ominous and suggest the possibility of perforation. Similarly, the loss of the hepatic dullness to percussion suggests pneumoperitoneum. These findings should urgently prompt an abdominal obstructive series and computed tomography (CT) scan if there is a high index of suspicion.

b. Pallor and tachycardia may reflect anemia and dehydration, while fever and tachycardia may represent toxicity as well.

c. Peripheral edema may be found in patients with hypoalbuminemia secondary to malnutrition and intestinal protein loss.

d. Physical findings of extraintestinal manifestations may be present (see below).

4. Laboratory Features

a. Anemia may be multifactorial; while iron deficiency from blood loss is usually the chief cause, anemia of chronic disease may be present in chronically active colitis. Anemia may also be secondary to the bone marrow suppressing effect of the medications 6-mercaptopurine or azathioprine. These drugs may also be responsible for leukopenia and (rarely) thrombocytopenia.

b. The ESR may be elevated and be used as a disease marker in some but not all patients.

c. Hypokalemia and hypomagnesemia may result from stool losses and contribute to muscle weakness.

    d. Hypoalbuminemia is a marker for the malnutrition and intestinal protein loss seen in patients with severe disease.

    e. Hypocholesterolemia is a similar marker of malnutrition and is of clinical significance in patients to be treated with cyclosporine, since hypocholesterolemia increases the risk of neurotoxicity, including seizures in these patients.

    f. Liver function tests may indicate cholestasis in patients with primary sclerosing cholangitis.

5. Clinical Course
    a. Outcome of first attack
        i. In 20% to 25% of patients, the first attack of ulcerative colitis is mild (three to four bowel movements/day with some blood, mild abdominal cramping, absence of tachycardia or fever, minimal abdominal tenderness), moderate in 50% to 75%, and severe (10 or more bloody bowel movements/day with significant abdominal pain, abnormal vital signs, anemia, and significant abdominal tenderness) in 10% to 20%.

        ii. More than 85% of patients with mild or moderate disease will go into remission after the first attack.

        iii. Older studies noted only 40% of patients with severe disease entering remission after the first attack. Newer therapies, such as cyclosporine, may raise that percentage to over 80%.

    b. Clinical course after first attack
        i. Remission/relapse

1. The vast majority (approximately 90%) of patients with ulcerative colitis experience a relapsing course of disease with long-term follow-up. Fewer than 10% of patients will have a completely relapse-free course, while less than 1% will experience continuously active disease.

2. Relapses are generally unpredictable. However, patients with disease activity in the preceding 2 years have a 70% to 80% probability that the disease activity will continue in the following year.

3. The probability of relapse increases with duration of the disease.

4. Despite the frequent relapses, half of the patients with ulcerative colitis are in remission at any given time.

5. After the first year of disease, 90% of patients are fully capable of work.

6. Overall mortality due to ulcerative colitis is low (less than 1%), and is highest in patients with severe disease in the first year of diagnosis, usually due to complications (see below).

ii. Disease extension

1. Half of patients with proctitis will develop more extensive inflammatory disease. Usually, the disease extends only to the sigmoid or descending colon, with less than 10% extending proximal to the splenic flexure. The majority of proximal extension in proctitis occurs in the first 5 years but has been documented as occurring up to 10 years after initial diagnosis.

2. In left-sided colitis inflammation will extend to the proximal colon in 30% to 50% of patients.

iii. The need for surgery

1. In a community-based study, the need for colectomy was 9% during the first year of disease, 3% per year during years 2 to 5, and 1% yearly thereafter, with 30% of patients requiring colectomy within 15 years of diagnosis. Series reporting higher rates of surgery have been reported from tertiary care centers and must be interpreted with caution because of significant referral bias.

2. The indications for colectomy vary with disease duration. Early in the disease course, colectomy is usually performed for refractory disease or due to complications of disease, whereas patients with long-standing colitis require colectomy more frequently for dysplasia or cancer.

iv. Intestinal complications

1. Perforation occurs in up to one-third of patients with toxic megacolon (see below) but can occur in severe colitis even in the absence of megacolon. Perforation may be suspected on physical examination by loss of hepatic dullness on percussion or diagnosed with abdominal x-rays or CT scan. Perforation occurs more frequently during the initial episode of colitis.

2. *Toxic megacolon* refers to a dilated and ahaustral colon occurring in the setting of an acutely ill patient with fever, tachycardia, and abdominal distention. Toxic megacolon must be suspected in a patient with moderate to severe colitis who has progressive abdominal distention or an abrupt decrease in the number of bowel movements without other general clinical signs of improvement. Abdominal x-rays reveal a dilated and ahaustral colon, often with thumbprinting. The area of greatest dilation is usually the transverse colon due to its anterior position in the abdomen. Treatment consists of keeping the patient on a nothing-by-mouth diet, with aggressive fluid replacement. Rotating the patient's position from side-to-side, with time spent lying prone to distribute the colonic gas, may help. It is important to promptly recognize mega-

Table 3-4

COMMON EXTRAINTESTINAL MANIFESTATIONS

Extraintestinal Manifestation	Symptom	Sign	Association With Colitis Activity
Aphthous ulcer, stomatitis	Oral pain	Oral ulcers on palate, tongue, or buccal mucosa	+++
Uveitis	Painful eye, visual blurring, photophobia, headache	Iridospasm, abnormal pupillary response to light, possible loss of visual acuity; slit lamp exam reveals perilimbic edema	++
Episcleritis	Painless red eye	Hyperemia of the sclera and conjunctiva; no change in visual acuity	+++
Erythema nodosum	Painful red nodules	Hot, tender nodules, usually symmetrically distributed on the subcutaneous; usually on extensor surfaces of the lower legs but may also occur on thighs and arms	++++

continued on next page

colon because mortality rates in patients with perforation due to toxic megacolon are nearly 40%.

3. Hemorrhage in ulcerative colitis rarely presents with massive exsanguination, unless a coexisting bleeding disorder is present. This complication occurs in less than 1% of patients with ulcerative colitis and is managed with a colectomy.

v. Extraintestinal manifestations

1. Extraintestinal manifestations (EIM) are described in more detail in Chapter 6. The most common EIMs are described in Table 3-4, which lists the typical symptoms and signs that should suggest these diagnoses and indicates whether the activity of the EIM is associated with the activity of the colitis.

Table 3-4 continued

COMMON EXTRAINTESTINAL MANIFESTATIONS

Extraintestinal Manifestation	Symptom	Sign	Association With Colitis Activity
Pyoderma gangrenosum	Painful ulcers, often with discharge; often at sites of recent trauma (even minor)	Usually begins as pustules or fluctuant nodules that undermine adjacent skin and then ulcerate with violaceous edges; occur most commonly on lower extremities but may also be found on trunk, arms, and even face	++
Reactive arthritis	Joint pain and swelling	Nondeforming edema and occasional limitation in range of motion; involving joints in an asymmetric and migratory pattern, most commonly involves knees, ankles, wrists, elbows, and less frequently hands and shoulders	++++
Ankylosing spondylitis and sacroiliitis	Pelvic girdle, back pain, and stiffness	Loss of lumber lordosis and thoracic kyphosis	–
Primary sclerosing	Asymptomatic (detected because of cholestatic liver enzymes) or pruritus	Excoriations, jaundice late in course	–

REFERENCE

1. Truelove SC, Witts LJ. Cortisone in ulcerative colitis. Final report on a therapeutic trial. *Br Med J.* 1955;2:1041.

BIBLIOGRAPHY

Andres PG, Friedman LS. Epidemiology and natural course of inflammatory bowel disease. *Gastroenterol Clin North Am.* 1999;28:255.

Ayres RC, Gillen CD, Walmsley RS, et al. Progression of ulcerative proctosigmoiditis: incidence and risk factors influencing progression. *Eur J Gastroenterol Hepatol.* 1996;8:555.

Cima RR, Pemberton JH. Surgical management of inflammatory bowel disease. *Curr Treat Opt Gastroenterol.* 2001;4:215.

Edwards FC, Truelove SC. The course and prognosis of ulcerative colitis. *Gut.* 1963;4:299.

Farmer RG, Easley KA, Rankin GB. Clinical patterns, natural history, and progression of ulcerative colitis. A long-term follow-up of 1116 patients. *Dig Dis Sci.* 1993;38:1137.

Greenstein AJ, Barth JA, Sachar DB, et al. Free colonic perforation without dilatation in ulcerative colitis. *Am J Surg.* 1986;152:272.

Greenstein AJ, Janowitz HD, Sachar DB. Extra-intestinal complications of Crohn's disease and ulcerative colitis: study of 700 patients. *Medicine.* 1979;55:401.

Heppell J, Farkouh E, Dube S, et al. Toxic megacolon: an analysis of 70 cases. *Dis Colon Rectum.* 1986;29:789.

Langholz E, Munckholm P, Davidsen M, et al. Course of ulcerative colitis: analysis of changes in disease activity over years. *Gastroenterology.* 1994;107:3.

Lennard-Jones J, Ritchie J, Hilser W, et al. Assessment of severity in colitis: a preliminary study. *Gut.* 1975;16:579.

Lichtiger S, Present DH, Kornbluth A, et al. Cyclosporine in severe ulcerative colitis refractory to steroid therapy. *New Engl J Med.* 1994;330:1841.

Meucci G, Vecchi M, Astegiano M, et al. The natural history of ulcerative proctitis: a multicenter, retrospective study. *Am J Gastroenterol.* 2000;95:469.

Pardi DS, Loftus EV, Tremaine WJ, et al. Acute major gastrointestinal hemorrhage in inflammatory bowel disease. *Gastrointest Endosc.* 1999;49:153.

Raj V, Lichtenstein DR. Hepatobiliary manifestations of inflammatory bowel disease. *Gastroenterol Clin North Am.* 1999;28:491.

Robert JH, Sachar DB, Aufses AH, et al. Management of severe hemorrhage in ulcerative colitis. *Am J Surg.* 1990;159:550.

Sinclair TS, Brunt PW, Mowat NAG. Nonspecific proctocolitis in northeastern Scotland: a community study. *Gastroenterology.* 1983;85:1.

Sutherland LR, Martin F, Greer S, et al. 5-aminosalicylic acid enema in the treatment of distal ulcerative colitis, proctosigmoiditis, and proctitis. *Gastroenterology.* 1987;92:1894.

Von Bodegraven AA, Dijkmans BAC, Lips P, et al. Extraintestinal complications of inflammatory bowel disease. *Curr Treat Opt Gastroenterol.* 2001;4:227.

chapter 4

Clinical Features, Course, and Laboratory Findings in Crohn's Disease

Brian Brauer, MD and Joshua R. Korzenik, MD

The protean manifestations of Crohn's disease (CD) can afflict any part of the gastrointestinal tract from the mouth to the anus, resulting in a variety of clinical dilemmas. In addition, symptoms and patterns of disease vary greatly from patient to patient. Recognition of the differences in the clinical features and presentations in subgroups of patients is critical to optimal care, guiding the evaluation, treatment, and education of Crohn's patients. The characteristic segmental, transmural inflammation does not always result in the hallmark symptoms of abdominal pain, diarrhea, fever, and fatigue. Abscesses, intestinal stricturing, perianal disease, fistula, postoperative changes, reactions to medications, and extraintestinal manifestations can alter the clinical presentation, torment the patient, and challenge the physician.

SUBGROUPS OF CROHN'S DISEASE

Due to its heterogeneity, CD management necessitates identification of distinct subgroups. Different classifications have been proposed. While none allows for a clean distinction of subgroups, each is useful in understanding the clinical aspects of the disease. Working groups have developed systems of classifying the clinical pattern of CD: anatomic location and behavior (stricturing, penetrating-fistulizing, and nonpenetrating-nonstricturing). Other categories include age of onset (before or after 40 years), extent of disease, and operative history. These modifiers and their variables will be discussed in detail.

LOCATION: UPPER GASTROINTESTINAL DISEASE

Esophagus

CD of the esophagus occurs infrequently, with a cited range of 0.75% to 7%, but it is most likely found in 1% to 2% of CD patients. Isolated esophageal Crohn's would be rare, and concomitant disease usually affects the small bowel and/or colon. The most common presenting symptom is progressive painful dysphagia, but odynophagia, substernal chest pain, epigastric discomfort, and gastroesophageal reflux disease (GERD)-like symptoms are frequent. Weight loss may also be evident. Oral aphthous ulcers are frequent in patients with esophageal CD. While some professionals consider the presence of aphthous ulcers indication for endoscopy, they most commonly occur without esophageal disease.

CD of the esophagus is divided into two stages. In stage I, inflammation and erosive ulcerations predominate and stricture formation is generally absent. Stage II is characterized by stricture formation, the most concerning complication of esophageal CD, and is likely related to longstanding disease. Fistula formation occurs but is rare in esophageal CD. Stage II frequently requires dilation or surgical resection.

The diagnosis of esophageal CD is challenging because it may mimic other diseases and may be consequently misdiagnosed. The differential diagnosis includes reflux esophagitis, viral and fungal infections, drug-induced ulcerations, and Behçet's syndrome. Radiographic findings include cobblestoning, thickened mucosal folds, ulcerations, and stricture and fistula formation in late disease. Endoscopically, esophageal CD appears as mucosal thickening, hyperemia, friability, ulcerations, cobblestoning, and strictures. Aphthous-appearing lesions of the esophagus are felt to be early lesions, and their presence should cause suspicion.

Generally, the presence of noncaseating granulomas in the absence of other systemic granulomatous disease is considered a histologic indication of CD. However, as granulomas are only seen infrequently in endoscopic biopsy specimens of the esophagus, their presence is not necessarily needed to establish the diagnosis.

Stomach and Duodenum

Gastroduodenal CD is infrequent, with a reported frequency between 0.5% and 5%, with the higher figure likely being more accurate. Symptoms include abdominal pain, weight loss, dyspepsia, nausea and vomiting, and gastrointestinal hemorrhage. Abdominal pain is present in a majority of cases, while hemorrhage is relatively rare. Frequently, the symptoms mimic peptic ulcer disease, and gastroduodenal CD is diagnosed only after a failure to respond to acid suppression. Rarely, patients may be asymptomatic.

The average age of onset is generally in the late 20s but is variable. Most patients have disease elsewhere, but isolated gastroduodenal disease has been reported and may be misdiagnosed. Many patients initially found to have isolated gastroduodenal disease will go on to develop more distal disease. The most frequent site of involvement of the stomach is the antrum, and in the duodenum, the bulb. It is seen less commonly in the second, third, and fourth portions of the duodenum and anywhere in the stomach besides the antrum.

Early radiographic features of gastroduodenal CD include mucosal thickening, edema, ulceration, and cobblestoning. The disease, once advanced, will often show signs of stenosis, usually in the antrum and proximal duodenum. A "ram's horn" sign (ie, a thickened stomach with a funnel-shaped stenosis of the antrum) is the classic radiographic finding.

Endoscopic findings include granular- or nodular-appearing mucosa of involved areas, which is frequently friable. Superficial ulcerations and aphthous ulcers are also common. Decreased distensibility, stenosis, and the inability to traverse the pylorus with the endoscope are seen as well. As in esophageal disease, fistula formation is rare, and when present usually originates from the distal small intestine or colon. Similarly, gastroduodenal CD may eventuate in stricturing and gastric outlet obstruction.

Pathologic features include inflammation, lymphoid aggregates, ulceration, and noncaseating granulomas. Granulomas are present in only a small percentage of endoscopic biopsies, so multiple biopsies are essential to establish the diagnosis. Conversely, granulomas are sometimes seen in endoscopically normal appearing mucosa as well. Because of the low frequency of granulomas in endoscopic biopsies and its overlap with other diseases, strict pathologic criteria for gastroduodenal CD have been suggested.

The differential diagnosis of gastroduodenal CD includes peptic ulcer disease with or without *Helicobacter pylori* infection, erosive gastritis, gastric cancer, and other neoplasms, such as lymphomas. Systemic granulomatous disease must be excluded as well. Patients with the disease in this location usually respond well to medical therapy, but 10% to 40% eventually require surgery, most commonly for obstruction or hemorrhage.

Jejunum

CD of the jejunum alone is rare, with most reported cases representing diffuse jejunoileitis. Patients with jejunoileitis related to CD present at a younger age, usually in their mid 20s. Most patients with this disease distribution present with diffuse jejunoileitis at the time of diagnosis, but some patients had pre-existing disease elsewhere. The most common symptoms include colicky abdominal pain, weight loss, and diarrhea. Laboratory findings include anemia, hypoalbuminemia, and increased markers of inflammation.

Radiographic features include single or multiple strictures. Diffuse jejunoileitis has a high rate of surgery, with 82% of reported cases requiring one or more operations. Generally, surgery is considered after three to four episodes of severe obstructive symptoms. Severity does tend to lessen with time, and the operation rate decreases markedly 1 year after diagnosis.

Ileum

The most common site of CD is the terminal ileum, with over 70% having disease evident. Inflammation extends into the cecum and ascending colon in approximately 40% of patients, while 30% of patients have isolated small bowel disease including diffuse jejunoileitis, mentioned previously. The clinical presentation varies, as does the age of onset. Recurrent crampy abdominal pain, nausea, vomiting, and weight loss are frequent symptoms. Diarrhea is less severe in isolated ileal disease in comparison to colonic disease and may be absent in 10% to 15% of patients. In addition, ileocecal disease may mimic acute appendicitis, presenting with fever, right lower quadrant tenderness, anorexia, nausea, and vomiting, with the initial diagnosis made at the time of surgery. Occasionally, a right lower quadrant mass, which may or may not represent an abscess, can be a presenting sign. The presence of fevers increases concern for an abscess.

Long-standing disease and severe inflammation may manifest themselves as malabsorption, malnutrition, or anemia. Other complications of ileal disease include vitamin B_{12} deficiency, even without a history of ileal resections and bile salt diarrhea. Osteopenia, more common in CD patients even in the absence of steroid use, is associated with disease activity, ileal resection, and a younger age of diagnosis.

Radiographic findings in Crohn's ileitis include ulceration, single or multiple strictures, fistulas, and masses. Endoscopic findings include aphthous ulceration, long ulcerations, skip lesions, and strictures. Histologic features include transmural inflammation with lymphoid aggregates around lymphatic and blood vessels and the presence of noncaseating granulomas. Other nonspecific histologic findings, such as fibrosis, are often present as well.

In a large series by Bernell et al,[1] 87% of patients with ileocecal disease eventually required resection, 61% within the first year of diagnosis. The most common indication for surgery was obstruction, but acute abdominal pain, mass or abscess, fistula formation, and failure of medical therapy were also common indications for surgery. The need for surgery and the frequency of postoperative recurrence will be discussed in more detail later.

Colon

Approximately 25% of patients have predominately colonic involvement, and another 40% have ileocecal disease. Symptoms of Crohn's colitis include abdominal pain, diarrhea, hematochezia, and weight loss. The diarrhea tends to be less voluminous, and the amount of hematochezia is often less than that occurring in ulcerative colitis (UC).

Three clinical forms of Crohn's colitis exist. The first is ileocolitis, as mentioned above. The second, distal or left-sided colitis, usually presents with diarrhea and may also have associated rectal bleeding. The usual locations are the descending colon and the sigmoid. The differential diagnosis includes ischemic colitis, which may have a similar clinical presentation.

Total, or extensive, colitis is the third form of Crohn's colitis. As the name suggests, this variant affects large portions of the colon and may range from fulminant colitis to segmental colitis with characteristic skip lesions. While rectal sparing is a classic finding of CD, rectal involvement is common. Clinical symptoms include diarrhea, weight loss, and lethargy. Hematochezia may be present.

The distinction between Crohn's colitis and UC can be difficult but is important because treatment options differ, especially if surgery is contemplated. The presence of perianal disease or small bowel disease makes the diagnosis of Crohn's more likely. Approximately 10% of patients with inflammatory colitis will carry a diagnosis of indeterminate colitis in which a clear diagnosis of CD or UC cannot be made.

Endoscopic findings of Crohn's colitis include cobblestoning, ulceration, and inflammation. Involvement may be diffuse or discontinuous. Pseudopolyp formation may also be present. Although pseudopolyp formation is more classically associated with UC, and cobblestoning with CD, each can be seen in either disease. In addition, discontinuous involvement can be seen in partially treated UC, but skip lesions are characteristic of CD. Rectal sparing, once thought a feature unique to Crohn's, can also be seen occasionally in UC.

Endoscopic appearances of UC with CD may overlap, and even histology may not clarify the diagnosis. However, criteria for histologic diagnosis of CD have been established based on four features: transmural inflammation, serositis, microscopic fissures, and submucosal lymphedema. Granulomas are helpful in the diagnosis, but are only present in about half of biopsy specimens.

In another large series, 44% of patients required surgery, including total, subtotal, and segmental colectomy, a median of 2.1 years following diagnosis. The most common indication for surgery was failure of medical therapy, but obstruction was frequent as well. Other studies have supported these numbers, indicating that approximately one-half of all patients will undergo surgical resection within the first 10 years after the initial diagnosis, and approximately 25% of patients with Crohn's colitis will eventually require colectomy with ileostomy.

Rectum

Sole involvement of the rectum with CD is rare, but it is frequently implicated in perianal or colonic disease, with some fistulas extending into the rectum. Although rectal sparing is classically associated with CD of the colon in comparison to UC, rectal disease is present in as many as 60% of patients with Crohn's colitis. As many as 27% of patients that initially have rectal sparing will eventually develop rectal involvement.

Anus and Perineum

Approximately 30% of CD patients will develop perianal disease sometime during their life. As many as 5% will develop isolated perianal disease, although most will eventually develop the disease elsewhere. Patients with colonic involvement are much more likely to have perianal disease than those with only small bowel involvement. In one series, nearly one-half of the patients who presented with perianal disease had the disease limited to the colon, while only 18% of patients had small bowel disease. One-third of the patients had ileocolic disease. The perianal complications of CD can be divided into three distinct entities: skin tags, fissures, and fistulas/abscesses.

Skin tags are usually asymptomatic, consisting of edematous skin. During the acute phase, they are soft and edematous often with a bluish hue. Inactive or long-standing skin tags can become hard and fibrous. Fibrous skin tags rarely cause complications or symptoms, but if they interfere with hygiene, they can usually be safely excised. Soft, edematous skin tags should not be removed, as healing is delayed and infection can occur, leading to more complicated disease.

Anal fissures, much like skin tags, are generally asymptomatic or associated with only mild discomfort but can be severe. The presence of severe pain with a fissure is suggestive of an underlying abscess and warrants further investigation. Fissures usually occur in the midline. Local therapy and hygiene, such as sitz baths, are often the only treatment required. As many as 80% of fissures will heal spontaneously.

The presence of pain should cause suspicion for an underlying abscess. The treatment of abscesses requires prompt identification and drainage. A careful perineal and rectal examination should be performed. If the patient has a low threshold to pain, perform the examination under anesthesia. The early involvement of an experienced colorectal surgeon is essential. At the initial drainage of an abscess, it is not necessary to search endlessly for a fistula, as only half of drained abscesses recur. However, if the abscess fails to resolve after drainage or does recur, a fistula should be suspected. Exact operations and their rationale will be discussed in a separate chapter.

Fistulas range from superficial and simple to deep and complex and are probably the most difficult perianal complication of CD. Fistulas in general are classified by their location in relation to the anal sphincter. As previously stated, severe pain indicates the presence of an abscess and warrants immediate investigation and drainage, in particular when a previously asymptomatic fistula becomes painful.

Anatomic locations of perianal fistulas include submucosal, intersphincteric, transsphincteric, suprasphincteric, and extrasphincteric. Intersphincteric and submucosal fistulas are considered simple or superficial, with most of the anal sphincter lying above the fistulous tract. Traditionally, these lesions have been observed and surgery performed only when abscesses or symptomatic fistulas are present. Recent studies have shown good results with early surgical therapy in simple fistulas with minimal sphincter involvement, and many authors now advocate an early surgical approach to simple fistulas.

High fistulas (ie, those located above the sphincter) are often complex and more difficult to treat. Active rectal disease complicates their management. In addition, fistulas with multiple openings and recurrent fistulas are also considered complex, as well as those with internal extension and internal openings above the dentate line. Careful inspection, including exam under anesthesia, and a combined medical and surgical approach are essential to their management.

Rectovaginal fistulas occur in 3% to 10% of women with CD. Their classification is similar to perianal fistulas, and many are actually anovaginal fistulas. Most patients are asymptomatic or complain of occasional vaginal discharge or passage of flatus through the vagina. Some women have dyspareunia, perineal pain, and recurrent vaginal infections, but severe complications are rare. The treatment of rectovaginal fistulas does not differ greatly from perianal fistulas, and the same principles are generally followed.

Most perianal fistulas do heal, with a median time to healing of approximately 1 year, even with pre-infliximab therapy. In one series, 15% healed at 6 months, 30% at 1 year, and 69% at 3 years. Unfortunately, nearly one-half of fistulas recur by 18 months. Less than 20% will eventually require proctectomy. Approximately one-half of patients with perianal disease will develop an abscess during the course of their disease.

Anal stenosis is a frequent finding in perianal CD but rarely causes problems, since most patients with CD have loose stools. The occasional symptomatic stenosis or stricture usually responds to single finger dilatation. Sphincterotomy should be avoided.

BEHAVIOR

In an attempt to characterize the primary complications of CD in a particular patient, three categories of behavior have been described: inflammatory (nonstricturing/nonpenetrating), penetrating/perforating, and fibrostenotic/stricturing. Though these three behaviors may coexist in the same patient, the predominant feature of the disease is used for classification.

Inflammatory (Nonstricturing-Nonpenetrating) Disease

Inflammatory disease, also called nonstricturing-nonpenetrating, generally consists of superficial ulceration and inflammation. Fistula and abscess formation are not significant features. Typical symptoms include abdominal pain and diarrhea. Nonstricturing-nonpenetrating is probably a better term, as all three classes of behavior have some degree of inflammation present. Recent studies have suggested that many patients who initially present with nonstricturing-nonpenetrating disease will eventually develop either penetrating or stricturing complications over time.

Perforating (Penetrating) Disease

Perforating, or penetrating, CD is characterized by fistulas and complications of perforation through the bowel wall. This subgroup includes three clinical presentations: acute free perforation (less common), subacute perforation with abscess formation, and fistula formation. Fistulas include internal fistulas, in which a fistula connects to another internal organ (eg, enteroenteric fistulas) and external fistulas, which terminate on the surface of the body (eg, enterocutaneous fistulas). Some consider abscesses to be blind internal fistulas. The lifetime risk of fistula formation in CD ranges from 20% to 40%. Patients who present with an acute perforation are at an increased risk for a subsequent similar complication.

ENTEROENTERIC AND ENTEROCOLIC FISTULAS

Enteroenteric and enterocolic fistulas occur between adjacent bowel. Ileocolic fistulas are the most common, many of which occur in the ileocecal area or between the ileum and sigmoid. Often found only after imaging has been performed, many enteroenteric fistulas are asymptomatic and do not require surgical therapy. Depending on the location, fistulas have the potential to cause significant diarrhea and even weight loss if a large portion of intestine is bypassed by a fistula, such as a gastrocolic or duodenocolic fistula, both of which are uncommon.

ENTEROURINARY FISTULAS

Enterovesical and enterourethral fistulas account for most enterourinary fistulas. Symptoms include dysuria, recurrent urinary tract infections, and occasionally pneumaturia and fecaluria. Some of these findings may not be volunteered by the patient, so the clinician should question the patient. A minority present with sepsis and require prompt antibiotic therapy. Therapeutic goals include control of septic complications and closure of the fistulas. Emergent surgery is usually not necessary, and medical therapy for the underlying CD can be safely instituted in most cases.

RECTOVAGINAL FISTULAS

Many rectovaginal fistulas are actually anovaginal fistulas and are relatively superficial, with minimal involvement of the sphincter. They occur in as many as 10% of women with CD and are more frequent in women who have had an episiotomy. Presenting symptoms include intermittent vaginal discharge, vaginal infections, and occasional vaginal flatus. Some women will have severe inflammation and discomfort. Severe pain suggests an underlying abscess and warrants further investigation and, if necessary, drainage.

PERIANAL FISTULAS

Perianal fistulas are managed in much the same manner as rectovaginal fistulas and classified based on their location relative to the anal sphincter. Severe pain may indicate an underlying abscess, which requires further examination and drainage. The clinician should perform the examination under anesthesia if the patient has a low pain threshold.

ENTEROCUTANEOUS FISTULAS

Enterocutaneous fistulas result from the inflamed intestine forming a fistulous tract with the body wall. Most enterocutaneous fistulas occur following an operation, usually either a resection or stricturoplasty.

Patients with a postoperative enterocutaneous fistula usually present with succus (intestinal contents) drainage through their incision 7 to 10 days postoperatively. Increased pain and fever may be present.

Spontaneous enterocutaneous fistulas usually occur through a previous surgical incision and rarely occur through an unoperated abdominal wall. Erythema, pain, and swelling usually occur under a healed surgical scar. The patient may have a fever and malaise out of proportion to his or her usual CD symptoms. Incision of the inflamed area will often reveal pus. The development of an enterocutaneous fistula requires a careful evaluation of the anatomy, consideration of recurrence of disease and intestinal stricture formation, and a search for occult abscesses. Recent studies have shown the incidence of postoperative enterocutaneous fistula as low as 6% in the hands of experienced surgeons.

PELVIC AND INTRA-ABDOMINAL ABSCESSES

As many as 25% of patients with CD will develop an abscess during their lifetime. An abscess, which is a walled-off collection of pus, usually results from intestinal perforation, however small. Intra-abdominal abscesses are most common in patients with ileocecal or ileocolic disease and less frequent in patients with isolated ileal or colonic disease. The majority of abscesses (over 80% in one series) are located in the right lower quadrant. Presenting signs and symptoms may include fever, abdominal pain, nausea, vomiting, diarrhea, and, in some cases, a palpable mass. An abscess may result in an ileus and present with symptoms consistent with obstruction. Pain out of proportion to the patient's usual pattern of pain and a fever over 100.5°F, should cause suspicion of an intra-abdominal abscess. Because many of these symptoms are typical of CD, suspicion of an abscess warrants early abdominal imaging. The abdominal computed tomography (CT) scan is usually the modality of choice. Further imaging to locate a perforation or fistulous tract may be warranted.

Fibrostenotic (Stricturing) Disease

Fibrostenotic, or stricturing, disease is characterized by stricture formation and obstruction. By definition, there is a constant luminal narrowing demonstrated by endoscopic, radiographic, or surgical examination in conjunction with dilation proximal to the narrowed region, and/or obstructive symptoms. Patients with stricturing disease may often present postoperatively with recurrent strictures.

AGE OF ONSET

The Vienna classification system also classifies patients by age at diagnosis, either before age 40 or after age 40. The important element in this classification is the age at diagnosis, not the present age of the patient. An earlier age of onset is more likely to be associated with a family history of CD, small bowel involvement, and complications of small bowel disease, such as abscesses and stricture formation. Older onset is more likely associated with colonic disease and less likely to have an associated fistula or obstruction.

DISEASE SEVERITY

An ideal index of CD activity would be an objective measurement of inflammation and symptoms, be easy to use, and encompass the variability of CD signs and symptoms. Such an index would hopefully guide the clinician in selecting the appropriate therapy and on measuring response. Inflammatory activity, as measured by several laboratory tests, does not necessarily correlate with a distinct set of physical symptoms or severity. The many different indexes described have been developed for use primarily in clinical studies to characterize activity and response to therapy, with reproducibility from institution to institution.

These indexes range in spectrum from mostly clinical, relying heavily on subjective assessments and physical findings, to largely laboratory-based determinations. No index replaces or enhances a basic guided clinical history. (Laboratory findings will be described in more detail later in this chapter.)

CROHN'S DISEASE ACTIVITY INDEX

The CD Activity Index (CDAI) was developed by Best and colleagues[2] in 1975 as part of the National Cooperative CD Study and is the gold standard for any clinical trial. A primarily clinical index, it uses eight variables found to be good predictors of disease activity. The variables include number of stools, abdominal pain, general well-being, opiate use for diarrhea control, abdominal mass palpated on exam, hematocrit, body weight, and a panel of six systemic manifestations. Each variable is then assigned a weight, and a total is then calculated. The number of stools, abdominal pain, and general well-being are recorded in a patient diary for 7 consecutive days prior to the office visit. A score of <150 corresponds with relatively quiescent disease, while values above 200 to 220 are considered moderate disease, and a score above 450 indicates severe disease. A decrease in greater than 70 points is used by convention to indicate a significant improvement in disease activity.

In general, the CDAI is thought to be a reliable representation of disease activity and is reproducible. Its main drawbacks include the complexity of calculation on the physician's part, the requirement for the patient to keep a diary of symptoms for 7 consecutive days, and its reliance on subjective measures. In addition, it requires the measure of the hematocrit. Its use in routine clinical evaluation of a patient is impractical but is essential to understand in a critical appraisal of therapeutic trials in CD.

SIMPLE INDEX (HARVEY-BRADSHAW INDEX)

In contrast to the CDAI, the Simple Index (SI), also called the Harvey-Bradshaw Index, was developed as a simplified index in comparison to the CDAI, using just five variables recorded on one occasion. The items include general well-being, abdominal pain, abdominal mass, number of liquid stools, and systemic complications. The day prior to the office visit is used. Each variable is weighted equally.

The Harvey-Bradshaw Index correlates well with the CDAI, is easier to calculate, and requires no laboratory studies. The Harvey-Bradshaw Index records symptoms for a single day, so a symptom diary is not required. The index can easily be calculated by recall.

DUTCH ACTIVITY INDEX (VAN HEES INDEX)

The Dutch Activity Index (DAI) was developed by Van Hees as an alternative to the CDAI in an attempt to develop a more objective scale. The DAI consists of nine criteria, including serum albumin, erythrocyte sedimentation rate (ESR), quetelet count (a weight:height ratio), abdominal mass, gender, temperature, stool consistency, history of resection, and extraintestinal lesions. Each variable is then multiplied by a regression coefficient to give a total score. The DAI showed better correlation with independent physician assessment than the CDAI in the initial series, but the complexity of the required calculations limits its utility in clinical practice.

INFLAMMATORY BOWEL DISEASE QUESTIONNAIRE AND SHORT INFLAMMATORY BOWEL DISEASE QUESTIONNAIRE

The inflammatory bowel disease questionnaire (IBDQ) aims to assess overall quality of life and disease related dysfunction in patients with inflammatory bowel disease. By nature a subjective test, its design better assesses the patient's symptoms, emotional response to symptoms, and quality of life than the more objective indices previously mentioned.

The IBDQ consists of 32 questions divided into four categories: symptoms related to the primary bowel disturbance, systemic symptoms, emotional function, and social function. Each item is then answered on a seven-point scale, each with a numerical value from one to seven, from which a total is calculated. Total score can range from 32 to 224, with a higher number indicating a better quality of life. A score greater than 170 is considered a good quality of life. The IBDQ has good correlation with other indices, has been shown to be a reliable and valid tool in clinical trials, and can be used in both UC and CD. Its main drawbacks are the time it takes to complete, which is usually 10 to 30 minutes, and the fact that it can be cumbersome for the physician to score.

The short inflammatory bowel disease questionnaire (SIBDQ) is a simplified version of the IBDQ, containing 10 questions covering the same four categories as the IBDQ. The same responses are used as in the IBDQ, with scores ranging from 10 to 70, a higher score again indicating a better quality of life. The SIBDQ is quicker to administer and score, and in early studies has shown good correlation with the IBDQ and other indices.

LABORATORY INDICATORS OF DISEASE ACTIVITY

In an effort to find an objective and reproducible measure of disease activity, numerous laboratory measures, mostly acute phase reactants, have been studied. The utility of these tests as a routine, frequent assessment of an individual patient is an area of debate.

ERYTHROCYTE SEDIMENTATION RATE

A simple and quick parameter to obtain, the ESR is a nonspecific assessment of inflammation. It is an indirect measure of proteins in the blood, many of which are acute phase reactants.

A positive correlation has been demonstrated in patients with predominantly Crohn's colitis, although separation of mild and moderate disease is difficult. The correlation is poor in ileitis and, in some instances, a negative correlation exists. In addition, the ESR does not reflect intestinal inflammation alone. In order to be useful, the patients should have a baseline value when the disease is under good control. Some of the acute phase reactants have a relatively long half-life, and ESR may stay elevated despite clinical improvement.

C-REACTIVE PROTEIN AND SERUM AMYLOID A

C-reactive protein (CRP) and serum amyloid A (SAA), which are also acute phase reactants, are released by the liver in response to injury and inflammation. Levels rise rapidly following acute injury and reach high peaks. Levels peak within 24 to 48 hours, with a rapid decline following resolution of injury or inflammation, providing some utility in judging response to therapy during an acute flare.

CRP and SAA both reach higher levels in CD than UC, and levels tend to correlate with disease severity. The one caveat is that symptoms must be caused by inflammation in order to cause an elevation. A high-grade obstruction caused by a fibrous stricture may yield relatively normal values. Both values have good correlation with CDAI and are useful in predicting treatment failure and relapse, but recent studies have shown SAA to correlate slightly better with the CDAI than CRP, though SAA is not commonly used in routine clinical practice.

ANTINEUTROPHIL CYTOPLASMIC ANTIBODIES (ANCA)

Antineutrophil cytoplasmic antibody (ANCA) is an autoantibody traditionally utilized in the diagnosis of Wegener's granulomatosis, but it has recently received attention recently in IBD. ANCA is present in 10% to 30% of CD patients and has been reported in up to 65% of UC patients. While ANCA is much more prevalent in UC, a subgroup of CD patients with primarily left-sided colitis have a high frequency of ANCA positivity. These patients tend to have a clinical course similar to UC and many are initially diagnosed with UC. While this group of patients may have severe colonic disease and require operation for refractory disease, the frequency of small bowel involvement and fistula formation is much less. In addition, studies have suggested these patients are likely to have a poor response to infliximab, a monoclonal antibody against tumor necrosis factor (TNF).

ANTI-Saccharomyces cerevisiae ANTIBODIES

Anti-*Saccharomyces cerevisiae* antibodies (ASCA), antibodies against oligomanosidic epitopes of *S. cerevisiae* (a yeast) are present in 60% to 70% of CD patients and less than 15% of UC patients. ASCA are rarely present in patients with non-IBD bowel disorders. Patients positive for both IgG and IgA ASCA, considered double-ASCA positive, are highly predictive of CD. Likewise, Crohn's colitis patients with UC-like disease are much less likely to be double-ASCA positive.

The combination of perinuclear antineutrophil cytoplasmic antibodies (pANCA) and ASCA appears to predict disease behavior. Patients who are double-ASCA positive and pANCA negative are more likely to have stricturing or penetrating disease, while those who are double-ASCA negative and pANCA positive are much more likely to have UC-like left-sided colon disease and are unlikely to have stricturing or penetrating complications (nonstricturing-nonpenetrating behavior). ASCA are more likely positive in ileal than colonic disease and wanes over time after a surgical remission. The precise role for this test in clinical practice is yet to be determined.

CLINICAL COURSE

CD is a chronic inflammatory disease characterized by frequent relapses. Disease severity varies greatly between individuals, as some follow a rather indolent course while others suffer from frequent relapses or even persistent disease.

OUTCOME OF FIRST ATTACK

The course of CD is very unpredictable. Spontaneous remissions have been reported between 8% to 44% and may be long lasting in as many as 20%. A small percentage of CD patients never achieve remission. Two recent studies of large populations of patients with primarily ileocecal disease or colitis indicate that about 18% of patients with colonic disease required colonic resection in relation to their first flare, while 74% attained a clinical remission. In contrast, 61% of patients with ileocecal disease required surgical resection within 1 year of diagnosis.

CLINICAL COURSE AFTER THE FIRST ATTACK

Clinical Relapse

As mentioned previously, approximately 20% of CD patients will have indolent disease, with long-lasting remissions after just one or two flares. Of the remaining patients, approximately 30% will relapse within 1 year and 40% will relapse within 2 years. A small percentage never reach a clinical remission. Munkholm[3] followed a large cohort of patients and found that 58% of patients who achieved remission relapsed within 2 years and 88% at 10 years.

In a recent series of patients treated with mesalamine, relapse was classified by location. In patients with ileal disease, 26% relapsed within 1 year, 85% within 2 years, and all had relapsed by 5 years. In ileocecal disease, 39% relapsed within 1 year, 89% in 2 years, and all had relapsed within 4 years of enrollment. Of the patients with colonic disease, one-third relapsed within 1 year, 71% at 2 years, and all had relapsed by 6 years.

The Need for Surgery

The need for surgery is very dependent on location, as is the recurrence time following a surgical remission. Up to 74% of patients will eventually require surgery for CD; the frequency varies with location. Whether newer therapies will alter the course of disease is not yet established.

Patients with ileocecal disease carry the highest risk for surgery, with 87% to 90% eventually requiring surgery. In a recent series, 87% required surgery, 61% within the first year of diagnosis. Sixty-nine percent underwent ileocecal resection, and 23% underwent a right hemicolectomy. Forty-three percent relapsed postoperatively, with a median time to relapse of 6.8 years. The main risk factors for a higher rate of recurrence were the presence of perianal disease and a resected portion of ileum greater than 50 cm. Smoking also increases the recurrence rate. There was also a trend toward a lower relapse rate in patients diagnosed and treated later in the study period, which may reflect advances in medical therapy, as the study included patients over a span of 35 years. Relapse rates were 28% and 36% at 5 and 10 years, respectively, which may be at the lower end of the spectrum. Other studies suggest a relapse rate of 10% to 15% per year.

Colorectal disease is associated with a lower risk of surgery, with approximately 50% to 58% eventually requiring surgery. Patients with disease in the proximal (ascending) colon are much more likely to require surgery than those with left-sided disease. The rate of relapse depends on the type of surgery performed, with segmental colectomy and ileorectal anastomoses having higher relapse rates. Overall, relapse rates range from 24% to 58%, with subtotal colectomy and ileostomy having the lowest relapse rate.

Small bowel disease, usually involving the terminal ileum, has a risk of surgery slightly higher than colonic disease, but much less than ileocecal disease. Approximately two-thirds of patients will eventually require surgery, with a majority requiring surgery for obstruction.

More than 70% of patients who achieve remission following surgical resection will have endoscopic evidence of recurrence within 1 year, but only 20% are associated with clinical symptoms. While there is a tendency for the disease to progress distally prior to surgery, recurrences after surgery are usually on the proximal side of the anastomosis.

Noninflammatory Complications

While recurrent inflammatory disease is often the most difficult therapeutic challenge, noninflammatory complications, such as bile salt diarrhea, bacterial overgrowth, or short gut syndrome, may mimic exacerbations of CD and should be considered.

Acute Hemorrhage

Although bleeding is relatively frequent in CD, the incidence of major gastrointestinal hemorrhage is low. When it does occur, it can be an indication for emergent surgery. Major lower gastrointestinal hemorrhage has been reported in up to 6% of patients, but the lack of criteria for major hemorrhage makes the data difficult to interpret. Major hemorrhage is more frequent in colonic disease than ileal disease. Acute hemorrhage was the initial presentation in nearly one-fourth of the CD patients in a recent case series. Sixty-five percent of patients in this series had quiescent pre-existing disease at the time of hemorrhage.

Therapy for acute hemorrhage varies from primary surgery to angiography, endoscopy, or medical therapy alone. Good results have been reported with endoscopic therapy, but a lower incidence of rebleeding is reported in patients treated with surgery.

More Proximal Progression of the Disease

Approximately 25% of patients with colorectal disease will eventually develop small bowel disease, a majority in the ileum. In addition, patients who undergo small bowel or ileocolonic resection usually have recurrences proximal to the anastomosis within 25 cm.

Risk Factors for Recurrence

Identification of risk factors for recurrence and a more aggressive course continue to be debated. Smoking is generally agreed upon as a risk factor for more aggressive disease behavior. Smokers have an increased rate of recurrence following both medically and surgically induced remissions and also tend to have an increased incidence of perforating complications. A recent study by Cosnes at al[4] showed ex-smokers had disease behavior similar to nonsmokers as little as 1 year after cessation, while those who continued to smoke had a more aggressive course.

The clinical challenges presented by CD can be best responded to by understanding the behavior of these subgroups. The advances in genetics, immunology, and therapeutics will hopefully lead to better identification of subgroups and enable the clinician to alter the natural history of this disease.

REFERENCES

1. Bernell O, Lapidus A, Hellers G. Recurrence after colectomy in Crohn's colitis. *Dis Colon Rectum.* 2001;44:647-654.

2. Best WR, Becktel JM, Singleton JW, Kern F. Development of a Crohn's disease activity index. *Gastroenterology.* 1976;70:439-444.

3. Munkholm P. Crohn's disease-occurrence, course, and prognosis. *Danish Medical Bulletin.* 1997;44:287-301.

4. Cosnes J, Beaugerie L, Carbonnel F, Gendre JP. Smoking cessation and the course of Crohn's disease: an intervention study. *Gastroenterology.* 2001;120:1093-1099.

BIBLIOGRAPHY

Abreu MT, Vasiliauskas EA, Kam LY, Dubinsky MC. Use of serologic tests in Crohn's disease. *Clinical Perspectives in Gastroenterology.* 2001;4:155-164.

Belaiche J, Louis E, D'Haens G, et al. Acute lower gastrointestinal bleeding in Crohn's disease: characteristics of a unique series of 34 patients. *Am J Gastroenterol.* 1999;94:2177-2181.

Bernell O, Lapidus A, Hellers G. Risk factors for surgery and recurrence in 907 patients with primary ileocecal Crohn's disease. *Br J Surg.* 2000;87:1697-1701.

Breschi G, Parisi G, Bertoni M, Masolino P, Scatena F, Capria A. Does the initial location of Crohn's disease have an influence on the time-to-relapse in patients under maintenance treatment with oral mesalamine? *J Clin Gastroenterol.* 2000;31:147-151.

Cary ER, Tremaine WJ, Banks PM, Nagorney DM. Isolated Crohn's disease of the stomach. *Mayo Clin Proc.* 1989;64:776-779.

Gasche C. Complications of inflammatory bowel disease. *Hepato-Gastroenterology.* 2000;47:49-56.

Gasche C, Scholmerich J, Brynskov J, et al. A simple classification of Crohn's disease: report of the working party for the world congresses of gastroenterology, Vienna 1998. *Inflamm Bowel Dis.* 2000;6:8-15.

Geboes K, Janssens J, Rutgeerts P, Vantrappen G. Crohn's disease of the esophagus. *J Clin Gastroenterol.* 1986;8:31-37.

Geboes K, Janssens J, Rutgeerts P, et al. Risk factors for surgery and recurrence in 907 patients with primary ileocecal Crohn's disease. *Br J Surg.* 2000;87:1697-1701.

Hofer B, Böttger T, Hernandes-Richter T, Seifert JK, Juninger T. The impact of clinical types of disease manifestation on the risk of early postoperative recurrence in Crohn's disease. *Hepato-Gastroenterology.* 2001;48:152-155.

Lapidus A, Bernell O, Hellers G, Lofberg R. Clinical course of colorectal Crohn's disease: a 35-year follow-up study of 507 patients. *Gastroenterology.* 1998;114:1151-1160.

Lichtenstein GR. Treatment of fistulizing Crohn's disease. *Gastroenterology.* 2000;119:1132-1147.

McClane SJ, Rombeau, JL. Anorectal Crohn's disease. *Surg Clin North Am.* 2001;81:169-183.

Mankowiec F, Jehle EC, Starlinger M. Clinical course of perianal fistulas in Crohn's disease. *Gut.* 1995;37:696-701.

Marshak RH, Maklansky D, Kurzban JD, Lindner AE. Crohn's disease of the stomach and duodenum. *Am J Gastroenterol.* 1982;77:340-343.

Nugent FW, Roy MA. Duodenal Crohn's disease: an analysis of 89 cases. *Am J Gastroenterol.* 1989;84:249-254.

Papi C, Ciaco A, Bianchi M, Montanti S, Koch M, Capurso L. Correlation of various Crohn's disease activity indexes in subgroups of patients with primarily inflammatory or fibrostenosing characteristics. *J Clin Gastroenterol.* 1996;23:40-43.

Raab Y, Bergstrom R, Ejerblad S, Graf W, Pahlman L. Factors influencing recurrence in Crohn's disease: an analysis of a consecutive series of 353 patients treated with primary surgery. *Dis Colon Rectum.* 1996;39:918-925.

Robert JR, Sachar DB, Greenstein AJ. Severe gastrointestinal hemorrhage in Crohn's disease. *Ann Surg.* 1991;213:207-211.

Sachar DB, Andrews HA, Farmer PG, et al. Proposed classification of patient subgroups in Crohn's disease. *Gastroenterology International.* 1992;5:141-154.

Sachar DB, Subramani K, Mauer K, et al. Patterns of postoperative recurrence in fistulizing and stenotic Crohn's disease: a retrospective cohort study of 71 patients. *J Clin Gastroenterol.* 1996;22:114-116.

Schoon EJ, van Neunen AB, Wouters RSME, Stockbrugger RW, Russel MGVM. Osteopenia and osteoporosis in Crohn's disease: prevalence in a Dutch population-based cohort. *Scand J Gastroenterol Suppl.* 2000;232:43-47.

Tan WC, Allan RN. Diffuse jejunoileitis of Crohn's disease. *Gut.* 1993;34:1374-1378.

Yamamoto T, Allan R, Keighley MRB. An audit of gastroduodenal Crohn's disease: clinicopathologic features and management. *Scand J Gastroenterol.* 1999;34:1019-1024.

chapter 5

Postoperative Recurrence of Crohn's Disease

Mohammed Al Haddad, MD and Jean-Paul Achkar, MD

INTRODUCTION

Crohn's disease is a chronic inflammatory condition of the gastrointestinal tract with reported prevalence rates in North America ranging between 26 and 199 per 100,000 persons. Approximately 70% of Crohn's disease patients will require surgical resection at some point in their disease course. However, surgery for Crohn's disease is usually only a temporary intervention because of the high rate of recurrence. Therefore, it can be seen that postoperative recurrence poses a significant problem in the management of patients with Crohn's disease.

The frequency of postoperative recurrence depends on how recurrence is defined. Recurrence is typically first detected on endoscopic or radiologic studies and has been noted as early as 3 months postoperatively (ie, *endoscopic recurrence*). Some studies have suggested endoscopic recurrence rates as high as 72% to 93% in the first year after surgery, while a more recent study suggested lower recurrence rates of 28% at 1 year and 77% at 3 years. There is a progression of endoscopic lesions, from scattered aphthous ulcers to severe ulcerations and strictures, which is predictive of the subsequent clinical course. Recurrence of symptoms has been reported to be as high as 55% at 5 years and

76% at 15 years (ie, *clinical recurrence*). The need for further surgical resection, which can be considered the most severe form of recurrence, is fortunately much less (ie, *surgical recurrence*). Approximately one-third of patients require further surgical intervention within 10 years of their initial surgery.

In this chapter, we will try to shed some light on current theories regarding the pathogenesis of postoperative Crohn's disease recurrence, predisposing risk factors, and, finally, we will discuss the role of medical prophylaxis in modifying postoperative disease recurrence.

PATHOPHYSIOLOGY

PROPOSED THEORIES

It has long been known that a diverting ileostomy can lead to improvement of symptoms in patients with active Crohn's colitis. In addition, recurrence rates after surgical resection are higher for patients undergoing anastomotic procedures than those for patients requiring end ileostomies. In a long-term follow-up (mean period of 15 years) of a single surgeon's practice conducted by Goligher,[1] outcomes for 207 patients undergoing excisional surgery for Crohn's disease of the colon were assessed. The definition of recurrence was not stated but presumably consisted of endoscopic and/or clinical endpoints. Recurrence developed in 15% of patients who underwent proctocolectomy with end ileostomy compared to 71% of those who underwent subtotal colectomy with ileorectal anastomosis. In patients with an ileorectal anastomosis who developed recurrence, the location of recurrent disease was the rectum in 44%, the ileum proximal to the anastomosis in 31%, and both the rectum and ileum in 22%. Of note, however, is the fact that this study only included patients with colonic Crohn's disease. There is evidence that the preoperative site of disease has an impact on risk of recurrence in patients undergoing resection with ileostomy. Ho et al[2] evaluated outcomes in 182 Crohn's disease patients with end ileostomies. Preoperative disease extent included both ileum and colon in 117 patients and colon alone in 65 patients. Using the Kaplan-Meier life-table analysis, the authors demonstrated that surgical recurrence rates were significantly higher in patients who underwent ileostomy for ileocolonic disease (42% at 10 years) than those for patients with isolated colonic disease (15% at 10 years); p<0.01.

These studies suggest that fecal stream and bowel continuity play important etiologic roles in the postoperative recurrence of Crohn's disease. Further support for this theory comes from studies that demonstrate that mucosal lesions and histologic changes begin to appear rapidly after exposure to intestinal fluid if intestinal continuity is restored after an initial diverting ileostomy procedure. In a Belgium study, five patients who had undergone surgical resection with a diverting ileostomy proximal to an ileocolic anastomosis were studied. These patients had no endoscopic or histological evidence of anastomotic disease 6 months after surgery compared to an endoscopic recurrence rate of

71% at 6 months among 75 patients who underwent surgical resection without a diverting ileostomy proximal to an ileocolic anastomosis. Six months after takedown of the diverting ileostomy, all five patients developed endoscopic and histological evidence of recurrent disease. These authors subsequently studied three patients with a diverting ileostomy proximal to an ileocolic anastomosis whose ileal effluents were infused daily into the distal limb of the ileostomy. The three patients were examined endoscopically with collection of six biopsy specimens at the ileal side and two biopsy specimens at the colonic side of the anastomosis. All biopsies were entirely normal at baseline. However, within 8 days of daily infusion of the ileal effluent, there was histological evidence of mucosal inflammation in the neoterminal ileum, which manifested as moderate to severe increase of mononuclear cells and eosinophils in the lamina propria and a moderate increase of polymorphonuclear cells in the lamina propria as well as in small vessels and in the epithelium. Although no crypt abscesses or cryptitis were present, edema, blunting of villi, and even loss of villous surface epithelial cells were noticed. Immunologic evidence of inflammation was demonstrated by increased epithelial HLA-DR expression and expression of the KP-1 antigen associated with activation by mononuclear cells. In addition, marked up regulation of intercellular adhesion molecule-1 and lymphocyte function-associated antigen-1 was observed reflecting epithelial and transendothelial lymphocyte recruitment.

Specific toxins or antigens that cause this association between fecal stream and postoperative disease recurrence have not been identified, but possible factors include intestinal bacteria and dietary components. The role of intestinal bacteria in the pathogenesis of inflammatory bowel disease as a whole has been suggested by the finding that luminal bacteria appear to be the main stimulus for experimental models of colitis. In humans, both *Bacteroides fragilis* and *Escherichia coli* concentrations are increased in Crohn's disease ileal resection specimens. The potential pathogenic role of bacteria in the postoperative setting is suggested by a study that demonstrated heavy colonization by a colonic-like bacterial flora in the neoterminal ileum following ileocolonic resection. In addition, as discussed in further detail below, metronidazole and probiotics have both been shown to reduce the risk of postoperative disease recurrence.

The role of the cytokines in mediating the postoperative inflammatory response also needs to be further defined. An imbalance of the cytokine system in the intestinal tract is believed to herald postoperative inflammatory changes. In active Crohn's disease, a typical T helper-1 (TH-1) pattern of cytokines is typically observed, with tumor necrosis factor (TNF), interleukin-1 (IL-1), and interferon (INF) being present in abundance in the inflamed mucosa. However, in one study, the pattern observed in early postoperative ileal Crohn's lesions was different, with an abundance of IL-4 and low levels of IFN, a pattern more typical for the immunoregulatory Th-2 cytokines. IL-4 induces changes in the intestinal epithelium and may enhance penetration of noxious agents.

PREDILECTION TO NEOTERMINAL ILEUM

It has been well recognized that recurrence of Crohn's disease most commonly develops in the ileal segment immediately proximal to the ileocolonic anastomosis, referred to as the *neoterminal ileum*. Studies have shown that recurrence typically develops proximal to the anastomosis after resection of ileal disease, while resection for ileocolonic disease is associated with recurrence on both sides of the anastomosis. Rutgeerts et al[3] performed colonoscopies to document the natural history of recurrence at the ileocolic anastomosis. The earliest evidence of recurrence consisted of aphthous ulceration in the neoterminal ileum, a finding seen in 72% of patients within 1 year of resection. One to 3 years after surgery, more advanced lesions were seen, including thickening of the mucosal folds and larger coalescing ulcers. These changes progressed with ulceration extending across the anastomosis to involve colonic mucosa and also stenosis at the site of the anastomosis.

Electron microscopy studies have shown that changes including goblet cell hyperplasia, epithelial bridge formation, and mucosal architectural alterations take place in both affected as well as unaffected proximal ileal section margins. Progression of theses changes leads to endoscopically recognizable recurrence at a later stage.

The pathophysiologic basis for predilection of recurrent disease to the neoterminal ileum is unclear, but reflux of colonic contents, bacterial overgrowth, and stasis may play key roles in this phenomenon.

RECURRENCE BEHAVIOR

The clinical course of recurrent Crohn's disease is often very similar to the original preoperative disease. For example, Sachar et al[4] found that patients with perforating disease (acute perforation, abscess, fistula) tended to manifest the same disease pattern when they required further surgery, while those with nonperforating disease (obstruction, medical intractability, hemorrhage) retained a nonperforating clinical pattern at diagnosis of postoperative recurrence. Other investigators have reported similar findings, although controversy does exist regarding the predictability and consistency of the "perforating" and "nonperforating" classification. Another study demonstrated that the length of ileal disease as assessed by small bowel radiographic studies before resection was similar to the length of disease at the time of clinical recurrence.

Furthermore, the preoperative course and indication for initial surgery may predict postoperative outcomes. One study reported that longer preoperative duration of disease was associated with prolonged recurrence-free survival. A retrospective analysis of surgical indications in 770 patients with Crohn's disease was done at Mount Sinai Hospital in New York. Operations for perforating indications were followed by reoperation approximately twice as fast as operations for nonperforating indications, whether going from first to second operation (perforating 4.7 years versus nonperforating 8.8 years, p<0.001) or from second to third (perforating 2.3 years versus nonperforating 5.2 years, p<0.005).

RISK FACTORS FOR RECURRENCE

PATIENT-RELATED FACTORS

Smoking

Smoking is a well-documented risk factor for Crohn's disease. Smoking has also been shown to increase the risk of postoperative recurrence. In one study, smoking was found to be associated with higher surgical recurrence rates, especially in females. The need for repeat surgery 5 and 10 years after the first intervention was found to be significantly lower in nonsmokers (20% and 41%) compared to smokers (36% and 70%). The odds ratio for postoperative recurrence in women who smoked was higher than that for men (4.2 versus 1.5). Similarly, Cottone et al[5] studied 182 patients who underwent surgery for Crohn's disease and reported that smoking was an independent risk factor for clinical, surgical, and endoscopic Crohn's disease recurrence (odds ratio, 2.2; 95% confidence interval [CI], 1.2 to 3.8). Postoperative counseling should focus on smoking cessation given the fact that this is a modifiable risk factor.

Age

Younger age at time of surgery may be associated with higher postoperative recurrence rates. A database of 692 patients with Crohn's disease who underwent surgery in Stockholm County in the period between 1955 and 1974 was reviewed. Patients were followed for a mean of 10.4 years after "curative" surgery (ie, resection of all macroscopically diseased areas with pathology reports indicating disease-free resection margins). In patients younger than 25 years of age, the cumulative recurrence rate after 10 years of follow-up was 55%, compared to 45% for patients aged between 25 and 40, and 40% in patients older than 40 years. The differences between the youngest and oldest age groups were significant ($p < 0.05$). By contrast, age at initial diagnosis of Crohn's disease does not seem to affect the rate of postoperative recurrence.

DISEASE-RELATED FACTORS

Studies have shown that the duration of the disease before surgery may be related to risk of postoperative recurrence. In one study, patients with preoperative disease history of greater than 9 years had lower rates of surgical recurrence compared to those with short preoperative disease duration. Lautenbach et al[6] reported that a longer preoperative duration of disease showed a borderline significant association with earlier median time to recurrence (5.0 versus 6.8 years; p = 0.064). This pattern was not reproduced in a pediatric study, in which shorter duration of symptoms before surgery was associated with delayed time to recurrence.

Another factor that has been studied is the location of the initial disease. Some studies have shown that patients with ileocolonic disease have a higher risk of recurrence compared to those with predominant ileal disease or those with isolated colonic disease. Another study showed that patients with either pure ileal or pure colonic involvement had a considerably longer period of time between diagnosis and the date of first surgery.

SURGICAL FACTORS

As previously discussed, the creation of an ileostomy is associated with lower recurrence rates when compared to anastomotic procedures. The effects of other surgical techniques have been evaluated. No significant differences in recurrence rates have been shown for several factors including extent of macroscopic resection margins and type of anastomosis used (end-to-side versus side-to-side anastomosis).

The influence of microscopic changes at resection margins on recurrence rates has been studied. The great bulk of evidence indicates that inflammatory changes at resection margins do not predict recurrence rates or severity. Other histological features, including granulomas in the resected bowel, have not been found to be predictive of disease recurrence.

The effect of the number of resections on recurrence rates is still unclear. However, Hellers et al[7] followed nearly 200 patients who had undergone previous resection and found that cumulative recurrence rates at 5 and 10 years were 45% and 65%, respectively. These were significantly higher than the recurrence rates after the initial resection, which were 30% and 50%, respectively.

MEDICAL THERAPY TO REDUCE POSTOPERATIVE RECURRENCE

Given the significant recurrence risk following surgical resection in Crohn's disease, identification of preventive measures to reduce these recurrences is important. The role of medical prophylaxis following surgery is entirely clear in part due to different diagnostic criteria, drugs, dosing, and duration of treatment and follow-up. The remainder of this chapter critically reviews the information available regarding medical prophylaxis of recurrence in patients with Crohn's disease undergoing surgical resection and outlines a proposed strategy for postoperative management.

SULFASALAZINE

Three trials have evaluated sulfasalazine alone, while a fourth trial studied the combination of sulfasalazine and low dose corticosteroids for the prevention of postoperative recurrence of Crohn's disease.

In a study from Sweden, 84 patients who underwent radical resection with 10 cm margins were randomized to receive either a combination of sulfasalazine (3 grams per day for 17 weeks, then 1.5 grams per day for 16 weeks) and prednisolone (15 mg per day for 2 weeks, then tapering to 5 mg over the next 31 weeks) or no postoperative treatment. Radiologic recurrence was found in 33% of the treatment group compared to 29% of the untreated group. An important consideration was the short period of postoperative therapy (33 weeks) despite the 3-year follow-up. It is possible that a difference in recurrence between the two groups would have been detected if treatment had been continued for the duration of the study.

A group from Denmark evaluated 66 patients undergoing their first surgical resection for Crohn's disease. They were randomized in double-blind fashion to postoperative treatment with sulfasalazine (3 grams per day) or placebo. Treatment was started within 1 month of surgery and was originally planned to continue for 12 months, but the authors subsequently extended the study for an additional 6 months in 26 patients. Recurrence was clinically based on symptoms and signs. At 12 months, 13% of the treatment group versus 15% of the placebo group had developed recurrent disease. However, actuarial analysis at 18 months of follow-up demonstrated that recurrence rates remained at 13% for the treatment group but had increased to 45% for the placebo group. Although this difference did not reach statistical significance, given the small number of patients, a type II error cannot be excluded.

The National Cooperative Crohn's Disease Study (NCCDS) included 48 asymptomatic patients with no evidence of recurrence by intestinal barium radiography after surgical resection. Patients were randomized to receive sulfasalazine (N = 15), prednisone (N = 12), azathioprine (N = 8), or placebo (N = 13). The patients in the placebo group had a statistically insignificant improved outcome rank compared to those receiving sulfasalazine. The small number of patients and a delay of up to 1 year prior to starting therapy limit the interpretation of these results. As previously noted, endoscopic recurrence rates as high as 93% at 1 year following surgery have been described; therefore, delaying therapy may have affected the results in this study.

Finally, Ewe et al[8] evaluated 232 patients who were randomized to treatment with either sulfasalazine (3 grams per day) or placebo. Medications were started prior to discharge and continued for the duration of the 3-year study. The measurement of recurrence rates in this study was a combination of endoscopic/radiologic recurrence and of clinical recurrence. At the end of 1 year, 16% of patients in the treatment group versus 28% of those in the placebo group developed recurrent disease (p<0.01). However, by the end of 3 years, the difference between the two groups was no longer significant. This may have been related to the fact that only 44 patients remained in the study.

In summary, except for the 1-year follow-up data from the study by Ewe et al,[8] sulfasalazine has not been shown to be statistically superior to placebo in preventing postoperative Crohn's disease recurrence. However, the study from Denmark suggests at least a trend toward its benefit. These two studies are similar in design and sulfasalazine dosing (3 grams per day), thus allowing analysis of combined data at 12 months for a total of 298 patients. Recurrence rates from this combined analysis are 15% in the sulfasalazine group and 25% in the placebo group, a difference that is statistically significant (p = 0.04 by Mantel-Haenszel statistic). Therefore, there may be a modest beneficial effect from treatment with sulfasalazine in the first 12 months following surgery, but definitive conclusions cannot be made based on these two studies alone.

Although the lack of a consistently demonstrable benefit with sulfasalazine may be due to methodological problems, one must also consider that there may not be a significant effect due to the pharmacological properties of sulfasalazine. Sulfasalazine delivers the active moiety 5-aminosalicylic acid (5-ASA) to the colon after bacterial breakdown of an azo bond linking the 5-ASA to sulfapyridine. Based on this property, little therapeutic effect would be expected in the neoterminal ileum, the most common site of disease recurrence. Due to the availability of other 5-ASA preparations capable of delivering mesalamine to the small bowel, it is unlikely that sulfasalazine will be studied in the future or used prophylactically for patients undergoing ileal or ileocolonic resection. Sulfasalazine would be of more theoretical benefit for patients undergoing segmental colonic resection for Crohn's disease.

MESALAMINE

In contrast to sulfasalazine, agents that deliver mesalamine to specific sites proximal to an anastomosis have a theoretical advantage for prevention of postoperative recurrence of Crohn's disease. Six published studies have reported on the use of mesalamine in this setting. Three studies evaluated clinical recurrence rates, two studies evaluated endoscopic and clinical recurrence rates, and one study measured endoscopic recurrence rates (Table 5-1).

The European Cooperative Crohn's Disease Study VI Group[9] performed a study with the largest number of patients of any therapeutic trial in the prevention of recurrent postoperative Crohn's disease to date. This study evaluated 318 patients undergoing surgical resection who were started on Pentasa (Ferring A/S, Vanlose, Denmark) (4 grams per day) or placebo within 10 days of surgery. Randomization was double blinded and therapy was continued for 18 months. The primary outcome parameter was clinical relapse assessed by changes in Crohn's Disease Activity Index (CDAI) scores. Cumulative recurrence rates were 24% in the mesalamine group and 31% in the placebo group at 18 months, a difference that was not statistically significant. Subgroup analysis demonstrated significant reduction in recurrences among patients with disease limited to the small intestine (22% for the mesalamine group versus 40% for the placebo group; $p = 0.002$), while no treatment effect was found for patients with disease including the colon. This study included a large number of patients and used a high dose of mesalamine that was initiated shortly after surgery and continued for 18 months. All these features suggest that the results of this study are reliable.

In an unblinded trial, Caprilli et al[10] randomized 110 patients to Asacol (Bracco SPA, Italy) (2.4 grams per day) or to no treatment within 2 weeks of surgery. Endoscopic recurrence rates were significantly lower in the treatment group at 6, 12, and 24 months ($p = 0.002$). At 24 months, endoscopic recurrence rates were 52% for the treatment group and 85% for the untreated group, while symptomatic recurrence occurred in 18% and 41%, respectively ($p = 0.006$). Of note, the results at 24 months were based on analysis of only 39 patients. The use of untreated controls rather than a placebo group represents a potential source of bias.

Table 5-1

SUMMARY OF MESALAMINE TRIALS FOR POSTOPERATIVE PROPHYLAXIS

Reference	N[a]	Treatment Duration	Measure of Recurrence	Date of Analysis[b]	Treatment Recurrence[c]	Placebo Recurrence[d]	p Value
Lochs et al[9]	318	18 months	Clinical	18 months	24%	31%	NS
			Subgroup[e]	18 months[e]	22%[e]	40%[e]	0.002[e]
Caprilli et al[10]	110	60 months	Endoscopic	24 months	52%	85%	0.002
			Clinical	24 months	18%	41%	0.006
Brignola et al[11]	87	12 months	Endoscopic	12 months	N/A[f]	N/A[f]	<0.008
			Clinical	12 months	16%	23%	NS
Florent et al[12]	126	3 months	Endoscopic	3 months	50%	63%	NS
McLeod et al[13]	163	72 months	Clinical	Variable[g]	31%	41%	0.031
Sutherland et al[14]	66	11 months	Clinical	11 months	10%	23%	NS

[a]Number of patients in the study
[b]Time after initiation of therapy at which recurrence data are reported
[c]Recurrence rate in treatment group
[d]Recurrence in placebo group
[e]Data from subgroup analysis of patients with small bowel disease
[f]Endoscopic scores used for analysis rather than recurrence rates
[g]Mean follow-up of 35 months in treatment group and of 29 months in placebo group

Brignola et al[11] randomized 87 patients to Pentasa (Yamanoichi Pharma SPA, Carugate-Milano, Italy) (3 grams per day) or to placebo within 1 month of surgery. The measured endpoint was endoscopic scoring of disease activity after one 1 of follow-up. A secondary outcome measure was that of clinical recurrence as defined by changes in CDAI scores and confirmed by radiologic or endoscopic testing. At 12 months the endoscopic scores of the treatment group were significantly lower than those of the placebo group (p <0.008). Additionally, recurrences were less severe in the treatment group (p <0.002). Although differences in clinical recurrence were not statistically significant between the two groups, logistic regression analysis revealed that the only factor affecting recurrence was treatment with mesalamine (odds ratio = 4.1; 95% CI = 2.7 to 6.3).

Florent et al[12] randomized 126 patients undergoing resection of all active Crohn's disease to Claversal (Smith Kline Beecham, Paris, France) (3 grams per day) or to placebo within 15 days of the operation. Endoscopic recurrence rates at 12 weeks were 50% in the treatment group and 63% in the placebo group (p = 0.16). This study is limited by very short follow-up time, which makes it difficult to assess the significance of the reported results. Since endoscopic recurrence rates as high as 93% at 1 year have previously been described, it is possible that a significant difference would have been noted if endoscopy had been done at a longer time interval following resection.

In a North American trial assessing clinical recurrence as its primary endpoint, McLeod et al[13] randomized 163 patients to treatment with mesalamine (Rowasa [Solvay, Marietta, Ga] or Salfolak [Axcan Pharma, Saint-Hilaire, Quebec] 3 grams per day) or placebo within 8 weeks of surgery. All grossly diseased bowel was resected but not all patients underwent anastomosis. Twenty-five patients underwent proctocolectomy (13 in treatment group and 12 in placebo group), while 10 patients had proctectomy (3 in treatment group and 7 in placebo group). Although not specifically stated, it is presumed that these patients had end ileostomies or colostomies created. As predicted, recurrence rates were much lower for patients without anastomoses. In addition to the primary outcome measure of symptomatic recurrence confirmed by radiologic or endoscopic studies, a secondary outcome of total recurrence (endoscopic, radiologic, or symptomatic) was also recorded. Mean follow-up was 34.8 months for the treatment group and 28.8 months for the placebo group with corresponding symptomatic recurrence rates of 31% and 41%, respectively (p = 0.031). The risk ratio for the development of recurrent disease in the treatment group was 0.628 (90% CI = 0.40 to 0.97). In contrast to the results from the European Cooperative Crohn's Disease Study,[9] the largest treatment effect was seen in patients with disease limited to the colon and the smallest effect was in those with disease limited to the small bowel. Endoscopic and radiologic recurrence rates were similarly decreased in the treatment group (risk ratio = 0.654; 90% CI = 0.47 to 0.91). Although McLeod's study[13] showed significant treatment effects, earlier initiation of therapy and exclusion of patients with nonanastomotic procedures may have allowed more discriminating treatment results in a more homogeneous patient population.

In another published trial evaluating mesalamine maintenance therapy for Crohn's disease, Sutherland et al[14] compared Pentasa (3 grams per day) to placebo. Of the 246 patients in the trial, 66 had achieved remission by "recent" surgical resection. The duration of remission (medical or surgical) was <180 days in approximately 75% of the patient population and the primary end-points were rate of clinical relapse and time to relapse. After 48 weeks of post-operative treatment, patients randomized to mesalamine had fewer relapses (10%) than patients receiving placebo (23%). This difference did not achieve statistical significance due to the small sample size. Furthermore, there was a significant delay in study entry after surgery that could have decreased potential benefits of therapy.

In summary, three of six studies showed a benefit for mesalamine in reduction of either endoscopic or clinical recurrence in patients with Crohn's disease undergoing surgical resection. Of the three other studies, all revealed trends in favor of therapy that was not statistically significant, and one study showed a significant benefit when subgroup analysis was performed. Although these results suggest that mesalamine may have some benefit in reducing the rate of postoperative Crohn's disease recurrence, it is difficult to draw definitive conclusions. However, a recent meta-analysis of the five published studies evaluating clinical recurrence concluded that mesalamine has a statistically significant effect on postoperative recurrence with a 10% decrease in pooled risk. The magnitude of the effect from mesalamine can also be estimated from analysis of the number needed to treat (NNT), a value which estimates how many patients would need to receive treatment in order to prevent one postoperative recurrence. The NNT for prevention of endoscopic recurrence is 3, whereas the NNT to prevent clinical recurrence in the published trials ranges between 4 and 10 (Table 5-2), and was 10 in the meta-analysis.

ANTIBIOTICS AND PROBIOTICS

Based on data regarding the impact of the fecal stream on postoperative recurrence, the use of postoperative antibiotics in this setting appears logical. A single trial that evaluated the effect of metronidazole on postoperative recurrence rates in Crohn's disease has been published. Sixty patients undergoing ileocolonic resection were randomized to treatment with metronidazole (20 mg/kg/day) or placebo within 1 week of surgery. Treatment was continued for a total of 12 weeks at which time a colonoscopy was performed. The endpoints of the study were endoscopic recurrence at 12 weeks and at 3 years, as well as clinical recurrence at 3 years. After 12 weeks, colonoscopy revealed recurrence in 52% of patients on metronidazole compared to 75% on placebo (p = 0.09). Severity of endoscopic lesions was also less severe in the metronidazole group (p = 0.02). By 3 years, however, endoscopic recurrences were equal in both groups (78% for metronidazole and 82% for placebo). There was a borderline significant effect of metronidazole at 1 year on clinical recurrence (4% for metronidazole versus 25% for placebo; p = 0.046). There was a trend toward lower clinical recurrence at 2 and 3 years after metronidazole, but these differences were not statistically significant. The positive results were offset by

Table 5-2

NUMBER NEEDED TO TREAT
IN MESALAMINE STUDIES

Reference	Measured Endpoint	Agent Used	NNT
Lochs et al[9]	Clinical recurrence	Pentasa 4 g/d	5.6[a]
Caprilli et al[10]	Endoscopic recurrence	Asacol 2.4 g/d	3.0[b]
	Clinical recurrence		4.3[b]
Brignola et al[11]	Endoscopic recurrence	Pentasa 3 g/d	3.1[c]
McLeod et al[13]	Clinical recurrence	Rowasa/Salfolak-3 g/d	10.0
Camma et al[15]	Meta-analysis	N/A	10.0

[a]Subgroup of patients with small bowel disease
[b]Data at 24 months
[c]Recurrence of endoscopically severe lesions (score of 3 to 4 on a 0-to-4 scale) or abnormal radiology

prominent side effects related to the high doses of metronidazole. Additional trials are needed to assess lower, more tolerable doses of metronidazole administered for longer periods after resection as well as to evaluate alternative antibiotics.

Probiotics are viable microorganisms that when ingested have a beneficial effect on human health. There has been recent interest in the use of probiotics for the management of inflammatory bowel disease. Proposed mechanisms of probiotic efficacy in inflammatory bowel disease include suppression of resident pathogenic bacteria, stimulation of mucin glycoprotein production by intestinal epithelial cells, prevention of adhesion of pathogenic strains to epithelial cells, and induction of host protective immune responses. A recent randomized trial of 40 patients, reported in abstract form, compared the combined use of an antibiotic (rifaximin) followed by a probiotic named VSL#3 versus mesalamine for prophylaxis of postoperative Crohn's disease recurrence. VSL#3 consists of four strains of *Lactobacillus*, three strains of *Bifidobacterium*, and one strain of *Streptococcus salivarius* at high concentrations of 300 billion viable bacteria per gram. Evidence of severe endoscopic recurrence at 1 year was found in 20% of the antibiotic/probiotic group compared to 40% for the mesalamine group. These preliminary results are promising, but final assessment should await knowledge of full study details.

6-MERCAPTOPURINE AND AZATHIOPRINE

6-mercaptopurine (6-MP) and azathioprine have been shown to maintain medically induced remissions in Crohn's disease. One could thus anticipate a similar benefit for patients with surgically induced remission.

The only controlled trial involving a large number of patients was reported in abstract form. The authors of this 2-year, five-center trial involving 131 patients studied the effects of 6-MP (50 mg per day) compared with mesalamine (Pentasa 3 grams per day) or placebo on the rate of postoperative clinical, endoscopic, and radiographic relapse. Life-table analyses demonstrated that 6-MP was statistically superior to placebo in decreasing clinical relapse and superior to both mesalamine and placebo in decreasing significant endoscopic relapse.

The only other controlled data regarding the use of 6-MP or azathioprine in the prevention of postoperative Crohn's disease comes from NCCDS. Only eight patients were randomized to treatment with azathioprine (1 mg/kg/day) and 13 patients to placebo within 1 year of surgical resection. After 1 year, patients on placebo had a significantly lower outcome ranking than those receiving azathioprine (p = 0.02). The significance of these results is unclear, given the small number of patients, the delay of up to 1 year prior to initiation of therapy, and the use of a relatively low dose of azathioprine.

Unlike the NCCDS results, data from two uncontrolled studies suggest a potential benefit of 6-MP or azathioprine in the prevention of postoperative recurrence. A recent retrospective study by Cuillerier et al[16] reported on 38 patients who received azathioprine and were followed for a median of 29 months after surgical resection. Clinical recurrence rates based on the Kaplan-Meier method were 9% at 1 year, 16% at 2 years, and 28% at 3 years. In 25 patients who underwent either radiologic or endoscopic evaluations during the follow-up period, endoscopic recurrence rates were 16% at 1 year, 36% at 2 years, and 59% at 3 years. Although there was no control group, these rates are lower than those reported for historical controls. Similarly, Korelitz et al[17] reported that 9 of 10 patients who were placed on 6-MP (no mean dose noted) after a second resection for Crohn's disease had not developed clinical recurrence after a mean follow-up of 41 months.

These preliminary results are encouraging, but additional controlled trials are needed to fully assess the dose response and long-term safety of 6-MP or azathioprine in the prevention of postoperative Crohn's disease recurrence.

CORTICOSTEROIDS

The previously described study from Sweden evaluated the combination of sulfasalazine and prednisolone (15 mg per day for 2 weeks, tapered to 5 mg over 31 weeks). There was no difference in radiographic evidence of recurrent disease when treated patients were compared to an untreated group. Again, the relatively short treatment period and lack of blinding limit interpretation of the results.

The NCCDS randomized 12 patients to treatment with prednisone (0.25 mg/kg/day) or placebo within 1 year of surgical resection. At the 1-year follow-up, patients on placebo had a significantly lower outcome ranking than those receiving prednisone (p = 0.05). The significance of these results is unclear given the small number of patients being evaluated and the delay of up to 1 year prior to initiation of therapy. Nevertheless, conventional corticosteroids have not been demonstrated to have a maintenance benefit for Crohn's disease.

In contrast to conventional steroids, budesonide has the potential advantages of potent topical anti-inflammatory activity due to high steroid receptor affinity, low systemic effects due to rapid first-pass hepatic metabolism, and the ability to develop pharmacological targeting to distal small bowel or colonic sites for drug delivery. A published trial from Europe described 129 patients randomized to treatment with a controlled ileal release budesonide formulation (6 mg once daily) or placebo within 14 days of surgical resection. No differences in endoscopic recurrence rates were found at 3 or 12 months. However, when subgroup analysis was performed, there was a trend toward decreased recurrence with budesonide for patients who had undergone surgery for "high disease activity." A second trial from Europe evaluated 83 patients who were randomized to budesonide (1 mg three times per day) versus placebo within 2 weeks of surgery. Endoscopic and/or clinical recurrence rates after 1 year were 57% for the budesonide treated group compared to 70% for the placebo group, but this difference was not statistically significant (p = 0.21). Based on these studies prophylactic treatment with budesonide in the postoperative setting cannot be recommended at this time. Further study of this agent, perhaps at higher doses, will be needed to better define its effect in decreasing postoperative recurrence.

INTERLEUKIN-10

The only other published controlled clinical trial evaluating medical therapy for the prevention of postoperative recurrence was a placebo-controlled trial of interleukin-10 (IL-10), an agent that has been shown to have anti-inflammatory immunologic effects. Sixty-five patients were randomized to IL-10 versus placebo within 2 weeks of resective surgery for Crohn's disease. After 12 weeks of therapy, there were no differences in endoscopic recurrence between the two groups (46% for the IL-10 group versus 52% for the placebo group). This was primarily a safety and tolerance study, thus it was not powered to fully evaluate the efficacy of IL-10 in this setting. However, the results at 12 weeks would suggest that IL-10 would not have a significant role in reduction of postoperative recurrence.

CONCLUSION

Patients with Crohn's disease who undergo surgical resection have a significant risk of developing recurrent disease, but medical therapy can help decrease this risk. There is an important need for identification of patients who may be at increased risk for the development of postoperative recurrence in order to maximize and better direct the use of medical therapy and possible preventive measures in this setting.

Our recommendations regarding prophylaxis of postoperative disease recurrence include counseling patients on smoking cessation because this the only known modifiable risk factor. Medical therapy considerations are as follows:

1. Mesalamine has a modest effect on prevention of postoperative recurrence rates of Crohn's disease and should at least be discussed with patients for postoperative prophylaxis.

2. Metronidazole and 6-MP/azathioprine appear to be of benefit in postoperative therapy but additional controlled studies are required to better define the efficacy and dose-response of these agents.

3. Probiotic therapy may be of benefit but further studies are needed.

4. Recommendations for individual patients should be based on the patient's willingness to take medications on a prophylactic basis and on the potential costs and side effects of treatment.

REFERENCES

1. Goligher JC, Dombal FT, Burton I. Recurrence of Crohn's disease after primary excisional surgery. *Gut.* 1971;12:519-527.

2. Ho I, Greenstein AJ, Bodain CA, et al. Recurrence of Crohn's disease in end ileostomies. Inflamm Bowel Dis. 1995;1:173-178.

3. Rutgeerts P, Goboes K, Vantrappen G, et al. Natural history in recurrent Crohn's disease at the ileocolonic anastomosis after curative surgery. *Gut.* 1984;25:665-672.

4. Sachar DB, Wolfson DM, Greenstein AJ, et al. Risk factors for postoperative recurrence of Crohn's disease. *Gastroenterology.* 1983;85:917-921.

5. Cottone M, Rosselli M, Orlando A, et al. Smoking habits and recurrence in Crohn's disease. *Gastroenterology.* 1994;106:643-648.

6. Lautenbach E, Berlin JA, Lichtenstein GR. Risk factors for early postoperative recurrence of Crohn's disease. *Gastroenterology.* 1998;115:259-267.

7. Hellers G, Cortot A, Jewell D, et al. Oral budesonide for prevention of postsurgical recurrence in Crohn's disease. *Gastroenterology.* 1999;116:294-300.

8. Ewe K, Bottger T, Buhr HJ, et al. Low-dose budesonide treatment for prevention of postoperative recurrence of Crohn's disease: a multicentre randomized placebo-controlled trial. *Eur J Gastroenterol Hepatol.* 1999;11:277-282.

9. Lochs H, Mayer M, Fleig WE, et al. Prophylaxis of postoperative relapse in Crohn's disease with mesalamine: European Cooperative Crohn's Disease Study VI. *Gastroenterology.* 2000;118:264-273.

10. Caprilli R, Andreoli A, Capurso L, et al. Oral mesalazine (Asacol) for the prevention of post-operative recurrence of Crohn's disease. *Aliment Pharmacol Ther.* 1994;8:35-43.

11. Brignola C, Cottone M, Pera A, et al. Mesalamine in the prevention of endoscopic recurrence after intestinal resection for Crohn's disease. *Gastroenterology.* 1995;108:345-349.

12. Florent C, Cortot A, Quandale P, et al. Placebo-controlled trial of mesalazine in the prevention of early endoscopic recurrence after "curative" resection for Crohn's disease. *Eur J Gastroenterol Hepatol.* 1996;8:229-233.

13. McLeod RS, Wolff BG, Steinhart AH, et al. Prophylactic mesalamine treatment decreases postoperative recurrence of Crohn's disease. *Gastroenterology.* 1995;109:404-413.

14. Sutherland LR, Martin F, Bailey RJ, et al. A randomized, placebo-controlled, double-blind trial of mesalamine in the maintenance of remission of Crohn's disease. *Gastroenterology.* 1997;112:1069-1077.

15. Camma C, Giunta M, Rosselli M, et al. 5-aminosalicylic acid in the maintenance of Crohn's disease: a meta-analysis adjusted for confounding variables. *Gastroenterology.* 1997;113:1465-1473.

16. Cuillerier E, Lemann M, Bouhnik Y, et al. Azathioprine for prevention of postoperative recurrence in Crohn's disease: a retrospective study. *Eur J Gastroenterol Hepatol.* 2001;13:1277-1279.

17. Korelitz B, Hanauer S, Rutgeerts P, et al. Post-operative prophylaxis with 6-MP, 5-ASA or placebo in Crohn's disease: a 2-year multicenter trial [abstract]. *Gastroenterology.* 1998;114:A1011.

SUGGESTED READING

Achkar JP, Hanauer SB. Medical therapy to reduce postoperative Crohn's disease recurrence. *Am J Gastroenterol.* 2000;95:1139-1146.

Cottone M, Camma C. Mesalamine and relapse prevention in Crohn's disease (letter). *Gastroenterology.* 2000;119:597.

D'Haens GR, Geboes K, Peeters M, et al. Early lesions of recurrent Crohn's disease caused by infusion of intestinal contents in excluded ileum. *Gastroenterology.* 1998;114:262-267.

D'Haens G, Rutgeerts P. Postoperative recurrence of Crohn's disease: pathophysiology and prevention. *Inflamm Bowel Dis.* 1999;5:295-303.

Greenstein AJ, Lachman P, Sachar DB, et al. Perforating and non-perforating indications for repeated operations in Crohn's disease: evidence for two clinical forms. *Gut.* 1988;29:588-592.

Janowitz HD, Croen EC, Sachar DB. The role of the fecal stream in Crohn's disease: a historical and analytic review. *Inflamm Bowel Dis.* 1998;4:29-39.

Rutgeerts P, Goboes K, Peeters M, et al. Effect of fecal stream diversion on recurrence of Crohn's disease in the neoterminal ileum. *Lancet.* 1991;338:771-774.

Rutgeerts P, Goboes K, Vantrappen G, et al. Predictability of the postoperative course of Crohn's disease. *Gastroenterology.* 1990;99:956-963.

Rutgeerts P, Hiele M, Geboes K, et al. Controlled trial of metronidazole treatment for prevention of Crohn's recurrence after ileal resection. *Gastroenterology.* 1995;108:1617-1621.

Sutherland LR, Ramcharan S, Bryant H, et al. Effect of cigarette smoking on recurrence of Crohn's disease. *Gastroenterology.* 1990;98:1123-1128.

Williams JG, Wong WD, Rothenberger DA, Goldberg SM. Recurrence of Crohn's disease after resection. *Br J Surg.* 1991;78(1):10-19.

chapter 6

Extraintestinal Manifestations of Inflammatory Bowel Disease

David G. Forcione, MD and Lawrence S. Friedman, MD

INTRODUCTION

It has become increasingly apparent that inflammatory bowel diseases (IBD) represent systemic illnesses with primarily gastrointestinal manifestations. There has been a growing literature describing a wide spectrum of extraintestinal manifestations (EIMs), with nearly every organ system affected (Table 6-1).

Extraintestinal manifestations may independently represent a source of morbidity and mortality for patients and may fail to improve with treatment directed against the underlying IBD, including bowel resection. Further, EIMs predate the formal diagnosis of either Crohn's disease or ulcerative colitis and thus point toward a diagnosis of IBD and may correlate with flares of the underlying IBD and, therefore, help predict disease relapse.

There have been few published epidemiologic surveys reporting on the prevalence and characteristics of the extraintestinal manifestations of IBD. In 1976, Greenstein and colleagues[1] reported on 700 IBD patients (9% with Crohn's colitis, 31% with Crohn's ileocolitis, 30% with Crohn's disease of the small bowel, and 30% with ulcerative colitis) evaluated at Mount Sinai Hospital from 1964 to 1973. Overall, 36% of patients had at least one extraintestinal manifestation. This analysis led to the classification of extraintestinal

Table 6-1

EXTRAINTESTINAL MANIFESTATIONS OF INFLAMMATORY BOWEL DISEASE

Hepatobiliary and Pancreatic

- Hepatic steatosis
- Cholelithiasis
- Chronic hepatitis
- Primary sclerosing cholangitis
- Cirrhosis
- Cholangiocarcinoma
- Hepatic granulomas
- Granulomatous hepatitis
- Acute and chronic pancreatitis
- Hemosiderosis
- Hepatic abscess

Musculoskeletal

- Enteropathic arthritis (pauciarticular and polyarticular)
- Spondylitis
- Sacroiliitis
- Hypertrophic osteoarthropathy
- Metastatic Crohn's disease of the bones, joints, and muscle
- Relapsing polychondritis
- Avascular necrosis
- Pelvic osteomyelitis

Dermatologic

- Erythema nodosum
- Pyoderma gangrenosum
- Pyoderma vegetans
- Vesiculopustular eruption of ulcerative colitis
- Cutaneous polyarteritis nodosa

- Metastatic Crohn's disease of the skin
- Epidermolysis bullosa acquisita
- Psoriasis
- Sweet's syndrome
- Perianal skin tags
- Erythema multiforme
- Stevens-Johnson syndrome
- Rosacea fulminans

Ocular

- Episcleritis
- Uveitis
- Central serous retinopathy
- Retinal artery and vein occlusion
- Retrobulbar neuritis
- Neuroretinitis
- Scleromalacia perforans
- Ischemic optic neuropathy
- Deep stromal inflammation
- Orbital cellulitis
- Papillitis
- Marginal corneal ulcers
- Orbital myositis
- Cataracts
- Glaucoma
- Ocular infections
- Exophthalmos

Urogenital and Renal

- Nephrolithiasis
- Amyloidosis
- Retroperitoneal abscess
- Noncalculous obstructive uropathy

continued on next page

Table 6-1 continued

EXTRAINTESTINAL MANIFESTATIONS OF INFLAMMATORY BOWEL DISEASE

- Fistulae
- Interstitial nephritis
- Renal tubular acidosis
- Glomerulonephritis
- Drug nephrotoxicity

Vascular and Hematologic

- Arterial and venous thromboembolism
- Nutritional anemia (iron, folate, vitamin B_{12} deficiency)
- Anemia of chronic disease
- Autoimmune hemolytic anemia
- Drug-induced bone marrow suppression

Cardiac

- Pericarditis
- Myocarditis
- Endocarditis

Pulmonary

- Bronchiolitis obliterans with organizing pneumonia (BOOP)
- Granulomatous pneumonitis
- Pulmonary eosinophilia with infiltrate
- Serositis
- Chronic bronchitis
- Necrobiotic parenchymal nodules

- Bronchiolitis
- Bronchiectasis
- Subglottic tracheal stenosis
- Colobronchial fistula

Endocrine and Metabolic

- Growth retardation
- Osteomalacia
- Osteopenia
- Osteoporosis
- Trace mineral and vitamin deficiencies
- Hypo- and hyperthyroidism

Neurologic

- Acute inflammatory demyelinating polyradiculopathy
- Mononeuritis multiplex
- Brachial plexopathy
- Melkersson-Rosenthal syndrome
- Vacuolar myopathy
- Myasthenia gravis
- Recurrent transient ischemic attacks
- Sinus venous thrombosis
- Myelopathy
- Sensorineural hearing loss
- Cerebrovascular accidents
- Leukoencephalitis
- Cerebellar degeneration
- Epilepsy
- Autonomic dysfunction

manifestations as associated primarily with colonic disease, small intestinal disease, or "nonspecific" disease. In this schema, colitis-related manifestations (36% of all patients) tended to be arthritic, dermatologic, oral, and ocular complications; small bowel-related manifestations (32% of all patients) were intestinal malabsorption, gallstones, and genitourinary complications (nephrolithiasis, noncalculous hydronephrosis, and enterovesical fistulae); and "nonspecific" disease-related manifestations (18% of all patients) included osteoporosis, liver disease, peptic ulcers, and amyloidosis. More recent surveys have included cardiovascular, pulmonary, hematologic, and neurologic complications in the nonspecific disease category.

In 1979, data from the National Cooperative Crohn's Disease Study (NCCDS) demonstrated that 24% of patients with Crohn's disease had at least one extraintestinal manifestation. In this series of 569 patients, the most common extraintestinal manifestations were arthritic (19%), dermatologic (4.6%), hepatobiliary (3.9%), and ocular (3.5%). Multiple extraintestinal manifestations were often found in the same patient (6% of all patients), with an occurrence that was more frequent than expected on the basis of a purely random distribution. Furthermore, there was a statistically significant association between the presence of perianal disease and extraintestinal manifestations.

In 1996, Veloso and colleagues[2] described the extraintestinal manifestations in a cohort of 792 patients with IBD followed prospectively over 20 years. In this study, 25.8% of patients had at least one extraintestinal manifestation, with a significantly higher rate among patients with Crohn's disease than among those with ulcerative colitis. As in the NCCDS, two or more extraintestinal manifestations occurred in the same patient more frequently than would be expected by chance alone. A number of concurrent autoimmune diseases including primary biliary cirrhosis (PBC), Sjögren's syndrome, alopecia areata, and Raynaud's disease were observed, although it is not clear if the frequency of these disorders was greater than that in the general population.

In 2001, Bernstein and colleagues[3] reported data from the University of Manitoba IBD Database, which includes nearly 5000 patients. In evaluating patients for six major extraintestinal manifestations (primary sclerosing cholangitis, ankylosing spondylitis, iritis/uveitis, pyoderma gangrenosum, and erythema nodosum), the investigators found that 6.2% of patients had at least one extraintestinal manifestation.

Despite advances in our understanding of the pathogenesis of IBD, the pathogenesis of extraintestinal manifestations remains unclear. In general, these manifestations are believed to arise from a state of generalized immune dysregulation, with formation of antibodies to various autoantigens. Circulating immune complexes containing autoantibodies have been found in some, but not all, patients with extraintestinal manifestations of IBD.

HEPATOBILIARY AND PANCREATIC MANIFESTATIONS

Since Thomas' description of fatty liver in a patient with ulcerative colitis in 1874,[4] a wide spectrum of hepatobiliary disorders have been found to coexist with IBD. Although up to 50% of patients with IBD have abnormal liver biochemical tests, less than 10% have clinically significant liver disease. Higher prevalence rates have been reported among patients undergoing wedge biopsy of the liver at the time of a bowel resection. In general, there is little correlation between the presence of hepatobiliary manifestations and the severity of the underlying IBD (Table 6-2).

Hepatic steatosis is the most common hepatobiliary manifestation of IBD and is seen in nearly one-half of abnormal liver biopsies. A review of 25 studies demonstrated that approximately 33% of all IBD patients have hepatic steatosis. Most affected patients are asymptomatic, although some may experience right upper quadrant discomfort due to hepatic distention. Laboratory studies often reveal a modest elevation of serum aminotransferase levels (up to ten times the upper limit of normal), with minimally elevated alkaline phosphatase levels. Hepatic synthetic function is nearly always preserved. Pathologic hallmarks include macrovesicular steatosis with minimal inflammatory changes. In some series, hepatic steatosis appeared to correlate with the disease severity of IBD and was found in nearly one half of patients requiring colectomy, 22% of nonoperated hospitalized patients, and only 5% of outpatients. Although the underlying pathogenesis remains obscure, multiple mechanisms appear to contribute, including chronic use of glucocorticoid and protein-calorie malnutrition. There is also increasing data from studies of leptin-deficient mice that elevated levels of tumor necrosis factor-α (TNF-α) and hyperinsulinemia play an important role in the pathogenesis of hepatic steatosis. In general, hepatic steatosis rarely causes hepatic fibrosis. Liver test abnormalities may normalize with improved control of IBD but not consistently. In general, liver histology does not appear to improve after colectomy.

Cholelithiasis represents the second most common hepatobiliary manifestation of IBD. Up to one-third of patients with Crohn's disease have gallstones, as compared to 10% to 15% of the general population. Although most Crohn's disease patients with gallstones have small bowel involvement (relative risk for gallstones of 4.5), patients with Crohn's colitis also have an increased risk (relative risk of 3.3). A recent Italian study of risk factors for gallstone formation among patients with Crohn's disease demonstrated that the risk was greatest in patients with a long duration of disease (>30 years), greater extent of ileal involvement (particularly >50 cm), older age (>45 years), and history of multiple bowel resections.

Although the exact mechanisms of the increased risk of cholelithiasis remain speculative, it is believed that ileal disease or resection results in bile salt malabsorption and consequent cholesterol supersaturation of bile. However, a recent study found a significantly lower cholesterol saturation in the bile of patients with Crohn's disease compared to controls. Thus, other factors have been explored.

A high glycine:taurine ratio and a decreased level of deoxycholate in bile increase the lithogenicity of the bile and have been implicated in gallstone formation in patients with Crohn's disease. Prolonged fasting and use of total parenteral nutrition (TPN) are associated with increased rates of biliary sludge formation, which is considered a prerequisite for gallstone formation. Finally,

Table 6-2

HEPATOBILIARY COMPLICATIONS OF INFLAMMATORY BOWEL DISEASE

Complication	Symptoms/ Signs	Liver Enzymes	Liver Biopsy
Steatosis	Rare hepatomegaly	Usually normal; occasional increased AP, ALT, and AST and decreased albumin	Centrilobular or periportal macrovesicular fat that displaces hepatocyte nucleus
Chronic hepatitis	Asymptomatic to liver failure	Moderate increased AST and ALT; variable increased AP and bilirubin	Chronic inflammatory hepatitis cells within the portal tracts and extending into the periportal region; bridging necrosis
Cirrhosis	Ascites, edema, jaundice; range of symptoms from asymptomatic to portal hypertension	Variable increased AST, ALT, AP, and bilirubin	Fibrosis with regenerative nodule formation
Granulomas	Rarely hepatomegaly and fever	Increased AP in 50%	Epithelioid and giant cells surrounded by lymphocytes within the portal tract or lobuli
Granulomatous hepatitis	Fever and jaundice	Significant increased AP and bilirubin	Lobular granulomas
Amyloid	Hepatomegaly	Occasional increased AP and bilirubin	Amyloid deposition in hepatic artery, venules, and bile ducts; Congo red-positive deposits

AP = alkaline phosphatase
ALT = alanine aminotransferase
AST = aspartate aminotransferase

there is evidence of gallbladder hypomotility in patients with IBD, possibly related to an imbalance in circulating levels of somatostatin and cholecystokinin.

In one study, 57% of gallstones in patients with Crohn's disease were pigment (calcium bilirubinate) stones. The mechanism of pigment stone formation in this population may relate to abnormal enterohepatic cycling of bilirubin.

Chronic hepatitis, often with features typical of autoimmune hepatitis, has been found in up to 13% of IBD patients, more commonly in those with ulcerative colitis than in those with Crohn's disease. In some series, chronic hepatitis has accounted for 10% to 15% of patients with abnormal liver biochemical tests in the setting of ulcerative colitis. Most affected patients are younger than age 40, and many are symptomatic with fever, abdominal pain, anorexia, rash, and arthropathy. Findings of liver disease may be seen on physical examination. Laboratory studies reveal mild to moderate elevations in serum aminotransferase levels with minimal elevations in alkaline phosphatase and bilirubin levels. Some patients have circulating antinuclear antibodies (ANA), smooth muscle antibodies, and elevated serum globulin levels. Endoscopic retrograde cholangiopancreatography (ERCP) is generally indicated in these patients because up to 40% may have associated primary sclerosing cholangitis (PSC) (see later discussion). Some patients with chronic hepatitis have associated autoimmune diseases, including polyarteritis nodosa, hypothyroidism, immune thrombocytopenic purpura, and glomerulonephritis. On liver biopsy, there is evidence of chronic portal inflammation, with bridging necrosis in some cases. Rarely, the disease may progress to cirrhosis. Glucocorticoids and azathioprine are used for treatment. Response rates are similar to those of patients with autoimmune hepatitis in the absence of IBD. The liver disease may improve after colectomy, as described in six patients who did not respond to glucocorticoids and azathioprine.

Primary sclerosing cholangitis (PSC), a chronic cholestatic disease of unknown etiology characterized by diffuse inflammation and fibrosis of the intrahepatic and extrahepatic bile ducts, has been reported in 3% to 8% of IBD patients, although the rate may be higher, as some patients with PSC have normal liver biochemical results. Nearly 75% of all patients with PSC have IBD, and over 80% of these have ulcerative colitis. Up to 10% of all patients with ulcerative colitis will develop PSC during their lifetime. Most patients are male (2.5:1 male:female ratio), with a median age of onset of 40 years.

Although the underlying pathogenesis of PSC is unknown, it is believed that portal bacteremia (as a result of bowel inflammation and increased permeability), excess lithocholic acid in bile, and immune dysregulation may play potential roles. Ischemic injury and infectious agents (eg, cytomegalovirus) produce PSC-like bile duct lesions in certain populations (after intra-arterial infusion of chemotherapy to the liver and among immunocompromised persons, respectively), but there is no evidence that they play a role in PSC. Patients with PSC frequently have elevated serum immunoglobulin levels, with elevations in IgM in 25% to 45%, IgA in 25% to 40%, and IgG in 10%. Antineutrophil cytoplasmic antibodies (ANCA) are found in 75% of affected patients, and 10% have a positive ANA, smooth muscle antibodies, or antimitochondrial antibodies (AMA). Certain human leukocyte antigen (HLA) alleles have also been associated with PSC.

Most patients with PSC will have symptoms for 2 years prior to diagnosis, including fatigue (75%), pruritus (70%), jaundice (65%), weight loss (40%), and fever (35%). Nearly one-half of patients have abnormal physical examination findings, including jaundice, hepatomegaly, right upper quadrant tenderness, and, less commonly, clubbing, xanthomas, and ascites. Up to 45% of patients present with asymptomatic elevations in liver biochemical test results. Rarely, patients can present with complications of portal hypertension, including the unique complication of peristomal varices among patients who have undergone colectomy with ileostomy. Bleeding from peristomal varices can be refractory to local treatments, and many patients will require portosystemic shunting. Ileoanal anastomoses are less susceptible to the development of bleeding varices. Patients with PSC are at increased risk of bacterial cholangitis, choledocholithiasis, and cholangiocarcinoma.

The diagnosis of PSC is based on a combination of clinical, biochemical, radiologic, and pathologic findings. Laboratory studies typically show an elevated serum alkaline phosphatase level and mild elevations in serum aminotransferase levels (two to five times above the upper limit of normal). Initially, serum bilirubin levels are normal, and a rising bilirubin may represent a harbinger of a dominant biliary stricture, cholangiocarcinoma, or frank cirrhosis. Cholangiography is the test of choice for making the diagnosis of PSC. Traditionally, ERCP (Figure 6-1) or possibly transhepatic cholangiography (THC) has been used, but increasingly magnetic resonance cholangiopancreatography (MRCP) is being used for diagnosis. Findings on cholangiography include diffuse multifocal annular strictures of intrahepatic and extrahepatic bile ducts. Most patients (approximately 80%) with PSC have involvement of both the intrahepatic and extrahepatic bile ducts; 20% of patients have involvement limited to the intrahepatic and proximal extrahepatic biliary tree. On liver biopsy, characteristic findings include periductal fibrosis (so called "onion-skin" fibrosis), bile ductile proliferation, and portal tract inflammation.

There does not appear to be any association between onset, duration, activity, or extent of IBD and the occurrence of PSC. PSC is usually diagnosed after the IBD is diagnosed and can even present years after colectomy. In most patients, cirrhosis develops after 5 to 10 years. Patients with PSC are at an increased risk for cholangiocarcinoma, with an estimated frequency of 4% to 20% and up to 42% in some autopsy series. Weight loss, anorexia, abdominal pain, or rising liver biochemistries should prompt an evaluation for cholangiocarcinoma in a patient with PSC. Serum CA 19-9 has been used as a screening test for cholangiocarcinoma; levels >100 U/mL predict the presence of cholangiocarcinoma with sensitivity and specificity rates that approach 90%. PSC also seems to be associated with an increased risk of colonic dysplasia and cancer in ulcerative colitis patients.

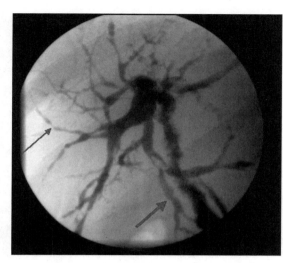

Figure 6-1. Endoscopic retrograde cholangiogram in a patient with primary sclerosing cholangitis. There is evidence of pruning in the intrahepatic bile ducts (thin arrow) and beading of the extrahepatic bile ducts (thick arrow) (courtesy of Robert H. Shapiro, MD, Massachusetts General Hospital, Boston, Mass).

In the majority of cases, progression of PSC occurs over a period of years. The median survival is 10 to 12 years. Older age, elevated serum bilirubin, low serum albumin, elevated aspartate aminotransferase (AST), hepatosplenomegaly, presence of IBD, histologic stage, and presence of variceal bleeding have all been identified as independent risk factors for a poor prognosis. The age-adjusted Child-Turcotte-Pugh model (Table 6-3) predicts survival before liver transplantation with an accuracy similar to that of the Mayo PSC mathematical model of survival probability (Table 6-4).

Medical therapy options for PSC are limited. Use of antibiotics and endoscopic dilation with short-term stent placement has made a significant impact on the morbidity and mortality associated with recurrent cholangitis and bile duct strictures. Ursodeoxycholic acid has not been shown to alter the natural history of PSC but may improve liver biochemical test results. Use of high doses (20 to 25 mg/kg/day) may have some benefit and is under study. There does not appear to be any benefit to glucocorticoids or colectomy. PSC remains one of the most common indications for orthotopic liver transplantation in the United States. In addition to end-stage liver disease, indications for transplantation include a serum bilirubin level >10 mg/dL, recurrent variceal bleeding, recurrent cholangitis, and severe osteomalacia. In approximately 10% of patients, cholangiocarcinoma is detected in the explanted liver. A preoperative diagnosis of cholangiocarcinoma generally precludes liver transplantation because of unacceptably high recurrence rates. Five-year survival rates after transplantation approach 85%. Recurrence of PSC after liver transplantation has been reported.

The term *pericholangitis* was used in the past to describe a subset of patients with inflammation involving the small bile ducts only. The term *small-duct*

Table 6-3

CHILD-TURCOTTE-PUGH CLASSIFICATION
OF SEVERITY OF LIVER DISEASE

Parameter	*Points* 1	2	3
Ascites	Absent	Slight	Moderate
Bilirubin (mg/dL)	<2	2 to 3	>3
Albumin (g/dL)	>3.5	2.8 to 3.5	<2.8
INR	<1.7	1.8 to 2.3	>2.3
Encephalopathy	None	Grades I to II	Grades III to IV

Note: A total score of 5 to 6 is considered class A (well-compensated cirrhosis; 1 year survival of 100%), 7 to 9 is class B (significant functional compromise; 1 year survival of 80%), and 10 to 15 is class C (decompensated disease; 1 year survival of 45%).

INR = International normalized ratio

Table 6-4

MAYO MODEL FOR SURVIVAL PROBABILITY
IN PRIMARY SCLEROSING CHOLANGITIS

R = 0.03 (age [years])
+ 0.54 $\log_e$ (bilirubin [mg/dL])
+ 0.54 $\log_e$ (AST [IU/L])
+ 1.24 (variceal bleed [0 = no, 1 = yes])
- 0.84 (albumin [g/dL])

Survival function coefficient [$S_0^{(t)}$] at

1 year	= 0.963	3 years	= 0.873
2 years	= 0.919	4 years	= 0.833

Probability of patient survival at time (t) year = $[S_0^{(t)}]^{(R-1.00)}$

A web-based calculator can be found at www.mayo.edu/int-med/gi/model/mayomodl.htm

AST = aspartate aminotransferase

Adapted from Kim WR, Therneau TM, Weisner RH, et al. A revised natural history model for primary sclerosing cholangitis. *Mayo Clin Proc.* 2000;75(7):688.

PSC is now used to describe such patients. It may occur in up to 30% of IBD patients, with similar rates among patients with Crohn's disease, usually in patients with primarily colonic involvement, and patients with ulcerative colitis. The severity and course of small-duct PSC seem to be independent of those of the underlying IBD. Most patients have an elevated serum alkaline phosphatase level. In a study by Wee and Ludwig[5] involving 1067 patients with ulcerative colitis and hepatobiliary disease, 37 had *pericholangitis*. Of these, 50% later developed PSC.

An association between cholangiocarcinoma and ulcerative colitis was first described in 1954. The estimated frequency has been reported to be 0.4% to 1.4%, which is 20 to 30 times that of the general population. The mean age at diagnosis is 40, which is 20 years younger than the mean age in patients without ulcerative colitis. It is more common in men than women (1.6:1). Cholangiocarcinoma almost always develops in patients with pre-existing PSC. The majority of patients with ulcerative colitis in whom cholangiocarcinoma develops will have had ulcerative colitis, usually pancolitis, for at least 15 years. Cholangiocarcinoma may also develop after proctocolectomy. Patients with cholangiocarcinoma usually present with fever, pain, jaundice, and weight loss. Diagnosis is generally made by computed tomography (CT) scan or ERCP, although up to 25% of cases are diagnosed at autopsy. Cholangiocarcinoma is a contraindication to liver transplantation because of the high probability of recurrence.

Cryptogenic cirrhosis occurs in up to 11% of IBD patients. The diagnosis usually follows that of the underlying IBD. In general, most affected patients have pancolitis. Autoimmune hepatitis or PSC is the suspected cause of cirrhosis in most cases. Patients with IBD and cirrhosis tend to have lower survival rates than patients with either IBD or cirrhosis alone. In order to avoid peristomal varices, patients with cirrhosis who undergo colectomy should have an ileal pouch-anal anastomosis created. Standard surveillance for hepatocellular carcinoma is recommended.

Hepatic granulomas may be found in up to 8% of all IBD patients, with Crohn's disease patients predominating. Other causes of hepatic granulomas should be considered, including drugs, sarcoidosis, and tuberculosis. Pathologically, noncaseating granulomas are found in the portal tracts or lobuli. Clinically, patients may range from being asymptomatic to having hepatomegaly, fever, and jaundice. Elevations in serum alkaline phosphatase and bilirubin levels can be seen in up to 50% of cases. Affected patients may respond to glucocorticoids and, in some cases, to bowel resection.

Granulomatous hepatitis is seen in 1% of all IBD patients. In these cases, granulomas are found in hepatic lobuli but not in portal tracts. Clinically, patients may exhibit fever and jaundice, often with elevated serum alkaline phosphatase and bilirubin levels.

Drug hepatotoxicity, specifically granulomatous hepatitis, has been reported with sulfasalazine, usually at doses greater than 4 g/day and rarely with mesalamine. Generally, the sulfapyridine moiety is believed to account for this reaction. Most cases develop 1 to 4 weeks after initiation of therapy. Azathioprine and 6-mercaptopurine have been associated with cholestasis, peliosis hepatitis, and hepatic veno-occlusive disease. Patients on chronic TPN are at increased risk of chronic cholestasis, steatohepatitis, and cholelithiasis.

There are several uncommon hepatobiliary manifestations of IBD. A *necrotizing arteritis* has been associated with ulcerative colitis and may respond to colectomy. *Hemosiderosis* has rarely been seen in patients who have received multiple blood transfusions. *Hepatic abscesses* have been reported primarily among patients with fistulizing Crohn's disease. *Primary biliary cirrhosis* was seen in only 0.2% of patients with ulcerative colitis in one recent study and does not appear to be associated with Crohn's disease at all.

IBD patients also appear to have an increased risk of developing acute and chronic *pancreatitis*. There are a number of postmortem reports describing pancreatic fibrosis. Most cases of acute pancreatitis in the IBD population are related to drugs, particularly azathioprine or 6-mercaptopurine. There are also reports of pancreatitis in the setting of Crohn's involvement of the duodenum with resulting ampullary obstruction. There are several reports of idiopathic pancreatitis as well.

The etiology of chronic pancreatitis associated with IBD remains unclear in most cases. Symptoms of pancreatic exocrine insufficiency may develop over time. Chronic pancreatitis associated with ulcerative colitis differs from that observed in Crohn's disease by the presence of more frequent bile duct involvement, weight loss, and pancreatic duct stenosis, possibly giving a pseudotumor appearance. Chronic pancreatitis precedes ulcerative colitis in 58% of affected patients. In contrast, the pancreatitis appears after the onset of Crohn's disease in 56% of cases. Pancreatitis in patients with ulcerative colitis has been associated with pancolitis (42%) and the need for colectomy. Granulomas in the pancreas have been found in some patients with Crohn's disease who have undergone surgery for chronic pancreatitis.

MUSCULOSKELETAL MANIFESTATIONS

Musculoskeletal complications are probably the most common extraintestinal manifestations of IBD, with a reported frequency of up to 23%. An association between arthritis and IBD was first reported in 1935 when Hench[6] described a patient with peripheral joint arthritis and ulcerative colitis. In the subsequent decades, numerous reports described arthritis as a symptom of the underlying IBD. It was not until 1959 that investigators described a distinct form of arthritis occurring in patients with IBD.

The most common form of arthritis in IBD is the so-called *enteropathic arthritis*, which is seen in 15% to 20% of IBD patients. It is more common in patients with Crohn's disease (20%) than in those with ulcerative colitis (12%). In one series, enteropathic arthritis among patients with Crohn's disease was seen in 16% of patients with colonic disease, 4% of those with small bowel involvement, and 3.6% of those with ileocolonic disease. The average age at diagnosis is 30, and males and females are affected equally.

Clinically, enteropathic arthritis is characterized by inflammation of larger joints. The most common joints involved are the knees, ankles, elbows, and wrists, followed by the small joints of the hands and feet. A pauciarticular pattern of involvement (<5 joints) tends to be acute and self-limited. Over 90% of flares, however, are polyarticular, and in nearly one-half of affected patients, the pattern of involvement is migratory. Typically, patients present with joint pain and swelling with decreased range of motion; the severity of symptoms peaks within 24 hours. Flares tend to correlate with the activity of the underlying IBD. Arthritic symptoms usually begin concurrently with or after the diagnosis of IBD, although there have been cases in which arthritis has predated the diagnosis of IBD. Enteropathic arthritis often occurs in association with other extraintestinal manifestations of IBD, particularly erythema nodosum, pyoderma gangrenosum, aphthous ulcers, and uveitis (see later discussion). Rheumatoid factor and HLA-B27 are generally not found. Radiologic evaluation of the affected joints shows evidence of soft tissue edema and joint effusions. Less than 20% of patients have bony erosions. Arthrocentesis of joint effusions typically reveals a white blood cell count of 5000 to 12,000 cells/mL and synovial complement and protein levels may be low. If a synovial biopsy is performed, it often demonstrates nonspecific inflammation. Approximately 50% of flares last less than 1 month, and less than 5% of patients have chronic symptoms. Chronic joint deformities and flexion contractures are quite rare.

Treatment strategies include glucocorticoids (both systemic and intra-articular), nonsteroidal anti-inflammatory drugs (NSAIDs), and physical therapy with both active and passive motion regimens. Bowel resection seems to have a more favorable effect on arthritis in patients with ulcerative colitis than in those with Crohn's disease.

Two forms of axial arthropathy can be seen in patients with IBD: spondylitis and isolated sacroiliitis. They occur with equal frequency among patients with Crohn's disease and ulcerative colitis. Axial arthropathy can predate the diagnosis of IBD, although it occurs most often after the onset of bowel symptoms. Spondylitis affects as many as 11% of IBD patients, although most studies demonstrate a frequency of approximately 4%. *Spondylitis* associated with IBD is clinically indistinguishable from idiopathic ankylosing spondylitis. However, unlike idiopathic ankylosing spondylitis, in which the mean age at diagnosis is in the twenties, IBD-associated spondylitis can occur at any age.

Males are affected slightly more commonly than females, with a male:female ratio of 1.5:1. Many patients have concurrent iritis. Approximately two thirds of patients are positive for HLA-B27, as compared to 90% of patients with idiopathic ankylosing spondylitis. Clinically, spondylitis is characterized by lower back pain, which is insidious in nature and characterized by morning stiffness. The pain is typically relieved with exercise and worsened with rest. Some patients also manifest pelvic, shoulder, and knee symptoms. There is limited spinal flexion, reduced chest wall expansion, and often sacroiliac pain on examination. Early radiologic hallmarks (Figure 6-2) are symmetric sacroiliac erosions with sclerosis. Later, as the disease progresses, bony bridging can be seen to progress from lumbar to cervical spine with ligamentous ossification, vertebral squaring, and osteitis pubis. In some patients,

Figure 6-2. Lumbosacral spinal x-ray of a patient with ulcerative colitis and ankylosing spondylitis. There is evidence of bony bridging between the vertebrae (arrows) (courtesy of Leon Ryback, MD, Massachusetts General Hospital, Boston, Mass).

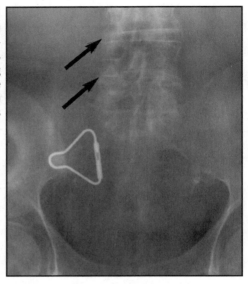

Figure 6-3. Pelvic x-ray of a patient with ulcerative colitis and sacroiliitis. There is evidence of bilateral sacroiliac joint narrowing and sclerosis (arrows) (courtesy of Leon Ryback, MD, Massachusetts General Hospital, Boston, Mass).

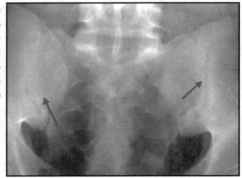

arthritis may also involve the hip and shoulder joints. These changes can lead to severe disability over several decades. There does not appear to be any correlation between the severity, extent, location, and duration of the underlying IBD and the course of spondylitis. NSAIDs and physical therapy are the mainstays of therapy, as glucocorticoids and bowel resection do not seem to affect the course significantly.

Isolated sacroiliitis (Figure 6-3) is also common in IBD patients and has been noted radiologically in up to 25% of IBD patients; the vast majority of these patients have no back pain. Unlike spondylitis, sacroiliitis is not associated with HLA-B27. Its course is independent of that of the underlying IBD. Treatment strategies involve analgesics and physical therapy.

Hypertrophic osteoarthropathy is seen in up to 58% of patients with Crohn's disease, primarily in those with small bowel involvement. The first case was described in 1968.[7] Typical clinical features include clubbing (33% to 58% of patients with Crohn's disease and 15% of patients with ulcerative colitis) and periostitis associated with bone pain (particularly along the anterior tibia, metacarpal, and distal femur). Rarely, patients may have asymptomatic involvement of multiple bone groups. In most affected patients, symptoms of bowel disease precede the diagnosis of hypertrophic osteoarthropathy by many years, and in the majority of patients the diagnosis of Crohn's disease is made before the age of 25. The correlation between bowel manifestations and activity of the osteoarthropathy is poor.

Rare extraintestinal manifestations include *metastatic Crohn's disease*, with noncaseating epithelioid granulomas of the synovium, muscle, and bone. Patients typically present with pain, difficulty ambulating, and, at times, induration over the affected area. These lesions are usually responsive to glucocorticoids. *Clinical vasculitis* is a relatively rare extraintestinal manifestation, even though granulomatous vasculitis is often seen microscopically in resected bowel specimens from patients with Crohn's disease. There are reports of granulomatous vasculitis involving the vessels of the aortic arch, mesentery, kidney, retina (leading to ischemic optic neuropathy), and muscle beds, including five cases involving the gastrocnemius muscle.

Relapsing polychondritis has been reported in association with both ulcerative colitis and Crohn's disease, although it is reported more commonly with the former. Classically, relapsing polychondritis is characterized by at least three of the following: bilateral auricular chondritis, nonerosive seronegative arthritis, nasal chondritis, ocular inflammation, laryngeal or tracheal chondritis, and cochlear or vestibular injury resulting in tinnitus and hearing loss. About one-half of patients have circulating antibodies to type II collagen. Most cases are diagnosed after the development of bowel symptoms. In a few reported cases, there appears to have been a correlation with bowel disease activity. Initial treatment includes local skin care and NSAIDs. In more severe cases, systemic glucocorticoids, dapsone, methotrexate, and cyclosporine have been used.

Other reported musculoskeletal associations with IBD include *avascular necrosis of the hips* (which may also be a complication of glucocorticoid therapy) and *pelvic osteomyelitis*.

Dermatologic Manifestations

Dermatologic manifestations occur in up to 15% of patients with IBD. In general, they are more common in female patients and in patients with colonic Crohn's disease. The two most common manifestations—erythema nodosum and pyoderma gangrenosum—are rarely seen in the same patient.

Erythema nodosum (EN) was first described in association with IBD in 1929 and can be found in up to 15% of patients with Crohn's disease and 10% of those with ulcerative colitis. Clinically, EN is characterized by tender, erythematous raised nodules that measure 1 to 5 cm in diameter and are found most typically on the anterior tibia and less commonly on the ankles, calves, thighs, and arms. Biopsy of the nodules shows fibrinoid degeneration without evidence of vasculitis. EN is usually diagnosed after the diagnosis of IBD is made, although there have been patients in whom EN preceded IBD. Approximately 80% of patients with EN are diagnosed in the setting of an acute bowel flare, with most patients having left colonic involvement. For most patients, there will be only a single episode of EN. Recurrent episodes of EN tend to correlate less specifically with the extent or severity of colitis. Rarely, a first episode of EN can be seen after colectomy. Approximately 70% of patients with EN also have enteropathic arthritis. Treatment may include glucocorticoids, potassium iodide, NSAIDs, and colchicine. After adequate treatment, the lesions may involute, often leaving areas of hyperpigmentation behind.

Pyoderma gangrenosum (PG) was described initially in 1916 by Brocq.[8] Over 500 cases have now been reported in the literature. PG is an ulcerative disease of the skin that is associated in 30% to 50% of IBD cases (Figure 6-4). Other associations include hematologic malignancies, chronic hepatitis, rheumatoid arthritis, and Takayasu's arteritis. Conversely, PG occurs in up to 12% of patients with ulcerative colitis and in only 1% to 2% of patients with Crohn's disease; the latter rate is similar to that seen in elderly persons without IBD. When PG does occur in patients with Crohn's disease, it is almost exclusively found in those with purely colonic involvement. There is a slight female predominance in most series.

PG typically begins as a pustule or fluctuant nodule anywhere on the body, although classically on the dorsum of the foot. Parastomal involvement may also be seen in up to 13% of cases. Lesions may be single or multiple and range in size from 1 to 30 cm. The lesions may coalesce and then ulcerate within a few days. An atypical bullous variant has also been described. Pathergy is seen in up to 50% of affected patients. Moreover, a future site of PG may be tender for days to weeks before typical dermatologic manifestations appear. Biopsy of a lesion reveals dermal and epidermal necrosis and a chronic lymphocytic vasculitis. However, the decision to biopsy these lesions is controversial because there is a risk of poor healing.

PG tends to be found in ulcerative colitis patients who are diagnosed later in life (as compared to EN) and is most often diagnosed years after the underlying IBD. As in EN, 80% of patients are diagnosed with PG in the setting of an acute flare of their bowel disease, with most patients (85%) having pancolitis. Less than 25% of patients will have recurrent episodes of PG. Approximately 38% of patients also have enteropathic arthritis. PG usually runs a course independent of that of the underlying bowel disease, although in general it is seen more commonly in patients with severe IBD.

Aggressive medical therapy of the underlying IBD is generally warranted. Prevention of secondary skin infections with topical antibiotics and good skin

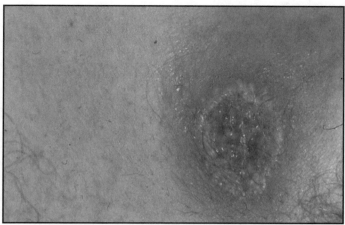

Figure 6-4. Pyoderma gangrenosum in a patient with ulcerative colitis. Note the violaceous margin around the ulcer bed (courtesy of Bonnie Mackool, MD, Massachusetts General Hospital, Boston, Mass).

care is critical. Therapeutic agents potentially useful in treating PG include glucocorticoids (systemic, topical, and intralesional), dapsone, sulfapyridine, minocycline, clofazimine, rifampin, systemic and topical tacrolimus, cyclosporine, 6-mercaptopurine, thalidomide, and infliximab. Unfortunately, lesions may heal with scar formation and sometimes remain painful. Debridement and placement of skin grafts are usually associated with delayed healing. Colectomy is often reserved for the most refractory cases.

Pyoderma vegetans and *vesiculopustular eruption of ulcerative colitis* have also been reported. These eruptions tend to be evanescent and correlate with activity of the underlying IBD. Pyoderma vegetans is a benign, rare disorder characterized by an oral pustular eruption and vegetating plaques anywhere on the body, particularly the inguinal and axillary folds. The disease may also manifest as multiple vesicles in intertriginous areas. Mucosal involvement can also be seen. On biopsy, dermal infiltration with polymorphonuclear cells and eosinophils and epidermal hyperplasia are seen. Immunofluorescence studies are negative. Vesiculopustular eruption of ulcerative colitis is characterized by the linear deposition of IgG along the basement membrane of the epidermis of the skin and neutrophilic abscesses. Lesions usually heal spontaneously over several months, usually with residual hyperpigmentation. Treatment of both disorders is directed against the underlying bowel disease.

Cutaneous polyarteritis nodosa (*PAN*) was first reported in association with Crohn's disease in the 1970s. Since then, there have been at least a dozen reports in the literature. Most patients have been men, with an average age of

30. Cutaneous PAN is characterized by painful nodules along the feet, legs, and, less commonly, the trunk and upper extremities; the lesions often go on to ulcerate. Biopsy shows a necrotizing small- and medium-vessel vasculitis at the dermal/subcutaneous junction with leukocytoclasis and fibrinoid necrosis. The disorder may follow a chronic, relapsing course but appears to behave independently of the underlying IBD. In the majority of cases, cutaneous PAN develops after the diagnosis of the underlying IBD. Treatment options include systemic glucocorticoids, sulfasalazine, azathioprine, and cyclophosphamide. Remission after bowel resection has also been reported, but the disease may relapse subsequently. Rare complications include tissue gangrene and large vessel thrombosis requiring anticoagulation.

Metastatic Crohn's disease of the skin was first described by Parks[9] in 1965. Lesions contain granulomas at the dermal/subcutaneous junction of skin noncontiguous to the gastrointestinal tract. Most of these reported cases have occurred in patients with known colonic involvement. However, 21% of metastatic Crohn's disease cases develop simultaneously with or precede by several months to years the gastrointestinal disease.

In 1997, Lucky and colleagues[10] published a retrospective review of 80 reported cases of metastatic Crohn's disease occurring between 1965 and 1995. Genital involvement was noted in 56% of cases, whereas nongenital sites, including extremities, trunk, face and lips, and intertriginous/flexural areas, constituted 44% of cases. Clinically, the nongenital lesions presented as painful nodules, ulcerations, lichenoid papules, pustules, and abscesses. Genital manifestations include tender perivulvar, perineal, and perirectal ulcerations; fissures; skin tags; and swelling. Microscopically, metastatic Crohn's disease is characterized by a noncaseating granulomatous infiltration of the dermis, with occasional extension into subcutaneous fat. The presence of lesions does not appear to correlate with the activity of the Crohn's disease.

Numerous therapies for the treatment of metastatic Crohn's disease have been attempted. Although most lesions spontaneously resolve, genital lesions appear to be especially recalcitrant to treatment. Systemic, intralesional, and topical glucocorticoids, dapsone, sulfasalazine, azathioprine, metronidazole, tetracycline, 6-mercaptopurine, and zinc supplementation are among the treatments purported to be of benefit. Surgical debridement, hyperbaric oxygen, and fecal diversion have been used in resistant cases.

Epidermolysis acquisita is characterized by blisters, excess scar formation, and milia. Approximately 25% of patients affected with epidermolysis acquisita have underlying IBD. There does not appear to be a relationship with bowel disease activity. Lesions may develop at sites of trauma. At biopsy, there is evidence of cleavage at the dermal/epidermal junction. Perilesional skin may also exhibit basement membrane deposition of immunoglobulins. Dapsone and glucocorticoids have been used to treat this disorder, but it is often refractory to therapy.

Psoriasis is seen more frequently in patients with IBD than in the general population; 6% and 11% of patients with ulcerative colitis and Crohn's disease, respectively, are affected, compared to 1% to 2% of the general population. The course of psoriasis appears to be unrelated to that of the underlying IBD.

Figure 6-5. Perianal disease in a patient with Crohn's disease (courtesy of Bonnie Mackool, MD, Massachusetts General Hospital, Boston, Mass).

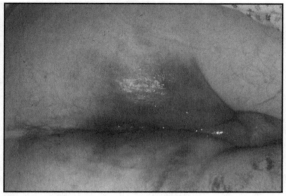

Sweet's syndrome, also known as acute febrile neutrophilic dermatosis, was first reported to be associated with IBD in 1988 and is an acute cutaneous illness characterized by raised erythematous plaques or nodules and occasionally pustules and vesicles. Most patients have fever, leukocytosis, and malaise. In addition to IBD, Sweet's syndrome has been associated with hematologic and genitourinary malignancies. Most affected IBD patients reported in the literature have been young females with colonic IBD. The disorder appears most often when bowel disease is active or shortly after colectomy. Treatment with glucocorticoids or metronidazole has been successful.

Perianal skin tags are seen most often in patients with Crohn's disease (75% to 80%), particularly those with Crohn's colitis (Figure 6-5). *Oral lesions* are found in up to 20% of patients with IBD and include aphthous stomatitis, glossitis, buccal cobblestoning, and lip fissures. *Nutritional deficiencies* may develop in the setting of intestinal malabsorption in patients with Crohn's disease. Zinc deficiency has been associated with perioral ulcerations and an extensor surface dermatitis. Nicotinic acid deficiency is associated with symmetric red plaques at sites of trauma and on sun-exposed surfaces (ie, elbows, dorsum of the hands, and anterior neck [V-shape]). *Erythema multiforme* and *Stevens-Johnson syndrome* have been reported in association with sulfasalazine use among IBD patients. *Rosacea fulminans*, a severe and potentially disfiguring form of acne rosacea, has been reported mostly in patients with ulcerative colitis.

OCULAR MANIFESTATIONS

There are many ocular manifestations of IBD. The most common include conjunctivitis, uveitis/iritis, and episcleritis. Ocular complications have been estimated to occur in up to 13% of patients with Crohn's disease and up to 11% of those with ulcerative colitis. Unfortunately, the precise prevalence rates

Figure 6-6. Episcleritis (courtesy of George Papaliodis, MD, Massachusetts Eye and Ear Infirmary, Boston, Mass).

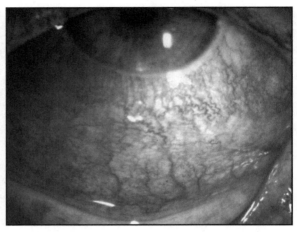

are unknown because most patients do not have scheduled eye examinations. Colonic involvement and the presence of arthritic extraintestinal manifestations are clear risk factors for ocular involvement. Most, if not all, ocular complaints in patients with IBD should prompt evaluation by an ophthalmologist.

Episcleritis occurs in 3% to 4% of all patients with IBD. However, it is more common in patients with Crohn's disease, particularly in those with involvement of the colon, than in those with ulcerative colitis. It appears to correlate with the activity of IBD. Clinically, episcleritis is characterized by burning, itching, and hyperemia of the sclera (Figure 6-6). Changes in visual acuity should prompt consideration of other diagnoses. Adequate control of ocular inflammation is achieved with topical and oral glucocorticoids, topical and oral NSAIDs, hydroxychloroquine, and azathioprine. Oral NSAIDs have been used to prevent attacks in some patients.

Uveitis accounts for up to 20% of all cases of blindness in the Western world. There is a 2% to 30% frequency of uveitis among patients with Crohn's disease and enteropathic arthritis. Episodes of uveitis may parallel the activity of the bowel disease, although not as closely as in episcleritis. Nearly one-half of IBD patients with uveitis are positive for HLA-B27. Uveitis usually presents with eye pain, red eye, blurred vision, headaches, photophobia, and abnormal pupillary responses to light (Figure 6-7). Subclinical uveitis is uncommon and has been reported in the pediatric IBD population only. Granulomatous uveitis is a rare variant found among patients with Crohn's disease. Suspected uveitis requires urgent ophthalmologic evaluation with a slit-lamp examination. Characteristic findings on slit-lamp examination include perilimbic erythema, cells in the anterior chamber, and "flare" resulting from proteinaceous deposits within the aqueous humor.

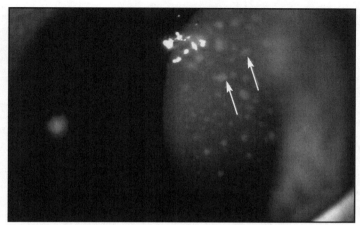

Figure 6-7. Uveitis (courtesy of George Papaliodis, MD, Massachusetts Eye and Ear Infirmary, Boston, Mass).

Prompt intervention is required in order to prevent iris atrophy, synechiae, and lens pigment deposits. Patients may require systemic or topical glucocorticoids. Rifampin and methotrexate have rarely been used in glucocorticoid-refractory cases in patients with Crohn's disease. Infliximab tends to not have a significant therapeutic benefit in uveitis. In general, patients who are HLA-B27 positive tend to be more refractory to glucocorticoids. Colectomy has been performed in patients with uveitis refractory to medical therapy, although some patients may experience further episodes of uveitis after colectomy.

Central serous retinopathy with bullous retinal detachment occurs in 1% of patients with IBD, typically patients with ileocolitis. They present with blurred vision and scotoma. Treatment involves the use of glucocorticoids (topical and systemic) and, less frequently, laser therapy. Spontaneous remissions rarely occur. *Retinal artery occlusion* and *retinal vein occlusion* have also been reported. On funduscopy, one can see capillary leak, cotton-wool spots, and retinal hemorrhages. Treatment is with topical glucocorticoids. Uncommon ocular manifestations of IBD include *orbital myositis* presenting with *proptosis, retrobulbar neuritis, neuroretinitis, scleromalacia perforans, ischemic optic neuropathy, deep stromal inflammation, orbital cellulitis, papillitis,* and *marginal corneal ulcers* (Figure 6-8). Specific complications, including *subcapsular cataracts, glaucoma, ocular infections,* and *exophthalmos,* may develop in patients on chronic glucocorticoid therapy.

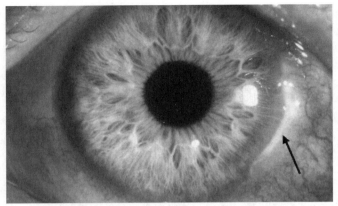

Figure 6-8. Marginal corneal ulcers. Note the ulcerated corneal margin (arrow) (courtesy of George Papaliodis, MD, Massachusetts Eye and Ear Infirmary, Boston, Mass).

UROGENITAL MANIFESTATIONS

Urogenital manifestations have been reported to affect 4% to 23% of IBD patients; patients with Crohn's disease are affected more often than those with ulcerative colitis. The most common complications are renal amyloidosis, nephrolithiasis, retroperitoneal abscess, periureteral fibrosis, cystitis, and fistulae.

Nephrolithiasis is the most common urogenital complication of IBD, affecting 8% to 19% of patients, compared to 0.1% of the general population. The highest frequency appears to be among patients with Crohn's disease who have had an ileal resection. Nephrolithiasis is more common in patients with ileo-colonic disease (9% to 17%) than in those with disease limited to the small bowel (6% to 8%) or colon (3% to 5%). Such patients are predisposed to the development of calcium oxalate, uric acid, and calcium phosphate stones. Stones are most commonly multiple and right sided.

Calcium oxalate stones are radiopaque and develop in the setting of hyperoxaluria. Hyperoxaluria results from increased intestinal absorption of dietary oxalate. Oxalate is found in many foods, including spinach, rhubarb, beets, nuts, tea, soda, chocolate, berries, wheat bran, yams, and celery. The following three theories have been proposed to account for the high prevalence of calcium oxalate stones in patients with IBD:

1. In the setting of ileal disease, nonabsorbed fatty acids reach the colon and bind luminal calcium, which is then unavailable to bind oxalate. The oxalate is then readily absorbed by the colonic mucosa.

2. *Oxalobacter formigenes,* an anaerobic bacterium in the colon that degrades oxalate, may be reduced in number in patients with Crohn's disease as a result of inhibition by poorly absorbed bile salts.

3. Increased mucosal permeability from low intraluminal calcium levels may allow increased oxalate absorption. In general, hyperoxaluria is rare when fecal fat excretion is <15 g/day or <30 cm of terminal ileum has been resected.

Patients with ileostomies are not at increased risk of calcium oxalate stones; an intact colon is required for oxalate stones to develop, except in cases related to chronic TPN, in which there may be increased endogenous oxalate synthesis. A contributing factor includes decreased urinary excretion of inhibitors of calcium urolithiasis, including magnesium, pyrophosphate, and citrate. Diminished urinary volume due to high stool water output may also predispose to urolithiasis. Treatment strategies include dietary restriction of oxalate-containing foods, use of calcium supplements (1 to 2 g/day) to bind luminal oxalate, use of cholestyramine (4 g/day) to bind luminal oxalate, and use of inhibitors, such as citrate and magnesium salts, to prevent urolithiasis. However, use of cholestyramine and magnesium supplements may actually promote diarrhea. Limiting fat intake (<50 g/day) while using medium chain triglycerides (which do not require bile salts for intestinal absorption) and increasing daily fluid intake may also decrease the risk of hyperoxaluria.

Uric acid stones may develop in patients with ileostomies or with copious diarrhea. Up to 5% of patients with ulcerative colitis develop uric acid stones. Uric acid stones, which are radiolucent, develop in the setting of excessive alkaline fluid losses from the gastrointestinal tract with resulting concentrated, acidified urine. At a pH of less than 5, 75% of uric acid is insoluble. Contributing factors include hyperuricemia; urinary tract infection; urinary tract obstruction; therapy with glucocorticoids; low urine levels of potassium, sodium, magnesium, and citrate; hypercalcemia; bed rest; and high gastrointestinal tract fluid output. Patients with recurrent episodes of urate nephrolithiasis may respond to bicarbonate and sodium supplementation.

The development of calcium phosphate stones is usually limited to pediatric IBD patients. The main risk factors for this form of nephrolithiasis include prolonged bed rest resulting in mobilization of skeletal calcium stores and use of glucocorticoids, which may not only increase calcium mobilization but also increase urinary excretion of calcium.

IBD accounts for up to 8% of cases of *secondary amyloidosis,* in which there is abnormal tissue deposition of serum amyloid-A protein, which is an acute phase reactant. Levels of serum amyloid-A protein are often chronically elevated in the serum of patients with IBD. In one series of 214 patients with Crohn's disease, the frequency of amyloidosis was 6%. Amyloidosis is much less frequent in patients with ulcerative colitis, with a frequency of <1%. Amyloidosis should be suspected when patients develop severe intestinal malabsorption, renal failure with nephrosis, or hepatomegaly (which may be associated with elevations in serum alkaline phosphatase and bilirubin levels). The majority of patients have renal involvement. In some autopsy series, nearly

25% of patients with Crohn's disease have had histologic evidence of renal amyloid. There is a 3.5:1 male:female ratio, and the mean age at diagnosis is 40. Most patients in whom amyloidosis develops have ileocolonic involvement. No correlation with suppurative complications or duration of IBD has been found in most studies. The progression of amyloidosis may be slowed by colchicine, usually at doses of 0.6 to 1.5 mg/day. Some patients with renal amyloidosis have also been treated with plasmapheresis and azathioprine. There are mixed data about the benefit of colectomy for reversing amyloid deposition. In general, surgery should be directed at ameliorating refractory bowel symptoms rather than attempting to reverse the amyloidosis. For patients with end-stage renal disease, kidney transplantation and aggressive immunosuppressive therapy can lead to long-term survival.

Retroperitoneal abscesses usually develop as a result of local extension of suppurative Crohn's disease. They may be located in the perinephric space, along the iliopsoas muscle, or in the deep pelvis. Extrinsic compression may cause ureteral or renal deviation and bladder deformity. Ureteral involvement ranges from periureteral fibrosis to complete obstruction. Although collections are typically right sided and occur in the setting of severe terminal ileal or cecal Crohn's disease, they have been reported in the left side of the abdomen in the setting of jejunal involvement. Clinically, patients may present with fever, abdominal pain, night sweats, and weight loss. Treatment includes catheter drainage and antibiotics, as well as control of bowel inflammation.

Noncalculous obstructive uropathy accounts for over one-half of the cases of ureteral obstruction in patients with Crohn's disease and ulcerative colitis and is unrelated to age, gender, duration of disease, extent of disease, and bowel disease activity. Obstructive uropathy has been found on intravenous pyelogram in up to 50% of asymptomatic patients with Crohn's disease. Most patients have few, if any, symptoms, including urinary urgency, frequency, dysuria, and fever. More than 75% of cases occur on the right side. Most cases of noncalculous obstructive uropathy result from retroperitoneal inflammation in association with ileal or ileocecal Crohn's involvement or retroperitoneal fibrosis from prior episodes of inflammation or near prior surgical sites, as also may occur in patients with ulcerative colitis. Colorectal cancer that develops in the setting of chronic ulcerative colitis has also been reported to cause noncalculous obstructive uropathy. Although most affected patients remain asymptomatic, there have been reports of recurrent pyelonephritis, hypertension, and pyonephrosis, which rarely require nephrectomy.

Initial treatment includes medical treatment of the underlying IBD. Ureteral stents are reserved for significant obstruction. Catheter drainage of focal abscesses is indicated. If there is no improvement with conservative therapies, bowel resection is indicated and usually leads to resolution of the obstructive uropathy. If complications continue to develop, ureterolysis and, uncommonly, nephrectomy may be necessary.

Fistulae, which may be enterovesical, enteroureteral, or enterovaginal, affect up to 8% of patients with Crohn's disease, approximately one-third the frequency of enteroenteric fistulae. After diverticulitis and malignancy, Crohn's disease is the most frequent cause of enterovesical fistulae, accounting for 5%

to 17% of all cases and 75% of cases in patients under the age of 40. Enterovesical fistulae arise from direct extension of transmural inflammation and most commonly involve the ileum and sigmoid colon. Most patients have well-established IBD at the time of fistula formation. The mean age of diagnosis is 50. Women are less affected than men because of the presence of the uterus and adnexa as intermediary structures.

Typically, patients present with persistent symptoms of cystitis including dysuria, urinary frequency, and urinary urgency. Pneumaturia and fecaluria, which are considered pathognomonic of an enterovesical fistula, have been in 38% to 94% and 17% to 63% of cases, respectively. Urorhea, the passage of urine via the rectum, is quite uncommon. Other uncommon clinical findings include epididymitis, hematuria, and prostatitis. Physical examination is usually normal, but abnormal findings may include fever, abdominal tenderness, and concomitant enterocutaneous fistulae. Over one-half of patients will have a positive urine culture, of which 33% will be polymicrobial.

Fistulae are difficult to identify. A high degree of suspicion must be maintained. Many patients are treated for chronic genitourinary infections for months to years before a diagnosis of fistula is made. Visualization of a fistula by direct endoscopic evaluation is limited. Cystoscopy can visualize a fistula in 6.7% to 67% of cases. CT scanning appears to be the most sensitive imaging modality. Findings may include air in the bladder, apposition of abnormal bowel to bladder, a paravesical mass or collection, and the detection of contrast medium in the bladder. Magnetic resonance imaging (MRI) has also been used to identify fistulae deep in the pelvis. Detection of barium in a centrifuged urine specimen after a barium study of the lower gastrointestinal tract (ie, Bourne test) may also provide a clue to the diagnosis of a fistula. Cystography is considered the best contrast study in these patients. More recently, endoscopic ultrasound has been particularly useful in characterizing perianorectal urinary fistulae.

Surgical debridement is usually indicated for enterovesical fistulae, although closure of the fistulae has been demonstrated with use of immunomodulatory agents (eg, glucocorticoids, azathioprine, 6-mercaptopurine) and rarely spontaneously. Most patients with Crohn's disease can be managed with a one-stage procedure. If resection is not possible, a diverting colostomy may allow closure of a rectovesical fistula, although it will not prevent urinary contamination.

Involvement of the external genitalia has also been reported in patients with IBD, including cases of direct extension from inflamed bowel, pyoderma gangrenosum, and metastatic (cutaneous) Crohn's disease. Pain, fever, and urethral discharge are typical symptoms, which may or may not parallel the activity of the underlying bowel disease. Treatment involves local wound care, antibiotics, systemic and topical glucocorticoids, systemic immunomodulatory agents, and, uncommonly, local resection of involved skin or bowel resection in refractory cases.

Markers of renal function are impaired in up to 45% of patients with Crohn's disease but less commonly in patients with ulcerative colitis. At autopsy, tubular degeneration has been described in 31% of patients with Crohn's disease and 23% with ulcerative colitis, although few patients had clinical manifestations detected during their life. *Interstitial nephritis* associated with aminosalicylate therapy, granulomatous involvement, hyperoxaluria, and prolonged hypokalemia has been reported.

Both *proximal* and *distal renal tubular acidosis* have also been described in association with IBD, including cases involving extensive small bowel resections, renal amyloidosis, secondary hyperparathyroidism, urinary obstruction, and chronic pyelonephritis.

Glomerulonephritis associated with IBD has been reported in patients with Crohn's disease and ulcerative colitis, although it is found primarily in the latter. A male preponderance has been identified. Most patients have active bowel disease at the time of diagnosis. Glomerulonephritis rarely precedes the diagnosis of the underlying IBD. Clinically, patients may present with rapidly progressive renal failure characterized by oliguria, proteinuria, an active urinary sediment, and elevated renal function tests (ie, blood urea nitrogen and serum creatinine level). Histologically, the disease is characterized by the deposition of immune complexes containing IgA and C3/C4 in glomeruli. Glucocorticoids are the mainstay of treatment, although bowel resection may be required to stabilize the disease.

Drug nephrotoxicity has been reported primarily with cyclosporine and 5-aminosalicylate (5-ASA, mesalamine) agents. With the latter, cases of nephrotic syndrome, interstitial nephritis, and glomerulonephritis have been reported. Of the 5-ASA agents in this class, sulfasalazine appears to be the least likely to result in nephrotoxicity. In most surveys, the frequency has been <1% of all treated patients. Most patients have been men. The duration of treatment typically has ranged from days to 4 years. Hypovolemia and pre-existing renal dysfunction appear to be risk factors. There does not appear to be a relationship between cumulative 5-ASA dose and risk of nephrotoxicity. Patients most commonly present with fever, anorexia, malaise, and night sweats. Renal function is usually reduced, although the urine sediment may be inactive. Pyuria and low specific gravity may be the earliest manifestations of 5-ASA nephrotoxicity. Although the mechanism is unclear, renal hypoxia resulting from antiprostaglandin properties of these agents is suspected. Most cases are reversible with hydration and cessation of therapy. Some authorities recommend checking a urinalysis and serum creatinine level periodically in all patients on 5-ASA.

Cyclosporine is most commonly used in refractory cases of fulminant ulcerative colitis but also may be used in the management of fistulae in Crohn's disease. Cyclosporine is associated with a dose-related nephrotoxicity. The mechanism of action appears to involve afferent arteriolar vasoconstriction. Multivariate analysis has shown that the risk of irreversible nephrotoxicity is low if the dose of cyclosporine is kept under 5 mg/kg/day and the serum creatinine level does not rise more than 30% above baseline. Risk factors for nephrotoxicity include use of other nephrotoxins, hypovolemia, and pre-existing renal dysfunction. Thus, the serum creatinine level must be monitored during therapy, and adjustments in the dose of cyclosporine must be made if renal function declines.

Neurogenic bladder and *impotence* may develop after iatrogenic injury to the pelvic nerves during complicated bowel resection. Neurogenic bladder is seen following <20% of proctocolectomies. Male sexual dysfunction, which may be temporary or permanent, may occur in as many as 27% of patients who undergo proctocolectomy. Risk factors include a difficult rectal dissection and older age of the patient. Fertility in women may also be impaired (see Chapter 10).

VASCULAR AND HEMATOLOGIC MANIFESTATIONS

Thromboembolic disease is a cause of substantial morbidity and mortality in patients with IBD. The association between thromboembolism and IBD has been recognized since a report by Bargen and Barker[11] in 1936 describing venous and arterial thrombosis complicating ulcerative colitis. Thromboembolism has been reported in 1.3% to 6.4% of IBD patients in clinical studies. In one autopsy study, 39% of patients were found to have venous thromboembolism, although only 6% had clinical evidence prior to death. Fewer than 1% of thromboembolic events necessitate hospital admission. The majority of patients are less than 50 years of age, and the absolute risk does not seem to be related to the site, extent, duration, or type of IBD or to the patient's gender. In a large clinical series of patients with thromboembolic events complicating IBD from the Mayo Clinic,[12] 67% had deep vein thrombosis with or without pulmonary embolism, 20% had a stroke, and 15% had arterial thromboses. Typically, arterial thrombosis developed in the postoperative period. Most of the patients in this series in whom peripheral venous thrombosis developed had active bowel disease (64%). There was a 25% mortality rate attributed to the first thromboembolic event. Fewer than 20% of affected patients have recurrent episodes of thrombosis. Thrombosis of the portal, hepatic, renal, and mesenteric veins is unusual. Central nervous system and retinal venous thromboses also may occur, typically in children.

Hypercoagulability itself also has been linked to the pathogenesis of IBD. Specifically, the risk of Crohn's disease is higher among patients who smoke or use oral contraceptive agents, whereas the risk of Crohn's disease is lower than expected among patients with von Willebrand's disease and hemophilia. Furthermore, microscopic evaluation of resected specimens from patients with Crohn's disease has demonstrated microvascular thromboses in association with small vessel inflammation. Some patients with ulcerative colitis appear to benefit from treatment with unfractionated and low molecular weight heparin, but a therapeutic role for heparin has not been confirmed in controlled trials.

All facets of the coagulation cascade likely play a role in the development of hypercoagulability (platelets, coagulation factors, and natural anticoagulants). Clearly, IBD patients are at risk of thrombosis on the basis of prolonged immobilization and surgery. Despite a higher frequency of anticardiolipin antibodies (up to 20% of patients with Crohn's disease versus 2.5% of controls), there does not appear to be any conclusive association between the presence of anticardiolipin antibodies and thrombosis in IBD. It is unclear if glucocorticoid-related inhibition of fibrinolysis plays a significant role in the risk of thrombosis. Recently, genetic markers, including the factor V Leiden mutation; prothrombin mutation G20210A; hyperhomocystinemia; factor V 4070G mutation; and deficiencies of protein C, protein S, and antithrombin III, have been examined. To date, deficiencies in protein S, protein C, or antithrombin III have not been found to occur more frequently among patients with IBD who experience thrombosis than in non-IBD patients with thrombosis. Factor V Leiden mutation leads to a hypercoagulable state by preventing degradation of prothrombin by activated protein C. This mutation is found in 5% of the general population and in 20% of persons with thrombosis. The frequency of factor V Leiden mutation in IBD patients with thrombosis (14.3%) has been found to be higher than that among IBD patients without thrombosis (0%), but similar to that in non-IBD patients with thrombosis (15.5%). Thus, although factor V Leiden mutation is not associated with IBD, per se, it increases the risk of thrombosis when present. Prothrombin mutation G20210A is associated with increased plasma prothrombin levels. After the factor V Leiden mutation, it is the second most common cause of genetic hypercoagulability. Several studies have shown no difference in the frequency of this mutation in IBD patients with thrombosis (14.3%) and non-IBD controls with thrombosis (11.8%), although the frequency is lower in IBD patients without thrombosis (1.7%). Factor V 4070G has not been shown to be more frequent among IBD patients, although some patients with thrombosis have been reported to have this mutation.

Hyperhomocystinemia has been reported to be present in up to 15% of IBD patients. Hyperhomocystinemia has been linked to both thrombosis and osteoporosis. Among IBD patients, the etiology of hyperhomocystinemia is probably multifactorial and includes genetic- (methyltetrahydrofolate reductase gene mutations [MTHFR]), nutritional- (folate, cobalamin, and pyridoxine deficiencies), and medication-related (glucocorticoids, methotrexate) factors. A few studies have demonstrated elevated levels of homocystine in IBD patients compared to controls. Nevertheless, several studies have failed to show a significant association between hyperhomocystinemia or mutations in MTHFR and thrombosis in patients with IBD.

The role of thrombocytosis and elevated levels of coagulation factors V and VIII, prothrombin fragments, D-dimers, and fibrinogen remains unclear. Some investigators have also described low endogenous tissue plasminogen activator and high plasminogen activator inhibitor levels in patients with IBD.

The treatment of thromboembolic complications is the same for patients with IBD as for those without IBD. In addition to anticoagulation, efforts should be directed at controlling the underlying IBD, cessation of smoking, and avoidance of oral contraceptives. For patients with evidence of the antiphospholipid antibody syndrome, the goal of anticoagulation with warfarin should be to achieve an international normalized ratio (INR) of 3.0 to 4.0 in order to prevent future thromboembolic episodes.

Anemia is common among IBD patients, with reported rates of 30% to 50%. Anemia accounts for substantial morbidity in IBD and is often associated with impairment in the quality of life due to fatigue, dyspnea, and irritability. Several studies have shown that treatment of IBD-associated anemia may have a significant impact on the quality of life of these patients. Only recently have the complexities of IBD-associated anemia begun to be understood. It is important for all patients with anemia to undergo evaluation of iron stores, cobalamin, and folate levels and a peripheral blood smear prior to beginning therapy for anemia. Combined deficiencies can be seen in this population.

Iron deficiency is the most common cause of anemia in IBD and will lead to microcytosis of the red blood cells. Iron deficiency may result from chronic gastrointestinal blood loss and less commonly from poor proximal small bowel malabsorption or diminished oral intake. Daily losses of only 10 mL of blood from the gastrointestinal tract may give rise to iron deficiency. Anemia of chronic disease is the next most common cause of anemia. It is associated with normal, or even supranormal, stores of iron but an inability to release these stores from the reticuloendothelial cells because of the inflammatory milieu created by increased circulating levels of interleukin-1 (IL-1) and TNF-α. As a result, there is reduced red blood cell (RBC) survival. In this setting, erythropoietin levels appear insufficient for the needed response, and the effect of erythropoietin on red blood cell progenitors in the bone marrow is blunted. Patients with IBD may have erythropoietin responses that are blunted to a greater degree than those of patients with anemia of equal severity from noninflammatory conditions and are thus inadequate for the degree of anemia. Patients treated with erythropoietin twice a week by subcutaneous injection and oral iron have higher mean hemoglobin concentrations than patients given oral iron alone (an increase in hemoglobin by 1 g/dL in 82% versus 24%). Interestingly, patients who respond poorly to erythropoietin also seem to have higher proinflammatory activity, as evidenced by clinical disease activity and in vitro measurement of IL-11B. In a recent trial, anemic patients with Crohn's disease who failed to respond to oral iron underwent treatment with intravenous iron saccharate followed by random assignment to erythropoietin or placebo. Eighty-five percent of patients responded to intravenous iron alone. However, the mean rise in hemoglobin was 1.6 g/dL greater in those who received erythropoietin than in those who received placebo. Among the nonresponders to oral iron, all had a rise in hemoglobin following the addition of parenteral erythropoietin (150 to 300 international units/kg subcutaneously three times/week). A recent evaluation of predictors of response to parenteral iron found that a serum erythropoietin level >166 international units/L, soluble transferring receptor level >75 nmol/L, and transferrin level >3.83 g/L were associated with adequate response to iron therapy alone. The high cost of erythropoietin precludes its use in all IBD patients with anemia. Therapy with erythropoietin should be limited to the small subset of patients with anemia that fail to improve with oral or parenteral iron supplementation.

Cobalamin (vitamin B_{12}) deficiency may lead to megaloblastic anemia, which develops most commonly in patients with terminal ileal disease or prior resection. Almost all patients who have undergone an ileal resection greater than 60 cm will malabsorb cobalamin, whereas only about one-half of those with a resection <60 cm will do so. Less commonly, small bowel bacterial overgrowth and gastric Crohn's disease can result in vitamin B_{12} deficiency. Folate deficiency also gives rise to megaloblastic anemia and may be seen in patients taking sulfasalazine or methotrexate. Other causes include poor oral intake and gastric or small bowel involvement by Crohn's disease.

An association between *autoimmune hemolytic anemia (AIHA)* and IBD was first described by Sheehy[13] in 1974. On the basis of several case series involving over 3000 IBD patients, the frequency of AIHA appears to range from 0.2% to 1.7%. The prevalence of a positive Coombs' test without hemolysis has been reported to be 2% among patients with ulcerative colitis. In most series of AIHA, females predominate, with a mean age of nearly 50 years. AIHA may precede, accompany, or follow the onset of the underlying colitis. In one study, the mean interval between a diagnosis of ulcerative colitis and the development of AIHA was 17 months. In most series, patients have active bowel disease, usually with pancolitis at the time of diagnosis of AIHA. The initial therapeutic approach is use of high-dose glucocorticoids. If this fails, use of adjunctive immunomodulatory therapies should be tried. Splenectomy and colectomy have each been successful in refractory cases. Sulfasalazine itself may cause hemolysis in patients with glucose-6-phosphate dehydrogenase (G6PD) deficiency. This entity is most common in African Americans and is characterized by the presence of Heinz bodies in the peripheral blood smear.

Finally, *drug-induced bone marrow suppression* may develop as a consequence of therapy with sulfasalazine, methotrexate, 6-mercaptopurine, or azathioprine.

CARDIAC MANIFESTATIONS

Cardiac manifestations of IBD are relatively uncommon. Pericardial involvement during the course of IBD was first described in 1967. Since then, it has been estimated that up to 36% of patients with IBD have at least one episode of *pericarditis* or *myocarditis* (or both) in their lifetimes. Patients with ulcerative colitis seem to be at higher risk than those with Crohn's disease. Patients with myopericarditis all have had colonic disease and often have active bowel disease at the time of diagnosis of myopericarditis. Rarely, the pericarditis may antedate the diagnosis. Constrictive pericarditis has also been recently reported in association with chronic ulcerative colitis. Treatment involves the use of NSAIDs, pericardial drainage, and rarely glucocorticoids. There are also several reports of atrioventricular block occurring in the setting of a relapse of IBD. The frequency of arrhythmias may also be increased in patients with IBD because of electrolyte imbalances during flares of IBD.

There appears to be an increased risk of *endocarditis* in patients with IBD. In one study of 213 patients with native valve endocarditis, 2.8% had IBD. On the basis of these data, IBD patients are estimated to have a 44-fold increased risk of bacterial endocarditis. It has been postulated that this risk derives from greater exposure to pathogens in the face of frequent bowel examinations (barium enemas and colonoscopies are associated with a 5% and 4%

frequency of bacteremia, respectively), increased mucosal permeability, and treatment with immunosuppressants. The increased risk of endocarditis suggests that antibiotic prophylaxis before endoscopy and other procedures should be considered.

PULMONARY MANIFESTATIONS

In 1976, Kraft and colleagues[14] described six patients with IBD in whom bronchiectasis developed. Since then, prospective studies have demonstrated pulmonary function test abnormalities in up to 60% of IBD patients. Impairment of pulmonary function is more pronounced in those patients with active bowel disease. The association of IBD with pulmonary involvement seems to be more common in patients with ulcerative colitis than in patients with Crohn's disease. The majority of patients are female and nonsmokers. Nearly 70% have other extraintestinal manifestations. Most often, pulmonary manifestations develop after the diagnosis of IBD has been made. Early recognition is important because pulmonary disease can be strikingly steroid responsive.

Veloso et al[2] have described four main pulmonary manifestations of IBD, including airway disease, interstitial lung disease, necrobiotic parenchymal nodules, and serositis. The majority (60%) of patients with pulmonary abnormalities have airway complications including subglottic tracheal stenosis, chronic bronchitis, bronchiectasis, and bronchiolitis. In addition, subclinical disease appears to be common. In one study, 65% of patients with Crohn's disease without pulmonary symptoms had elevated bronchial lymphocyte counts with high CD4+/CD8+ T cell ratios compared to age-matched controls. Typically, upper airway difficulties develop in the setting of more active bowel disease; however, bronchiectasis and bronchiolitis may worsen after colectomy and during remission of IBD. There does not seem to be any association between airway disease and use of sulfasalazine or 5-ASA compounds, as more than 80% of patients are not taking these medications at the onset of the lung disease.

The clinical presentations of airway disease are quite variable. Patients may present with a dry cough, dyspnea, and hemoptysis. Imaging may reveal infiltrates, effusions, nodules, and interstitial fibrosis. Histopathologic evaluation, often with video-assisted thoracoscopic surgery or open lung biopsy, remains the only certain way to make the diagnosis and exclude other possibilities, such as infectious pneumonitis.

Interstitial lung diseases associated with IBD include *bronchiolitis obliterans with organizing pneumonia (BOOP), granulomatous pneumonitis,* and *pulmonary eosinophilia with infiltrate,* which typically occurs in patients taking sulfasalazine. There have been case reports linking the use of 5-ASA in patients with ulcerative colitis to the development of BOOP.

Necrobiotic nodules are parenchymal lesions that are found to be sterile collections of polymorphonuclear leukocytes on biopsy. The differential diagnosis of these lesions is wide and includes septic pulmonary emboli, rheumatoid nodules, Wegener's granulomatosis, fungal infection, and neoplastic processes.

Serositis usually presents as a pleuropericarditis, often with an associated pleural or pericardial effusion. This manifestation typically occurs in the setting of active bowel symptoms. Most patients have not been on sulfasalazine therapy at the time of development of serositis. Glucocorticoids (systemic and inhaled) are the mainstay of therapy. NSAIDs have been used successfully in some cases of serositis. More recently, clinical resolution has been reported with infliximab.

There are also many reports of apparent overlap cases of Crohn's disease and *sarcoidosis*. In fact, in some studies, up to 50% of patients with Crohn's disease react to the Kveim antigen. *Colobronchial fistulae* represent a rare complication of fistulizing Crohn's disease.

ENDOCRINE AND METABOLIC MANIFESTATIONS

Growth retardation and delayed sexual maturation have been found in children with IBD, particularly those with Crohn's disease. Up to 40% of children with Crohn's disease and up to 20% of those with ulcerative colitis have a height below the third percentile. Mechanisms include inadequate caloric intake and intestinal malabsorption. Serum levels of growth hormone (GH) are normal in this population, although some investigators have reported low serum levels of insulin-like growth factor (IGF-1), which is thought to mediate the effects of GH. Although glucocorticoids are not thought to play a pathogenic role in growth retardation, some authorities recommend alternate-day glucocorticoid therapy for children with active IBD and impaired growth velocities.

Up to 30% of IBD patients meet criteria for osteoporosis by bone densitometry. In children with Crohn's disease, osteopenia has been seen in up to 41% of patients. At-risk subpopulations include patients who are amenorrheic, have disease of long duration, have had a small bowel resection, are on high doses of glucocorticoids for a long duration, have severe limitations in caloric intake, and already have a low bone mineral density at the time of the diagnosis of IBD. It is important to identify patients with low 25-OH vitamin D levels (which can lead to osteomalacia) because replacement therapy can mitigate the disease process. Minimizing glucocorticoid use, emphasizing smoking cessation and alcohol abstinence, and implementing a fitness regimen emphasizing weight bearing exercises have all been shown to limit the amount of bone mineral loss. Specific pharmacologic agents to prevent osteoporosis, including hormone replacement therapy and bisphosphonates, have not been adequately studied in this population.

Two epidemiologic surveys have found an increased frequency of clinically apparent thyroid disease in patients with ulcerative colitis compared to controls. In contrast, patients with Crohn's disease do not appear to have higher rates of hypo- or hyperthyroidism than that of the general population, although there are a few reports of Hashimoto's (autoimmune) thyroiditis among patients with Crohn's colitis. *Thyroid disease* has been reported to affect up to 3% of patients with ulcerative colitis and often precedes the diagnosis of IBD. Hyperthyroidism has been reported to be five times as common in patients with ulcerative colitis as in the general population. Physiologic studies have shown an increased frequency of iodine depletion in IBD patients, perhaps because of increased daily fractional turnover of thyroxine. In a recent Italian study evaluating thyroid morphology by ultrasound among 31 IBD patients and 50 controls, thyroid volume was increased by an average of 35% and the frequency of thyroid enlargement was three times higher in IBD patients than in controls. In this study, serum-free thyroxine levels were increased by nearly 50%, and 10% of patients had antithyroid antibodies. Finally, there are several reports of amyloid goiter in patients with Crohn's disease.

A number of *nutritional deficiencies* may develop in patients with chronic IBD, primarily those with substantial small bowel involvement or those on chronic TPN. Zinc deficiency is quite common. In one recent study, more than 50% of IBD patients with active disease had plasma zinc levels below the 15th percentile. In an inpatient series, 40% of patients with Crohn's disease had zinc deficiency. Zinc deficiency may result in poor wound healing, impaired growth, acrodermatitis, hypogonadism, diarrhea, dysgeusia, alopecia, and anorexia. Additional nutritional deficiencies can occur. Selenium deficiency can result in cardiac and skeletal myopathies. Chromium deficiency has been linked to impaired glucose intolerance and peripheral neuropathy. Manganese deficiency is associated with ataxia, retarded skeletal growth, and impaired fertility. Molybdenum deficiency is associated with headaches, night blindness, scotomata, lethargy, and rarely coma. In an inpatient series, 48% of patients with Crohn's disease and 5% of those with ulcerative colitis were found to be deficient in cobalamin. Cobalamin deficiency may result in peripheral neuropathy and macrocytic anemia (see earlier). Folate deficiency results in macrocytic anemia. Distal ileal disease or resection may result in deficiencies of fat soluble vitamins A, D, E, and K. Vitamin D deficiency, which can manifest as hypocalcemia and osteomalacia, is seen in up to 75% of inpatients with Crohn's disease. Vitamin A deficiency is seen in up to 50% of inpatients with Crohn's disease and may manifest as night blindness. Vitamin K deficiency, which manifests as coagulopathy, is relatively rare.

NEUROLOGIC MANIFESTATIONS

Neurologic involvement in patients with IBD rarely has been reported. In general, most series have shown a greater prevalence of peripheral nervous system involvement in patients with ulcerative colitis, whereas myopathy and myelopathy are more common in those with Crohn's disease. In a series from Germany, MRI disclosed focal white matter lesions in nearly one half of IBD patients, compared to 16% of age- and sex-matched controls.

A retrospective review of 638 patients with IBD in Israel over a 10-year period demonstrated a 3% prevalence of neurologic disease. There was equal occurrence patients with Crohn's disease and those with ulcerative colitis. The neurologic findings were unrelated to recognized iatrogenic causes or to a definable metabolic or nutritional deficiency. More than one-half of the patients with neurologic disease had other extraintestinal manifestations. In the vast majority of cases, neurologic disease was diagnosed after the development of IBD. The reported neurologic manifestations were quite varied and included *acute inflammatory demyelinating polyradiculopathy, mononeuritis multiplex, brachial plexopathy, Melkersson-Rosenthal syndrome (recurrent facial nerve palsy accompanied by tongue fissuring and noncaseating granulomas), dermatomyositis, vacuolar myopathy, myasthenia gravis, recurrent transient ischemic attacks, sinus venous thrombosis,* and *myelopathy.* Other series have reported less frequent associations with *sensorineural hearing loss, cerebrovascular accidents, leukoencephalitis,* and *cerebellar degeneration.* In some series, epilepsy has constituted 15% to 20% of the neurologic involvement in patients with IBD. *Autonomic dysfunction* has also been found to be common in IBD patients. In one prospective study, 48% of patients with Crohn's disease had evidence of autonomic dysfunction on the basis of noninvasive testing of heart rate variability.

REFERENCES

1. Greenstein AJ, Sachar DB, Panday AK, et al. Amyloidosis and inflammatory bowel disease. A 50 year experience with 25 patients. *Medicine.* 1992;71:261-270.

2. Veloso FT, Carvalho J, Magro F. Immune-related systemic manifestations of inflammatory bowel disease. A prospective study of 792 patients. *J Clin Gastroenterol.* 1996;23:29-34.

3. Bernstein CN, Blanchard JF, Rawsthorne P, et al. The prevalence of extraintestinal disease in inflammatory bowel disease: a population-based study. *Am J Gastroenterol.* 2001;96:1116-1121.

4. Dew MJ, Thompson H, Allan RN. The spectrum of hepatic dysfunction in inflammatory bowel disease. *Q J Med.* 1979;48:113-135.

5. Wee A, Ludwig J. Pericholangitis in chronic ulcerative colitis: primary sclerosing cholangitis of the small ducts? *Ann Int Med.* 1985;102:581-587.

6. Gravallese EM, Kantrowitz FG. Arthritic manifestations of inflammatory bowel disease. *Am J Gastroenterol.* 1988;83:703-709.

7. Oppenheimer DA, Jones HH. Hypertrophic osteoarthropathy of chronic inflammatory bowel disease. *Skeletal Radiology.* 1982;9:109-113.

8. Bennett ML, Jackson JM, Jorizzo JL, et al. Pyoderma gangrenosum. A comparison of typical and atypical forms with an emphasis on time to remission. Case review of 86 patients from 2 institutions. *Medicine.* 2000;79:37-46.

9. Parks AG, Morson BC, Pegum JS. Crohn's disease with cutaneous involvement. *Proc Roy Soc Med.* 1965;58:241.
10. Lucky A, Ploysangam T, Heubi J et al. Cutaneous Crohn's disease in children. *J Am Acad Dermatol.* 1997;36:697-704
11. Bargen JA, Barker NW. Extensive arterial and venous thrombosis complicating ulcerative colitis. *Arch Intern Med.* 1936;58:17-31.
12. Talbot RW, Heppell J, Dozois RR, Beart RW. Vascular complications of inflammatory bowel disease. *Mayo Clin Proc.* 1986;61:140-145.
13. Sheehy T, Cannon NJ. Hematologic complications of inflammatory bowel disease. *Journal of the Medical Association of the State of Alabama.* 1974;44:121-128.
14. Kraft SC, Earle RH, Roesler M, et al. Unexplained bronchopulmonary disease with inflammatory bowel disease. *Arch Intern Med.* 1976;136:454-459.

BIBLIOGRAPHY

Bianchi GP, Marchesini G, Gueli C, et al. Thyroid involvement in patients with active inflammatory bowel disease. *Ital J Gastroenterol.* 1995;27:291-295.

Camus P. The lung in inflammatory bowel disease. *Euro Resp J.* 2000;15:5-10.

Danzi JT. Extraintestinal manifestations of idiopathic inflammatory bowel disease. *Arch Intern Med.* 1988;148:297-302.

Fraquelli M, Losco A, Visentin S, et al. Gallstone disease and related risk factors in patients with Crohn's disease: analysis of 330 consecutive cases. *Arch Intern Med.* 2001;161:2201-2204.

Giannadaki E, Potamianos S, Roussomoustakaki M, et al. Autoimmune hemolytic anemia and positive Coombs' test associated with ulcerative colitis. *Am J Gastroenterol.* 1997;92:1872-1874.

Gravallese EM, Kantrowitz FG. Arthritic manifestations of inflammatory bowel disease. *Am J Gastroenterol.* 1988;83:703-709.

Han PD, Burke A, Baldassano RN, et al. Nutrition and inflammatory bowel disease. *Gastroenterol Clin North Am.* 1999;28:423-444.

Herrlinger KR. The pancreas and inflammatory bowel disease. *Int J Pancreatol.* 2000;27:171-179.

Herrlinger KR, Noftz K, Dalhoff K, et al. Alterations in pulmonary function in inflammatory bowel disease are frequent and persist during remission. *Am J Gastroenterol.* 2002;97:377-381.

Kastenberg DM, Friedman LS. Hepatobiliary complications of inflammatory bowel disease. In: Rustgi AN, Van Thiel DH, eds. *The Liver in Systemic Disease.* New York, NY: Raven Press; 1993:61-105.

Kuzela L. Pulmonary complications in patients with inflammatory bowel disease. *Hepato-Gastroenterol.* 1999;46:1714-1719.

Koutroubakis IE. Role of thrombotic vascular risk factors in inflammatory bowel disease. *Dig Dis.* 2000;18:161-167.

Kreuzpaintner G, Horstkotte D, Heyll A, et al. Increased risk of bacterial endocarditis in inflammatory bowel disease. *Am J Med.* 1992;92:391-395.

Levine JB, Lukawski-Trubish D. Extraintestinal considerations in inflammatory bowel disease. *Gastroenterol Clin North Am.* 1995;24:633-646.

Lossos A, River Y, Eliakim A, et al. Neurologic aspects of inflammatory bowel disease. *Neurology.* 1995;45:416-421.

Mahadeva R. Clinical and radiologic characteristics of lung disease in inflammatory bowel disease. *Euro Resp J.* 2000;15:41-48.

Pardi DS, Tremaine WJ, Sandborn WJ. Renal and urologic complications of inflammatory bowel disease. *Am J Gastroenterol.* 1998;93:504-514.

Raj V, Lichtenstein DR. Hepatobiliary manifestations of inflammatory bowel disease. *Gastroenterol Clin North Am.* 1999;28:491-513.

Rankin GB. Extraintestinal and systemic manifestations of inflammatory bowel disease. *Med Clin North Am.* 1990;74:39-50.

Rankin GB, Watts HD, Melnyl CS. National Cooperative Crohn's disease study: extraintestinal manifestations and perianal complications. *Gastroenterology.* 1979;77:914-920.

Rappaport A, Shaked M, Landau M. Sweet's syndrome in associations with Crohn's disease: report of a case and review of the literature. *Dis Col Rect.* 2001;44:1526-1529.

Retsky JE, Kraft SC. The extraintestinal manifestations of inflammatory bowel disease. In: Kirsner JB, ed. *Inflammatory Bowel Disease.* 5th ed. Philadelphia, Pa: WB Saunders; 1999:471-494.

Schreiber S, Howaldt S, Schnoor M. Recombinant erythropoietin for treatment of anemia in inflammatory bowel disease. *N Engl J Med.* 1996;334:619-623.

Shah S, Peppercorn MA, Pallotta JA. Autoimmune thyroiditis associated with Crohn's disease. *J Clin Gastroenterol.* 1998;26:117-120.

Soukiasan SH, Foster CS, Raizman MB. Treatment strategies for scleritis and uveitis associated with inflammatory bowel disease. *Am J Ophthalmol.* 1994;118:601-611.

chapter 7

Cancer in Inflammatory Bowel Disease

Bret A. Lashner, MD

Since the risk of colorectal cancer in inflammatory bowel disease (IBD) is elevated, cancer surveillance colonoscopy has evolved over the past 30 years to become the "standard of care" for high-risk patients, especially ulcerative colitis (UC) patients. To date, cancer surveillance colonoscopy is not the standard of care for patients with Crohn's colitis. Periodic colonoscopy to examine for asymptomatic cancer or the neoplastic lesion of dysplasia is routinely employed in most practices in the world but is costly and associated with some, albeit low, morbidity. It is incumbent on gastroenterologists to understand the principles of cancer surveillance colonoscopy and make an effort to minimize cost/effectiveness ratios so that this expensive form of cancer surveillance can be offered to as many patients as possible within the financial constraints of the health care system.

COLORECTAL CANCER IN ULCERATIVE COLITIS

RISK, MORTALITY, AND RISK FACTORS

The cumulative incidence of colorectal cancer (CRC) in UC patients ranges between 5% and 13% depending on the population studied. While this number is not very different from the colorectal cancer risk in an unaffected population, the younger age of CRC in UC makes age-specific relative risk estimates greater than three. Recent studies from Sweden, Denmark, Greece, Germany, and Japan have confirmed increased age-specific risks of CRC in UC populations.[1-5] As in sporadic CRC, cancer-related mortality in UC patients with CRC is approximately 50%. Some studies, though, have shown that mortality from rectal cancer in UC patients is higher than in sporadic rectal cancer.[6,7] Of note, while incidence rates for CRC in UC have been rising, CRC mortality rates have been declining.[8] Diverging incidence and mortality curves imply longer life expectancy in UC patients with CRC, likely related to better treatments and/or more effective cancer surveillance strategies.

The known risk factors for CRC in UC are increased extent and long duration of disease. Some studies have identified young age at symptom onset as an independent risk factor.[9] A recently identified important risk factor is primary sclerosing cholangitis (PSC). The small proportion of UC patients with PSC (approximately two) have a relative risk for CRC of at least three compared to a UC population without PSC.[10] PSC patients with IBD should be made aware of this increased risk and have surveillance examination performed more frequently than what would otherwise be done or be strongly considered for prophylactic colectomy before cancer or dysplasia is detected. One group in Seattle, Wash, has shown that altering bile acid composition in PSC patients with ursodeoxycholic acid can prevent cancer or dysplasia from occurring.[11] This chemoprevention strategy, as with any chemoprevention strategy, should not be used as a substitute for cancer surveillance.

THE BIOLOGY OF CANCER

An ideal marker of malignancy would be associated with a poor prognosis, be objective, be widespread throughout the colon, have a high sensitivity and specificity, and be inexpensive. Histologic dysplasia is not ideal because there is much interobserver variability, dysplasia tends to be focal, and there is imperfect sensitivity and specificity. Perhaps, in CRC surveillance in UC, dysplasia could be complemented with another premalignant marker that is objective, is associated with a poor prognosis, and improves the sensitivity and specificity of dysplasia. Of the available premalignant markers (ie, deoxyribonucleic acid [DNA] aneuploidy, DNA hypomethylation, oncogene mutations, abnormal mucin expression, microsatellite instability, and suppressor gene mutations and loss of heterozygosity), p53 suppressor gene mutations with detection of the mutated protein products using immunohistochemistry offer promising possibilities as a complementary test to dysplasia for use in cancer surveillance programs.[12] Testing for abnormal p53 immunohistochemistry is inexpensive, objective, associated with a poor prognosis, and can improve the sensitivity and specificity of testing when used as a complement to dysplasia.[13]

Suppressor genes, including p53, act as a G1 checkpoint in the cell replication cycle for cells with abnormal DNA until DNA repair can occur. If DNA damage is excessive, the p53 gene allows for programmed cell death (ie, apoptosis) to occur. Inactivation of suppressor gene function through mutations perpetuate abnormal DNA through loss of repair and/or apoptotic mechanisms, thus increasing the risk of malignant transformation.[14] While p53 abnormalities are a relatively late occurrence in sporadic colorectal cancer (few adenomas but many cancers have mutations), they are an early occurrence in UC-related colorectal cancer; p53 often is positive in both dysplastic lesions and malignant lesions.[15-20] While promising, use of abnormal p53 immunohistochemistry has not been sufficiently studied to be used in cancer surveillance currently.

EFFECTIVENESS OF CANCER SURVEILLANCE

Cancer surveillance colonoscopy programs that test for dysplasia are effective in reducing cancer-related mortality. Two case-control studies have shown a reduction in cancer-related mortality in UC patients who have had surveillance examinations, with only one study showing a larger reduction in those surveyed more often.[21,22] The strongest evidence, though, that cancer surveillance is effective comes from a decision analysis.[23] Using the best available data and applying it to a 30-year-old with panulcerative colitis for 10 years (and no PSC), 17 different cancer surveillance strategies were compared to both prophylactic colectomy and no surveillance (colectomy done when symptomatic cancer is detected). The estimated cumulative incidence of cancer in the no surveillance group was 7.45%, which was a reasonable rate. Performing cancer surveillance colonoscopy every 3 years and recommending colectomy for the detection of low-grade dysplasia or worse pathology (an often employed strategy) were associated with a lowering of the cumulative incidence of cancer to 0.47%. Of course, prophylactic colectomy eliminated the risk of developing CRC. The remaining life expectancy in this hypothetical 30-year-old was 46.07 years with no surveillance, 47.19 years if enrolled in a surveillance program, and 47.45 years if he or she had a prophylactic colectomy. If this model is accurate, cancer surveillance is effective in dramatically decreasing the cumulative incidence of cancer and increasing life expectancy, compared to the no surveillance strategy. Both cancer risk and life expectancy from cancer surveillance are nearly as good as that expected with prophylactic colectomy.

COST OF CANCER SURVEILLANCE

Of course, improved effectiveness of cancer surveillance and prophylactic colectomy comes with a cost that can be measured with number of colonoscopies performed, number of surgeries (both elective and urgent) performed, and decrease in the quality of life following colectomy. In the decision analysis presented above, the costs are listed in Table 7-1.[23] Therefore, compared to "no surveillance," both "surveillance" and "prophylactic colectomy" strategies have better effectiveness and higher cost. The differences in the cost/effectiveness ratio, though, is uncertain.

Table 7-1

COST RELATED TO NO SURVEILLANCE, SURVEILLANCE, AND PROPHYLACTIC COLECTOMY STRATEGIES

	Colonoscopies/ Patient	Elective Surgery	Urgent Surgery	% Life Expectancy After Surgery
No surveillance	2.01	25.5%	25.1%	25%
Surveillance	5.14	84.0%	8.9%	73%
Prophylactic colectomy	0	100%	0%	100%

Adapted from Provenzale D, Kowdley KV, Arora S, Wong JB. Prophylactic colectomy for surveillance for chronic ulcerative colitis? A decision analysis. *Gastroenterology.* 1995;109:1188-1196.

COST/EFFECTIVENESS OF CANCER SURVEILLANCE

The investigators that performed the above decision analysis also performed a cost/effectiveness analysis on their model.[24] In this cost/effectiveness analysis, all surveillance strategies had lower costs and better effectiveness than no surveillance. Therefore, a strategy of no surveillance is unacceptable. Furthermore, all surveillance strategies that used low-grade dysplasia as the criterion for a positive test that prompted a colectomy recommendation had lower costs and better effectiveness than identical strategies that used high-grade dysplasia as the criterion for a positive test.

Incremental cost/effectiveness ratios were calculated to compare different surveillance strategies and are shown in Table 7-2.[24] These incremental cost/effectiveness ratios favorably compare to incremental cost/effectiveness ratios of cancer surveillance that are accepted to be important for our society, such as mammography for breast cancer and Pap smears for cervical cancer. Surveillance colonoscopies in UC patients performed every 3 years (or using a variable interval based on a patient's individual risk) have acceptable incremental cost/effectiveness ratios. The effectiveness (decrease in cancer risk and increase in life expectancy) is worth the cost (costs of testing and surgery and decrease in quality of life following colectomy).

Another decision analysis compared costs (colonoscopy costs with testing every 2 years, surgery costs, and terminal care costs of patients dying from CRC) to effectiveness (life-years saved).[25] Compared to no surveillance, this surveillance strategy would become cost effective if the cumulative risk of

Table 7-2

INCREMENTAL COST/EFFECTIVENESS
OF SEVERAL SURVEILLANCE STRATEGIES

Surveillance Strategy	Incremental Cost/ Effectiveness
Every year versus every 2 years	$247,200/life-year gained
Every 2 years versus variable interval*	$159,500/life-year gained
Variable interval* versus every 3 years	$155,400/life-year gained
Every 3 years versus every 4 years	$111,600/life-year gained
Every 4 years versus every 5 years	$83,700/life-year gained
Every 5 years versus no surveillance	$4,700/life-year gained

*Surveillance colonoscopy every 3 years for the first 20 years of disease, every 2 years for the next 8 years, and annual testing thereafter.

Adapted from Provenzale D, Wong JB, Onken JE, Lipscomb J. Performing a cost-effectiveness analysis: surveillance of patients with ulcerative colitis. *Am J Gastroenterol.* 1998;93:872-880.

developing CRC were 27%. For testing every 3 years the threshold CRC risk is 19%, and for testing every 4 years the threshold risk is 14%. In this model, surveillance is not cost effective compared to no surveillance. However, the poor effectiveness of the no surveillance strategy makes this an unacceptable option.

IMPROVING COST EFFECTIVENESS

Since some decision analyses have demonstrated that cancer surveillance colonoscopies are cost effective compared to no surveillance, and it is generally perceived that cancer surveillance in ulcerative colitis is the standard of care that should be offered to eligible patients, it is incumbent on gastroenterologists to recommend surveillance with parameters that are the most effective in improving life expectancy at the most reasonable cost.

To minimize the cost/effectiveness ratio, careful attention should be paid to patient selection, the criterion for a positive test, and the testing interval. Cost/effectiveness ratios will be minimized if the population tested is limited to high-risk patients. In UC, high-risk patients are those who have had pancolitis for at least 7 years or PSC. Other IBD patients, such as left-sided UC patients, patients with UC of short duration, or patients with Crohn's colitis, have a lower risk of CRC and will have higher cost/effectiveness ratios than the high-risk patients. The choice of the criterion for a positive test also may alter cost/effectiveness. Recommending colectomy for low-grade dysplasia as opposed to high-grade dysplasia is likely to have a higher cost (increased number of colectomies) and a much higher effectiveness (increase number of life-years saved); the resultant cost/effectiveness ratio is lower. Annual testing is not cost effective nor is it an efficient use of scarce resources. As stated above, the marginal cost/effectiveness is reasonable when tests are performed every 3 years or when the testing interval is varied based on the patient's individual risk.[26] Such a recommendation, though, may not be appropriate when the CRC risk is exceedingly high, such as in PSC patients or in patients with extensive disease for more than 30 years; annual testing is appropriate in those patients.

SURVEILLANCE RECOMMENDATIONS

Summarizing the above discussion, cancer surveillance colonoscopies in UC should be performed on high-risk patients (ie, those with pancolitis of at least 7 years or patients with PSC). While surveillance may be performed on other lower risk populations, such as patients with left-sided disease or Crohn's colitis, the marginal cost effectiveness will be higher and possibly prohibitively high. To use scarce resources (ie, colonoscopy) efficiently, testing should be performed every 3 years for the first 20 years of disease, every 2 years for the next 8 years, and annually thereafter. Since the cancer risk in PSC patients is so high, annual surveillance should be performed throughout the course of their disease. At least 32 biopsies should be taken throughout the colon, and polypoid lesions suspicious for neoplasia should be carefully biopsied. Patients with dysplasia, low-grade dysplasia, or high-grade dysplasia on any biopsy of flat mucosa should have a colectomy recommended. Patients with a polypoid dysplastic lesion in an area involved with colitis or who are under age 50 (a population unlikely to have sporadic adenomas) should be advised to have colectomies.

SURVEILLANCE VERSUS PROPHYLACTIC COLECTOMY

A cancer surveillance colonoscopy program, no matter how cost effective, is not perfectly effective. For a variety of reasons, some patients who develop cancer will not have dysplasia detected at an earlier colonoscopy. Those patients who are averse to this risk of cancer and cannot accept the imperfect nature of cancer surveillance should have a prophylactic colectomy. The trade-off for eliminating the cancer risk is the resultant decrease in the quality of life following colectomy. This decision is very personal and not necessarily based on cost effectiveness.

CHEMOPREVENTION

Folic acid is a critical cofactor in one-carbon metabolism. Cells grown in folic acid-deficient media exhibit numerous DNA strand breaks at folic acid-sensitive fragile sites.[27-29] One such fragile site occurs in the "hot-spot" (ie, exons 5 to 8) of the p53 gene. DNA strand breaks and hypomethylation in exons 5 to 8 of the p53 gene, as well as impaired DNA excision repair, have been demonstrated in folic acid-deficient laboratory animals. Inaccurate repair of strand breaks by DNA repair enzymes could lead to p53 mutations.

Folic acid supplementation has been associated with a decreased risk of cancer or dysplasia in UC patients.[30-32] A dose-dependent protective effect of folic acid supplementation for cancer or dysplasia has been demonstrated. Also, higher red blood cell folic acid levels, a marker of medium-term stores, have a significant protective effect for cancer or dysplasia. Because patients with UC are particularly prone to develop folic acid deficiency due to intestinal losses, diminished intake, and competitive inhibition of folic acid absorption from the commonly used medication sulfasalazine, folic acid supplementation is an attractive chemopreventive agent for colorectal cancer. Because folic acid is inexpensive and has no appreciable side effects, it is recommended for chemoprevention in UC patients. Even with folic acid supplementation, cancer surveillance colonoscopy is necessary.

Other possible chemoprevention agents, some of which are effective for sporadic colorectal cancer such as calcium, nonsteroidal anti-inflammatory drugs, and antioxidant supplements, have not been studied in inflammatory bowel disease.

CANCER IN CROHN'S DISEASE

Adenocarcinoma of the small bowel or large bowel is a rarely reported complication of Crohn's disease. Hence, epidemiologic studies are few; only one paper on surveillance for colorectal cancer in Crohn's disease has been reported. Because information on cancer in Crohn's disease is limited, surveillance has not yet become the standard of care in the treatment of IBD patients. Surveillance should be performed only if it is understood by the patient and physician that it is not likely to be cost effective, and surgery for finding dysplasia likely will involve a total proctocolectomy with permanent ileostomy.

COLORECTAL CANCER

Crohn's disease affecting the colon may carry a risk of colon cancer similar to that of UC patients. A large cohort study from Winnipeg, Manitoba compared cancer rates in IBD patients (more than 40,000 person-years of follow-up) to controls.[33] The incidence rate ratio for colon cancer was 2.64 (95% confidence interval [CI] 1.69 to 4.12) for Crohn's disease and 2.75 (95% CI 1.91 to 3.97) for UC. UC patients, but not Crohn's disease patients, had an increased risk of rectal cancer. A report from a large Danish registry of 2645 Crohn's disease patients found the standardized incidence ratio of colorectal cancer to be 1.1 (95% CI 0.6 to 1.9).[34]

Investigators from the Cleveland Clinic report a series of 30 Crohn's disease patients with adenocarcinoma, 22 with colorectal cancer, and eight with small bowel cancer.[35] Interestingly, 86% of the colorectal cancers had adjacent dysplasia and 41% had dysplasia in distal segments, suggesting that there may be a role for cancer surveillance colonoscopy in this population of patients. Investigators from Mount Sinai Medical Center in New York reported experience with cancer surveillance colonoscopy among 259 patients with Crohn's disease affecting at least 30% of their colon.[36] Among 663 examinations on these patients, 23 were found to have low-grade dysplasia, four had high-grade dysplasia, and five developed cancer. By the third examination, the cumulative incidence of dysplasia or cancer was 10% (107 had at least three examinations), but by the fifth examination, the cumulative incidence was fully 20% (32 patients had at least five examinations). Colectomies were recommended for cancer, high-grade dysplasia, and recurrent or multifocal low-grade dysplasia. This approach appears to be effective because no patient died of colorectal cancer. The cost effectiveness, though, needs to be studied before surveillance can be recommended universally to Crohn's colitis patients.

SMALL BOWEL CANCER

The risk of small bowel adenocarcinoma is markedly increased in Crohn's disease. Contrary to what is seen with sporadic small bowel cancer, patients with Crohn's disease preferentially develop cancer in the distal small bowel and rarely in the duodenum. The distribution of small bowel cancer closely follows the distribution of Crohn's disease. Risk factors for small bowel cancer in Crohn's disease include excluded loops of bowel, chronic unresected disease, chronic fistula (especially in the perirectum), and possibly 6-mercaptopurine use.[37] It is rare that small bowel cancer is preoperatively diagnosed. More commonly, cancer is an unexpected finding at surgery for obstructive disease or is an unexpected finding made by the pathologists. Since strictureplasty surgery does not resect obstructed bowel, the surgeon should biopsy each stricture prior to performing the strictureplasty.[38] While there is no effective screening method for small bowel cancer, patients with long-standing, symptomatic unresected disease should have occasional small bowel x-rays to evaluate for a change in findings.

REFERENCES

1. Karlen P, Lofberg R, Brostrom O, Leijonmarck CE, Hellers G, Persson PG. Increased risk of cancer in ulcerative colitis: a population-based cohort study. *Am J Gastroenterol.* 1999;94:1047-1052.

2. Wandall EP, Damkier P, Moller Pedersen F, et al. Survival and incidence of colorectal cancer in patients with ulcerative colitis in Funen County diagnosed between 1973 and 1993. *Scand J Gastroenterol.* 2000;35:312-317.

3. Triantafillidis JK, Manousos ON, Pomonis E, Cheracakis P. Ulcerative colitis in Greece: clinicoepidemiological data, course, and prognostic factors in 413 consecutive patients. *J Clin Gastroenterol.* 1998;27:204-210.

4. Pohl C, Hombach A, Kruis W. Chronic inflammatory bowel disease and cancer. *Hepato-Gastroenterol.* 2000;47:57-70.

5. Ishibashi N, Hirota Y, Ikeda M, Hirohata T. Ulcerative colitis and colorectal cancer: a follow-up study in Fukuoka, Japan. *Int J Epidemiol.* 1999;28:609-613.

6. Palli D, Trallori G, Saieva C, et al. General and cancer specific mortality of a population based cohort of patients with inflammatory bowel disease: the Florence study. *Gut.* 1998;42:175-179.

7. Bansal P, Sonnenberg A. Risk factors for colorectal cancer in inflammatory bowel disease. *Am J Gastroenterol.* 1996;91:44-48.

8. Delco F, Sonnenberg A. Birth-cohort phenomenon in the time trends of mortality from ulcerative colitis. *Am J Epidemiol.* 1999;150:359-366.

9. Langholz E, Munkholm P, Krasilnikoff A, Binder V. Inflammatory bowel diseases with onset in childhood: clinical features, morbidity, and mortality in a regional cohort. *Scand J Gastroenterol.* 1997;32:139-147.

10. Shetty K, Rybicki L, Brzezinski A, Carey WD, Lashner BA. The risk of cancer or dysplasia in ulcerative colitis patients with primary sclerosing cholangitis. *Am J Gastroenterol.* 1999;94:1643-1649.

11. Tung BY, Emond MJ, Haggitt RC, et al. Ursodiol is associated with lower prevalence of colonic neoplasia in patients with ulcerative colitis and primary sclerosing cholangitis. *Ann Intern Med.* 2001;134:89-95.

12. Shapiro BD, Lashner BA. Cancer biology in ulcerative colitis and potential use in endoscopic surveillance. *Gastrointest Endosc Clin North Am.* 1997;7:453-468.

13. Lashner BA, Shapiro BD, Husain A, Goldblum JR. Evaluation of the usefulness of testing for p53 mutations in colorectal cancer surveillance for ulcerative colitis. *Am J Gastroenterol.* 1999;94:456-462.

14. Carson DA, Lois A. Cancer progression and p53. *Lancet.* 1995;346:1009-1011.

15. Brentnall TA, Crispin DA, Rabinovitch PS, et al. Mutations in the p53 gene: an early marker of neoplastic progression in ulcerative colitis. *Gastroenterology.* 1994;107:369-378.

16. Burmer GC, Rabinovitch PS, Haggitt RC, et al. Neoplastic progression in ulcerative colitis: histology, DNA content, and loss of a p53 allele. *Gastroenterology.* 1992;103:1602-1610.

17. Harpaz N, Peck AL, Yin J, et al. p53 protein expression in ulcerative colitis-associated colorectal dysplasia and carcinoma. *Hum Pathol.* 1994;25:1069-1074.

18. Taylor HW, Boyle M, Smith SC, Bustin S, Williams NS. Expression of p53 in colorectal cancer and dysplasia complicating ulcerative colitis. *Br J Surg.* 1993;80:442-444.

19. Yin J, Harpaz N, Tong Y, et al. p53 point mutations in dysplastic and cancerous ulcerative colitis lesions. *Gastroenterology.* 1993;104:1633-1639.

20. Ilyas M, Talbot IC. p53 expression in ulcerative colitis: a longitudinal study. *Gut.* 1995;37:802-804.

21. Eaden J, Abrams K, Ekbom A, Jackson E, Mayberry J. Colorectal cancer prevention in ulcerative colitis: a case-control study. *Aliment Pharmacol Ther.* 2000;14:145-151.

22. Karlen P, Kornfeld D, Brostrom O, et al. Is colonoscopic surveillance reducing colorectal cancer mortality in ulcerative colitis? A population based case control study. *Gut.* 1998;42:711-714.

23. Provenzale D, Kowdley KV, Arora S, Wong JB. Prophylactic colectomy for surveillance for chronic ulcerative colitis? A decision analysis. *Gastroenterology.* 1995;109:1188-1196.

24. Provenzale D, Wong JB, Onken JE, Lipscomb J. Performing a cost-effectiveness analysis: surveillance of patients with ulcerative colitis. *Am J Gastroenterol.* 1998;93:872-880.

25. Delco F, Sonnenberg A. A decision analysis of surveillance for colorectal cancer in ulcerative colitis. *Gut.* 2000;46:500-506.

26. Lashner BA, Hanauer SB, Silverstein MD. Optimal timing of colonoscopy to screen for cancer in ulcerative colitis. *Ann Intern Med.* 1988;108:274-278.

27. Kim YI, Pogribny IP, Basnakian AG, et al. Folate deficiency in rats induces DNA strand breaks and hypomethylation within the p53 tumor suppressor gene. *Am J Clin Nutr.* 1997;65:46-52.

28. Kim YI, Pogribny IP, Salomon RN, et al. Exon-specific DNA hypomethylation of the p53 gene of rat colon induced by dimethylhydrazine: modulation by dietary folate. *Am J Pathol.* 1996;149:1129-1137.

29. Choi SW, Kim YI, Weitzel JN, Mason JB. Folate depletion impairs DNA excision repair in the colon of the rat. *Gut.* 1998;43:93-99.

30. Lashner BA, Heidenreich PA, Su GL, Kane SV, Hanauer SB. Effect of folate supplementation on the incidence of dysplasia and cancer in chronic ulcerative colitis. *Gastroenterology.* 1989;97:255-259.

31. Lashner BA. Red blood cell folate is associated with the development of dysplasia and cancer in ulcerative colitis. *J Cancer Res Clin Oncol.* 1993;119:549-554.

32. Lashner BA, Provencher KS, Seidner DL, Knesebeck A, Brzezinski A. The effect of folic acid supplementation on the risk for cancer or dysplasia in ulcerative colitis. *Gastroenterology.* 1997;112:29-32.

33. Bernstein CN, Blanchard JF, Kliewer E, Wajda A. Cancer risk in patients with inflammatory bowel disease: a population-based study. *Cancer.* 2001;9:854-862.

34. Mellemkjaer L, Johansen C, Gridley G, et al. Crohn's disease and cancer risk. *Cancer Causes & Control.* 2000;11:145-150.

35. Sigel JE, Petras RE, Lashner BA, et al. Intestinal adenocarcinoma in Crohn's disease: a report of 30 cases with a focus on coexisting dysplasia. *Am J Surg Path.* 1999;23:651-655.

36. Friedman S, Rubin PH, Bodian C, et al. Screening and surveillance colonoscopy in chronic Crohn's colitis. *Gastroenterology.* 2001;120:820-826.

37. Korelitz BE, Mirsky FJ, Fleisher MR, et al. Malignant neoplasms subsequent to treatment of inflammatory bowel disease with 6-mercaptopurine. *Am J Gastroenterol.* 1999;94:3248-3253.

38. Jaskowiak NT, Michelassi F. Adenocarcinoma at a strictureplasty site in Crohn's disease. *Dis Colon Rectum.* 2001;44:284-287.

chapter 8

Complications of the Ileal Pouch-Anal Anastomosis

Thomas Lee, MD and Alan L. Buchman, MD, MSPH

Ulcerative colitis (UC) is primarily treated with medical therapy, but about 10% of chronic UC patients eventually require surgical intervention. Drug therapy with 5-aminosalicylic acid (5-ASA) compounds, corticosteroids, and other immunomodulating medications often controls symptoms. Patients with long-standing disease with an increased risk for colorectal cancer, severe flares that are not responsive to medical therapy, dysplasia or carcinoma, or significant medical complications may need surgical intervention. Proctocolectomy or colectomy with rectal mucosectomy completely removes both the mucosa at risk for neoplasia and inflamed mucosa causing UC symptoms. At the same time, by removing all colonic mucosa, proctocolectomy is curative for UC. Patients report an overall improvement in quality of life, but there are potential complications that cause significant morbidity after surgery.

Restorative proctocolectomy (RP) with ileal pouch-anal anastomosis (IPAA) is the surgical procedure of choice for the treatment of UC. This procedure removes all affected mucosa and maintains intestinal continuity. Alternatively, a total proctocolectomy with ileostomy can be performed, which also removes all affected mucosa but leaves the patient with an external appliance. IPAA can improve quality of life and patient satisfaction is high, especially in young patients who are unwilling to have the external appliance. Satisfaction is similar with or without an appliance.[1] Some of the different surgical procedures will be discussed in the text that follows.

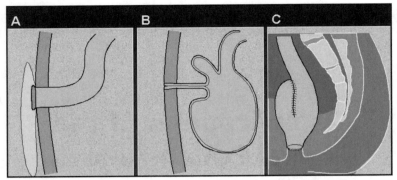

Figure 8-1. A. Brooke ileostomy. B. Kock pouch. C. Continent ileostomy (IPAA).

SURGERY IN CHRONIC ULCERATIVE COLITIS

ILEOSTOMY

The Brooke ileostomy (Figure 8-1A) is created by everting the ileal mucosa and sewing it to the skin so that the serosal surface of the intestine is not exposed to the bowel contents. This ileostomy is a free-flowing ostomy and an appliance must be worn to collect the contents that intermittently discharge throughout the day. In contrast to the Brooke ileostomy, the Kock pouch or "continent ileostomy" does not require an external bag (see Figure 8-1B). This procedure involves the creation of a nipple valve with ileal mucosa to make the ostomy continent. The ostomy is emptied several times each day by the insertion of a catheter to help expel the contents. Complications are high in this procedure compared to the Brooke ileostomy due to nipple valve failure, fistulas, strictures, and pouch dysfunction. The Kock pouch is rarely performed secondary to complication rates.

ILEAL POUCH-ANAL ANASTOMOSIS

Surgical therapy for chronic UC involves proctocolectomy, removal of the colon and mucosa of the distal rectum, and reanastomosis of the terminal ileum to the anus. Patients often desire this procedure because it retains continuity of the intestines and continence and does not require any appliances. Initially, the ileum was anastomosed directly to the anus without any pouch procedure. Complications of fecal urgency, frequency, and seepage frequently occurred. Therefore, a pouch was created to act as a reservoir to reduce these symptoms. There are several types of pouches that can be performed.

The J, W, and S pouches are shown in Figure 8-2. Differences are primarily in capacity and compliance of the reservoir. The procedure that is chosen

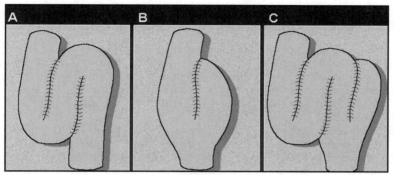

Figure 8-2. A. J pouch. B. S pouch. C. W pouch.

depends on the surgeon and institution preference. Patient satisfaction and complication rates are similar between pouches performed.[2]

A diverting ileostomy is generally performed and used for 2 to 3 months to allow the pouch and anastomosis to heal. After this period, the ileostomy is closed and the pouch is allowed to function as designed. Most patients have a two-stage procedure, while less than 10% have a one-stage operation. One-stage operations can be successfully performed in those patients who are not toxic, have not been on steroids, do not have diabetes mellitus, and have had the IPAA performed with excellent results. Patients undergoing one-stage operations must understand that they have an increased leakage rate from the anastomosis postoperatively, a longer hospital stay, and a longer recovery period.[3]

The colon normally absorbs about 1 liter of fluid from the stool; however, after a colectomy, the volume of stool that patients have will be higher than patients with an intact colon. Meagher et al studied 1310 patients with IPAAs and found that the mean number of stools was five during the day and one during the night after a mean follow-up of 6.5 years. Frequent incontinence occurred in 7% during the day and 12% at night.[4]

COMPLICATIONS OF IPAA

The results of the IPAA procedure are generally excellent and patient satisfaction is high. However, there can be significant morbidity after an IPAA. Perioperative complications can occur with an IPAA as with any abdominal or pelvic operation. Most of these complications will not be discussed further here, as they are beyond the scope of this text. Short-term complications such as pelvic sepsis and leakage from the anastomosis or pouch do occur. Long-term complications like intestinal obstruction, anastomotic strictures, sexual dysfunction, and pouchitis also occur.

CROHN'S DISEASE AND INDETERMINANT COLITIS

Patients with Crohn's disease (CD) who present with pancolitis, in the absence of endoscopic or radiographic evidence of small bowel involvement, may be misdiagnosed with UC. Up to 10% to 15% of patients fall into this category of indeterminant colitis. Due to the high rate of pouch failure, IPAA is not recommended for patients who have a known diagnosis of CD. Sagar et al studied 37 patients with CD who had an IPAA. They found a pouch failure rate of 45%.[5]

In contrast, patients with indeterminant colitis without any features of CD can probably undergo an IPAA with results similar to patients with UC. Hyman et al[6] looked at 25 patients who had an IPAA and were later diagnosed with CD. They found that 15 of 16 patients who had no features of CD preoperatively did well and maintained good pouch function. However, eight of the nine patients who did have a preoperative feature of CD did very poorly, with only one patient having a functioning pouch at a mean follow-up 38.1 months.[6]

PELVIC SEPSIS

Postoperative sepsis usually occurs in the setting of an anastomotic leak and is certainly one of the more serious complications of IPAA. The rate of sepsis is 6% to 37%, and treatment may require antibiotics, drainage, or prolonged ileostomy.[7] Pelvic sepsis is one of the more common causes of pouch failure.

INTESTINAL OBSTRUCTION

Small bowel obstruction (SBO) is a frequent complication and may occur in up to a quarter of IPAAs. SBOs commonly occur after the diverting ileostomy is closed, and the site of obstruction is often at the former ileostomy site. Only a minority of these cases require surgical intervention. MacLean et al studied 1178 patients and found that 23% had episodes of SBO over a mean follow-up of 8.7 years.[8] This study also found that 7.5% of these cases required surgical intervention.

STRICTURES

Anastomotic strictures may occur in up to 33% of patients undergoing routine pouchography[9]; however, clinically significant strictures may be closer to 5%.[10] These strictures can cause pouch dilatation and stasis, which can lead to bacterial overgrowth and symptoms similar to pouchitis (see below). These strictures can usually be successfully treated with finger dilatation. Strictures longer than 1 to 2 cm may require dilatation under anesthesia.

SEXUAL DYSFUNCTION

Impotence occurs in 1.5% of males undergoing IPAA, but retrograde ejaculation is reported more frequently in up to 10% of males. Dyspareunia can occur in 8% of females, as well as decreased fertility probably secondary to pelvic adhesions.[11] Postoperative vaginal dryness, pain interfering with the ability to feel sexual pleasure, and limited sexual activity due to fear of stool leakage have been reported.[12] In most patients, however, sexual function is significantly improved when compared with the period of active colitis prior to IPAA.[13]

DYSPLASIA

Dysplasia arising within the rectal cuff can occur. This dysplastic epithelium may arise from islands of retained colonic mucosa after colectomy and pouch construction. There have been reports of dysplasia occurring in the rectal cuff mucosa.[14] Screening should be considered in these patients, especially those patients who had cancer or dysplasia at the time of restorative proctocolectomy and IPAA.

POUCHITIS

Pouchitis is the most frequent long-term complication of IPAA. The incidence varies widely and depends upon the definition and length of patient follow-up. The diagnosis should be made using uniform criteria of symptoms, endoscopy, and histology, but previous studies have not used uniform criteria. These studies also have used differing lengths of follow-up, and the incidence of pouchitis does increase with longer duration of follow-up. Reported incidences range from about 6% to 50%.[15] The disease has been difficult to define and diagnose because symptoms do not necessarily correlate with disease activity endoscopically and/or histologically. One large series of patients had a cumulative probability of developing pouchitis of 18% at 1 year and 48% at 10 years.[4]

DEFINITION

Because of the confusion regarding the definition of pouchitis, the pouchitis disease activity index (PDAI) was created and helps clarify the presence and severity of the condition (Table 8-1). The PDAI takes clinical symptoms, endoscopic results, and histopathology into account. The score is weighted to account for more significant findings or symptoms. A score of 7 or higher indicates the presence of disease, while a score of less than 7 is defined as without pouchitis. Shen et al demonstrated that symptoms alone fail to reliably diagnose pouchitis. Twenty-five percent of the patients with symptoms suggestive of pouchitis had PDAI scores <7.[6] Endoscopy with biopsies should be performed in all patients suspected of having pouchitis.

Table 8-1

POUCHITIS DISEASE ACTIVITY INDEX

	Criteria	*Score*
Clinical		
Postoperative stool frequency	Usual	0
	1 to 2 stools/day more than usual	1
	3 or more stools/day more than usual	2
Rectal bleeding	None or rarely	0
	Present daily	1
Fecal urgency/ abdominal cramps	None	0
	Occasional	1
	Usual	2
Fever (>100°F)	Absent	0
	Present	1
Endoscopic		
	Edema	1
	Granularity	1
	Friability	1
	Loss of vascular pattern	1
	Mucus exudate	1
	Ulceration	1
Acute Histological		
Polymorph infiltration	Mild	1
	Moderate plus crypt abscess	2
	Severe plus crypt abscess	3
Ulceration per low-power field (average)	<25%	1
	≥25%, ≤50%	2
	>50%	3

Pouchitis is defined as a total score of ≥7.

Reprinted with permission from Sandborn WJ, Tremaine WJ, Batts KP, Pemberton JH, Phillips SF. Pouchitis following ileal pouch-anal anastomosis: a pouchitis disease activity index. *Mayo Clinic Proceedings.* 1994;69(5):409-415.

SYMPTOMS

Symptoms of pouchitis include increased stool frequency, hematochezia, abdominal pain, tenesmus, and fever. If the patient had a history of extraintestinal manifestations (eg, pyoderma gangrenosum, primary sclerosing cholangitis [PSC], arthralgias, etc) of ulcerative colitis, these often recur during an episode of pouchitis.

ENDOSCOPY

Endoscopy of the pouch is performed with a gastroscope. Endoscopic appearance of pouchitis includes friability, erythema, exudate, ulcers, loss of vascular pattern, and contact bleeding. The ileum just proximal to the pouch should appear normal in pouchitis.

HISTOPATHOLOGY

Chronic inflammation, crypt hyperplasia, and villous atrophy of the pouch are present in the majority of patients with IPAA and do not correlate with pouchitis. The inflammatory cells are predominantly lymphocytes and plasma cells, but eosinophils may also predominate. Acute inflammation with neutrophilic infiltration and ulceration is a finding consistent with pouchitis. Biopsies should be taken throughout the pouch to avoid sampling error. The posterior and inferior portions of the pouch are most often involved. This is thought to occur because the mucosa in those areas is more frequently in contact with stool; therefore, stasis and the anterior portion are often protected by gas.

RISK FACTORS

Gender

A retrospective review of 114 patients who had IPAAs performed concluded that women were more likely to develop pouchitis symptoms than men (74% versus 47%, respectively).[17] It is not clear why this was found in this study. The authors postulated that women may report pouchitis symptoms to their physician more frequently. This study did not use endoscopy or histology for diagnosis.

Serologic Tests

Perinuclear antineutrophil cytoplasmic antibody (pANCA) positivity is associated with UC, and whether this could be used as a predictor in the development of chronic pouchitis is currently uncertain. High levels of pANCA precolectomy have been reported to predict chronic pouchitis in one study[18]; however, several other studies do not show a correlation with pANCA and predict the development of pouchitis. At this point, pANCA should not be used in making management decisions about IPAA and pouchitis.

Smoking

Interestingly, smoking, which is associated with decreased rates of UC, has also been associated with decreased rates of pouchitis.[19]

DIFFERENTIAL DIAGNOSIS

Several other conditions must be considered and excluded in order to diagnose pouchitis. Bacterial infections with *Clostridium difficile, Campylobacter, Escherichia coli, Shigella,* and *Salmonella* can cause diarrheal illnesses that can be treated with appropriate antibiotics. Parasitic and viral infections may also be investigated.

Strictures at the IPAA can be successfully treated with gentle dilation. Longer strictures may need repeated dilation under anesthesia. Diagnosis can be made with videoproctography.

Primary bile acids can be dehydroxylated by bacteria, which makes them more lipophilic. These secondary bile acids, such as deoxycholic acid, may be more cytotoxic to colonic cell membranes. Damage to these cells may alter water and salt permeability and cause malabsorption.[20]

Unrecognized CD can present with similar symptoms to pouchitis, and the issue should be addressed but is often a difficult task. In order to diagnose CD of the pouch, the original colectomy specimen or examination of the proximal small bowel must be reviewed. Diagnosis based purely upon pouch findings (ie, endoscopy and pathology) may not be accurate, and these findings should not be used to diagnose CD.

RECURRENT IBD

CD of the pouch is one etiology for some patients, particularly those that were preoperatively diagnosed with indeterminant colitis. Diagnosis of CD requires histologic examination of the original colectomy specimen or proximal small intestine, not of the pouch itself. Indirect evidence that IBD plays some role in the pathogenesis of pouchitis is the appearance of extraintestinal manifestations of IBD, including PSC, arthralgias, uveitis, and pyoderma gangrenosum, can correlate with symptoms of pouchitis. A significant history for extraintestinal manifestations of IBD prior to proctocolectomy increases a person's risk for the development of pouchitis.[21]

IPAA patients may also have concomitant IBS. Results of stool studies/cultures, radiographic evaluation, endoscopy, and histopathology can be helpful in differentiating symptom etiology.

PATHOPHYSIOLOGY OF POUCHITIS

There are several theories on the pathophysiology of pouchitis, although no definitive etiology has been identified. Fecal stasis may play a central role in the development of the condition. Other etiologic factors that may play a role are bacterial infections or overgrowth, bile acid toxicity, short-chain fatty acid deficiency, recurrent inflammatory bowel disease (IBD), and ischemia. Of particular interest is that patients with IPAA for UC develop pouchitis more frequently than patients with familial adenomatous polyposis (FAP) who have an IPAA. The incidence of pouchitis ranges from 0% to 10% in patients with FAP versus 19% to 44% in patients with UC.[11] This suggests a possible IBD component to the development of pouchitis.

FECAL STASIS

The physiologic role of the ileum is for absorption of nutrients. After an IPAA is performed, the ileum's role changes from absorptive to storage. Several changes take place in order to adapt to this function. Pouches undergo a process of partial colonic metaplasia in which villous atrophy occurs and the depth of crypts increases.[22] The posterior portion of the pouch, which is the dependent portion, is the area most often affected by pouchitis. However, patients with FAP rarely develop pouchitis but most certainly have similar stasis.

BILE ACIDS

Stasis of fecal contents within the pouch may be an etiologic factor toward the development of pouchitis by the promotion of increased contact of the ileal mucosa to toxic or other potentially harmful substances. In the colon, bacteria normally deconjugate bile acids as well as convert primary bile acids to secondary bile acids through dehydroxylation. In the pouches, the bile acids are primarily deconjugated. These may be cytotoxic and cause chronic and acute inflammation of the pouch.[22]

BACTERIAL OVERGROWTH

Bacterial overgrowth may occur in the pouch. Microbial flora of pouches are intermediate to end ileostomy and colon flora.[23] However, bacterial flora and concentrations in patients with and without pouchitis have not been shown to differ.[11,24] The response to treatment with antibiotics favors a bacteriologic role for pathogenesis.

ROLE OF DIET

There is currently no evidence to suggest a role for dietary intake in either the pathogenesis or therapy of pouchitis. The limited available data suggest some high fiber foods, namely greens and fruits, are associated with increased frequency of bowel movements, although such is often the case in otherwise normal individuals. Self-imposed dietary restrictions are often encountered in patients with pouchitis.[29]

SHORT-CHAIN FATTY ACID DEFICIENCY

Bacterial metabolism of unabsorbed carbohydrates and starches in the colon normally provides short-chain fatty acids (SCFA) for the colonic mucosa. Acetate, propionate, and butyrate are preferred energy sources for the colon. In well-functioning pouches, SCFA concentrations are similar to normal controls, and decreased amounts of SCFAs were found in patients with pouchitis in two studies.[26,27] Investigations into whether low SCFA concentrations predict or are associated with pouchitis have yielded inconsistent results. It is unclear if the SCFA concentrations observed in patients with pouchitis were simply due to decreased soluble fiber and starch intake during a period of gastrointestinal distress.

SYSTEMIC IBD

There is evidence that pouchitis may be a manifestation of systemic disease. PSC is the extraintestinal manifestation of IBD most strongly associated with pouchitis. Cumulative risk for the development of pouchitis in patients with UC and PSC versus UC alone is 61% versus 36% at 5 years, and 79% versus 46% at 10 years, respectively, at 10 years at the Mayo Clinic.[28] This suggests that there might be a common pathophysiologic mechanism between PSC and pouchitis.

ISCHEMIA

Ischemia of the pouch mucosa seems like a reasonable cause of pouchitis given that mesenteric vessels are manipulated and divided in order to obtain low tension on the pouch and anastomosis. However, if this were the primary cause, one would expect patients with FAP to have similar rates of pouchitis, which is not the case. Ischemia likely does not play any major role in the pathogenesis of pouchitis.

DISEASE COURSE

In a Swedish study, the cumulative risk of developing one or more episodes of pouchitis was 51% over a 5-year period, and the median time to the first pouchitis episode was 12 months. Seventy-one percent of the patients who did develop pouchitis had their first occurrence within 2 years. The study also showed that most patients with pouchitis (76%) had one or a few episodes, while 18% had frequent recurrences that usually responded to therapy and 6% had severe chronic symptoms.[29] Approximately 5% to 10% of patients do develop chronic, refractory pouchitis.[30,31] These patients can be challenging to treat.

Another study demonstrated that the probability of having at least one episode of pouchitis was 18% at 1 year and 48% at 10 years. However, the diagnostic criteria used were patients' symptoms and response to therapy with metronidazole.[4]

TREATMENT

Antibiotics are the primary therapy used to treat pouchitis, and metronidazole is the initial treatment choice in most instances. In 1993, a double-blind crossover trial was performed to evaluate metronidazole treatment (400 mg three times a day [tid] for 7 days) versus placebo in chronic pouchitis.[32] Treatment resulted in the reduction in bowel movements by three per day versus one per day increase in frequency in the placebo group. Histologic inflammation, endoscopic findings, and symptomatic scores, however, were not significantly improved.

Reasonable metronidazole doses are 750 to 1500 mg per day for 7 to 10 days of therapy. Symptomatic response is usually seen in 1 or 2 days.[33] Patients may experience adverse reactions, such as peripheral neuropathy, at higher doses. Ciprofloxacin (1000 mg/day) has also shown benefit as alternative therapy for patients, especially those who have adverse reactions to metronidazole. Ciprofloxacin may actually be more effective, with a greater reduction in PDAI scores and less side effects.[34] Tetracyclines and amoxicillin/sulbactam can also be considered without significant evidence for their use. Combination antibiotic therapy with ciprofloxacin plus rifaximin as well as ciprofloxacin plus metronidazole has been successful.[35]

Most patients respond well to metronidazole therapy or other antibiotics, but recurrences are common, as discussed above.[36] If a partial response occurs or pouchitis recurs, another course of antibiotic therapy that includes metronidazole is recommended. If symptoms fail to improve, a trial of a different or additional antibiotic is generally warranted.

If symptoms persist following another course of antibiotics, alternative therapies should be considered. Probiotics, such as VSL#3 (Yovis, Sigma-Tau, Pomezia, Italy), which contains four strains of *Lactobacilli*, three strains of *Bifidobacterium*, and one strain of *Streptococcus salivarius*, may alter the flora of the pouch. VSL#3 has not been shown to induce remission of pouchitis but had promising results in the prevention of flares in a small trial.[37] Topical administration of anti-inflammatory agents, such as 5-ASA and steroid enemas, may also be effective in selected patients. Bismuth carbomer enemas, butyrate and glutamine suppositories, and allopurinol have not been shown to treat pouchitis effectively, but further research is needed to determine if these or other therapies may be beneficial for selected patients.

COMPLICATIONS OF POUCHITIS

DYSPLASIA IN THE POUCH

There may also be a small risk of dysplasia arising from the pouch mucosa itself. The risk is likely related to duration of follow-up and the presence of inflammation (ie, pouchitis). In one study, 106 patients with ileal pouches (Kock pouches were included) had pouch endoscopies, and the study found that there was one case of multifocal low grade dysplasia in the pouch.[38] There have been rare reports of adenocarcinoma arising from the pouch as well. One study found that pouches that contained severe villous atrophy had an increased incidence of dysplasia, although another study did not support this finding.[39] The exact amount of risk is unclear and warrants further study. Therefore, precise recommendations for surveillance endoscopy cannot conclusively be made.

POUCH FAILURE

Pouch failure occurs in about 10% of operations usually due to infection, leakage, pouchitis, or dysfunction. One large study of 1310 patients reported a cumulative probability of pouch failure at 1, 5, and 10 years of 2%, 5%, and 9%, respectively. Recalcitrant pouchitis itself results in pouch excision in less than 2% of patients with pouchitis. In the same study in which patients were followed for 10 years, the rate of pouch excision for pouchitis was 0.1%.[4] The overall rate of pouch failure in 187 patients with FAP in one study was 4%.[40]

CONCLUSION

UC is a disease that is managed with medical therapy. When medical therapy fails or when dysplasia and carcinoma arise, surgical intervention is often required. Restorative proctocolectomy with IPAA is the surgical procedure of choice. Many patients prefer the preservation of bowel continuity and are highly satisfied with the overall function of the pouch. As with all operations, complications do occur, and inflammation involving the pouch mucosa is a common problem. Several theories have been proposed for pouchitis, although the pathophysiology is not completely understood. Usually, pouchitis is mild and treatment with conventional medical therapy is straightforward, but some patients either do not respond or have frequent recurrences. Unremitting pouchitis causing pouch failure and removal of the pouch is rarely required. The risk of dysplasia and malignancy is unclear but likely small. Nevertheless, the IPAA has lead to a significant improvement in the management of UC and patients' quality of life. Figure 8-3 shows a treatment algorithm for the diagnosis and treatment of pouchitis.

REFERENCES

1. McLeod RS, Churchill DN, Lock AM, Vanderburgh S, Cohen Z. Quality of life of patients with ulcerative colitis preoperatively and postoperatively. *Gastroenterology.* 1991;101(5):1307-1313.

2. Pemberton JH, Phillips SF. Ileostomy and its alternatives. In: Feldman M, Scharschmidt BF, Sleisenger MH, eds. *Sleisenger & Fordtran's Gastrointestinal and Liver Disease.* Vol 2. 6th ed. Philadelphia, Pa: WB Saunders Company; 1998: 1765.

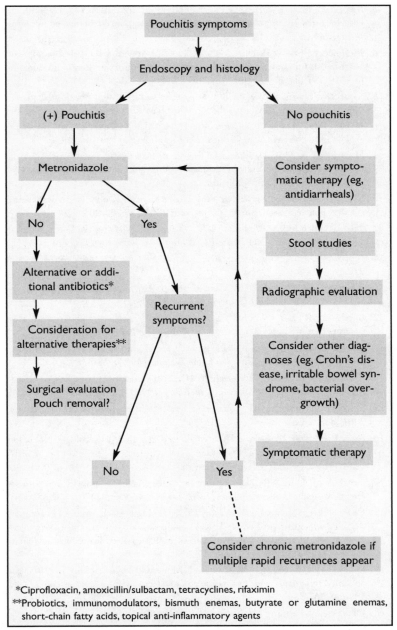

Figure 8-3. Treatment algorithm for diagnosis and treatment of pouchitis.

3. Remzi FH, Fazio VW. Ileoanal pouch anastomosis. In: Bayless TM, Hanauer SB, eds. *Advanced Therapy of Inflammatory Bowel Disease.* 2nd ed. Hamilton, Ontario: BC Decker Inc; 2001:197.

4. Meagher AP, Farouk R, Dozois RR, Kelly KA, Pemberton JH. J ileal pouch-anal anastomosis for chronic ulcerative colitis: complications and long-term outcome in 1310 patients. *Br J Surg.* 1998;85(6):800-803.

5. Sagar PM, Dozois RR, Wolff BG. Long-term results of ileal pouch-anal anastomosis in patients with Crohn's disease. *Dis Colon Rectum.* 1996;39(8):893-898.

6. Hyman NH, Fazio VW, Tuckson WB, Lavery IC. Consequences of ileal pouch-anal anastomosis for Crohn's colitis. *Dis Colon Rectum.* 1991;34(8):653-657.

7. Heuschen UA, Hinz U, Allemeyer EH, et al. Risk factors for ileoanal J pouch-related septic complications in ulcerative colitis and familial adenomatous polyposis. *Ann Surg.* 2002;235:207-216.

8. MacLean AR, Cohen Z, MacRae HM, et al. Risk of small bowel obstruction after the ileal pouch-anal anastomosis. *Ann Surg.* 2002;235:200-206.

9. Tsao JI, Galandiuk S, Pemberton JH. Pouchogram: predictor of clinical outcome following ileal pouch-anal anastomosis. *Dis Colon Rectum.* 1992;35(6):547-551.

10. Brostrom O. Prognosis in ulcerative colitis. *Med Clin No Am.* 1990;74(1):201-218.

11. Salemans JM, Nagengast FM. Clinical and physiological aspects of ileal pouch-anal anastomosis. *Scand J Gastroenterol Suppl.* 1995;212:3-12.

12. Bambrick M, Fazio VW, Hull TL, Pucel G. Sexual function following restorative proctocolectomy in women. *Dis Colon Rectum.* 1996;39:610-614.

13. Damgaard B, Wettergren A, Kirkegaard P. Social and sexual function following ileal pouch-anal anastomosis. *Dis Colon Rectum.* 1995;38:286-289.

14. Thompson-Fawcett MW, Mortensen NJ. Anal transitional zone and columnar cuff in restorative proctocolectomy. *Br J Surg.* 1996;83(8):1047-1055.

15. Stocchi L, Pemberton JH. Pouch and pouchitis. *Gastroenterol Clin North Am.* 2001;30:223-224.

16. Shen B, Achkar JP, Lashner BA, et al. Endoscopic and histologic evaluation together with symptom assessment are required to diagnose pouchitis. *Gastroenterology.* 2001;121:261-267.

17. Simchuk EJ, Thirlby RC. Risk factors and true incidence of pouchitis in patients after ileal pouch-anal anastomoses. *World Journal of Surgery.* 2000;24(7):851-856.

18. Fleshner PR, Vasiliauskas EA, Kam LY, et al. High level perinuclear antineutrophil cytoplasmic antibody (pANCA) in ulcerative colitis patients before colectomy predicts the development of chronic pouchitis after ileal pouch-anal anastomosis. *Gut.* 2001;49(5):671-677.

19. Merrett MN, Mortensen N, Kettlewell M, Jewell DO. Smoking may prevent pouchitis in patients with restorative proctocolectomy for ulcerative colitis. *Gut.* 1996;38:362-364.

20. Madden MV, Farthing MJ, Nicholls RJ. Inflammation in ileal reservoirs: 'pouchitis'. *Gut.* 1990;31(3):247-249.

21. Lohmuller JL, Pemberton JH, Dozois RR, Ilstrup D, van Heerden J. Pouchitis and extraintestinal manifestations of inflammatory bowel disease after ileal pouch-anal anastomosis. *Ann Surg.* 1990;211(5):622-627.

22. Lerch MM, Braun J, Harder M, Hofstadter F, Schumpelick V, Matern S. Postoperative adaptation of the small intestine after total colectomy and J-pouch-anal anastomosis. *Dis Colon Rectum.* 1989;32(7):600-608.

23. Shepherd NA, Hulten L, Tytgat GN, et al. Pouchitis. *International Journal of Colorectal Disease.* 1989;4(4):205-229.

24. Kmiot WA, Young D, Tudor R. Thompson H, Keighley MR. Mucosal morphology, cell proliferation and fecal bacteriology in acute pouchitis. *Br J Surg.* 1993;80(11):1445-1449.

25. Coffey JC, Winter DC, Neary P, et al. Quality of life after ileal pouch-anal anastomosis: an evaluation of diet and other factors using the Cleveland Clinic Global Quality of Life Instrument. *Dis Colon Rectum.* 2002;45:30-38.

26. Clausen MR, Tvede M, Mortensen PB. Short-chain fatty acids in pouch contents from patients with and without pouchitis after ileal pouch-anal anastomosis. *Gastroenterology.* 1992;103(4):1144-1153.

27. Sagar PM, Taylor BA, Godwin P, et al. Acute pouchitis and deficiencies of fuel. *Dis Colon Rectum.* 1995;38:488-493.

28. Penna C, Dozois R, Tremaine W, et al. Pouchitis after ileal pouch-anal anastomosis for ulcerative colitis occurs with increased frequency in patients with associated primary sclerosing cholangitis. *Gut.* 1996;38:234-239.

29. Svaninger G, Nordgren S, Oresland T, Hulten L. Incidence and characteristics of pouchitis in the Kock continent ileostomy and the pelvic pouch. *Scand J Gastroenterol.* 1993;28(8):695-700.

30. Mowschenson PM, Critchlow JF, Peppercorn MA. Ileoanal pouch operation: long-term outcome with or without diverting ileostomy. *Arch Surg.* 2000;135(4):463-465.

31. Hurst RD, Chung TP, Rubin M, Michelassi F. The implications of acute pouchitis on the long-term functional results after restorative proctocolectomy. *Inflamm Bowel Dis.* 1998;4(4):280-284.

32. Madden MV, McIntyre AS, Nicholls RJ. Double-blind crossover trial of metronidazole versus placebo in chronic unremitting pouchitis. *Dig Dis Sci.* 1994;39(6):1193-1196.

33. Sandborn WJ. Pouchitis following ileal pouch-anal anastomosis: definition, pathogenesis, and treatment. *Gastroenterology.* 1994;107(6):1856-1860.

34. Shen B, Achkar JP, Lashner B, et al. A randomized clinical trial of ciprofloxacin and metronidazole to treat acute pouchitis. *Inflamm Bowel Dis.* 2001;7(4):301-305.

35. Gionchetti P, Rizzello F, Venturi A, et al. Antibiotic combination therapy in patients with chronic, treatment-resistant pouchitis. *Aliment Pharmacol Ther.* 1999;13(6):713-718.

36. Sandborn WJ, McLeod R, Jewell DP. Medical therapy for induction and maintenance of remission in pouchitis: a systematic review. *Inflamm Bowel Dis.* 1999;5(1):33-39.

37. Gionchetti P, Rizzello F, Venturi A, et al. Oral bacteriotherapy as maintenance treatment in patients with chronic pouchitis: a double-blind, placebo-controlled trial. *Gastroenterology.* 2000;119:305-309.

38 Thompson-Fawcett MW, Marcus V, Redston M, Cohen Z, McLeod RS. Risk of dysplasia in long-term ileal pouches and pouches with chronic pouchitis. *Gastroenterology.* 2001;121(2):275-281.

39. Gullberg K, Stahlberg D, Liljeqvist L, et al. Neoplastic transformation of the pelvic pouch mucosa in patients with ulcerative colitis. *Gastroenterology.* 1997;112(5):1487-1492.

40. Nyam DC, Brillant PT, Dozois RR, Kelly KA, Pemberton JH, Wolff BG. Ileal pouch-anal canal anastomosis for familial adenomatous polyposis: early and late results. *Ann Surg.* 1997;226(4):514-519.

chapter 9

Nutritional Support in Inflammatory Bowel Disease

Alan L. Buchman, MD, MSPH and James S. Scolapio, MD

NUTRITIONAL ASSESSMENT

The nutritional management of a patient with inflammatory bowel disease (IBD) begins with appropriate nutritional assessment. Multiple factors contribute to malnutrition in both Crohn's disease and ulcerative colitis. It is reported that nutritional deficiencies are greater in Crohn's disease than ulcerative colitis. It is estimated that as many as 75% of hospitalized Crohn's patients are malnourished.[1] Reduced intake of food secondary to abdominal cramps, nausea, and diarrhea is a major cause of weight loss in IBD patients. Intestinal malabsorption also contributes to malnutrition in patients with active IBD. Extensive mucosal disease, bacterial overgrowth, and surgical resection all contribute to malabsorption and subsequent weight loss. Increased energy expenditure, as seen with fever, abscess, or sepsis, can also result in weight loss. Nutrient deficiency can result in altered cellular immunity with increased risk of infection, delayed wound healing, and growth retardation in children. Therefore, it is important to identify those patients that are at potential risk for malnutrition. Management goals should then include correction of nutritional deficits.

There is no gold standard or one laboratory test for measuring the malnutrition of a patient. All current assessment methods may be effected by the underlying illness and not necessary reflect the nutritional reserve of the patient. For example, serum albumin and prealbumin can be reduced in all inflammatory disorders including IBD without a history of weight loss or. other micronutrient deficiency as hepatic protein synthesis shifts to that of acute phase reactants. Likewise, extracellular fluid shifts can result in low serum albumin and prealbumin concentrations without a clinical history that suggests weight loss or malnutrition. Also delayed cutaneous hypersensitivity (DCH) is an unreliable marker of malnutrition because medications used in the treatment of IBD, including prednisone and immunosuppressants, can affect results. A history and physical examination is probably the best tool to access the gross nutritional status of an individual patient. Patients that have lost significant weight (defined as greater than 10%) and have had reduced oral caloric intake over a 2- to 24-week period are at risk of both macronutrient and micronutrient deficiencies. The important findings on physical examination besides an accurate weight include loss of subcutaneous fat, muscle wasting, dependent edema, and ascites. The subjective global assessment (SGA) is a clinical method of evaluating nutritional status that includes historical, symptomatic, and physical parameters of patients.[2] The findings from the history and physical examination are subjectively weighted to rank patients as being well nourished, moderately malnourished, or severely malnourished. The use of the SGA has been shown to give reproducible results with more than 80% agreement.[2] When to begin nutritional support and which method to use are discussed in the sections of this chapter that follow.

SPECIFIC NUTRIENT DEFICIENCIES

Deficiencies of vitamins, minerals, and trace elements may result from either inadequate intake or increased intestinal losses. Deficiencies are more common in Crohn's disease than ulcerative colitis given that the majority of micronutrients are absorbed in the small intestine. History and physical examination are useful tools in the diagnosis of specific nutrient deficiencies (Tables 9-1, 9-2, and 9-3).

Folic acid and vitamin B_{12} are the two most common water-soluble vitamin deficiencies that can occur. Deficiency of other water-soluble vitamins is rare. Folate deficiency may result from intestinal malabsorption when proximal jejunal disease is present, as well as interaction with sulfasalazine, which inhibits folate uptake. Approximately 30% of Crohn's patients have been reported to have low serum folate.[3] Replacement can be given with oral folic acid at a dose of 1.0 mg daily. Vitamin B_{12} absorption can be impaired if the distal 60 cm of the ileum is diseased or resected, which can occur with Crohn's disease.[4] Also bacterial overgrowth in the small intestine can reduce vitamin B_{12} absorption. One thousand ug monthly of subcutaneous vitamin B_{12} should be given to patients at risk.

Table 9-1

NUTRITIONAL ASSESSMENT

History and Physical Examination

History	Unusual dietary habits, medication/vitamin or mineral supplements, change in hair color or texture, poor night vision, dysguesia, dysphagia/odynophagia, abdominal pain/distention, diarrhea, bone pain, muscle pain/cramps/twitching, numbness/paresthesias, fatigue, diminished mental activity, weakness
Physical examination	Hair loss/texture, keratomalacia, cheilosis, glossitis, red tongue, parotid enlargement, dentition, skin rash/petechia/bruising, muscle wasting, hepatomegaly, edema, peripheral neuropathy

Anthropometrics

Ideal body weight (IBW)	Males: 48 kg + 2.3 kg for each inch >60
	Females: 45 kg + 2.7 kg for each inch >60
	Calculate % IBW: >5% weight loss in 1 month, >7.5% in 2 months, or >10% in 6 months are significant
	"Preferred" body weight for obese (Hamwi formula) = (ABW–IBW)(0.25) + IBW (Note: Used clinically, but not validated)

	Adjusted body weight for amputation:
	    Entire arm (-6.5%)
	    Upper arm (-3.5%)
	    Hand (-0.8%)
	    Forearm with hand (-3.1%)
	    Forearm without hand (-2.5%)
	    Entire leg (-18.6%)
	    Foot (-1.8%)

Muscle function	Handgrip strength, peak inspiratory pressure
Midarm circumference	Assess skeletal mass
Triceps skin fold thickness	Assess fat stores (Note: Operator-dependent variability, unreliable to assess short-term responses)

continued on next page

Table 9-1 continued

NUTRITIONAL ASSESSMENT

Laboratory Measurements

Nitrogen balance   N intake = grams protein/6.25
Balance = N intake − (24 urine urea nitrogen [UUN] + 4)
(Note: Requires sufficient calories as well as protein)

Indirect Calorimetry

Visceral proteins   Albumin, prealbumin, transferrin, retinol-binding protein
(Note: Affected by many non-nutritional conditions)

Immune function   Total lymphocyte count
Delayed hypersensitivity skin tests
(Note: Affected by many non-nutritional conditions)

Table 9-2

VITAMIN DEFICIENCY STATES AND THEIR DETECTION

Vitamin	Role	Deficiency State	Measurement
Water Soluble			
Thiamine (B_1)	Coenzyme in oxidative decarboxylation reactions	Beriberi (cardiomyopathy), peripheral neuropathy, encephalopathy	Erythrocyte transketolase with % enhancement resulting from added thiamin pyrophosphate
Riboflavin (B_2)	Coenzyme of flavoproteins (FMN and FAD) involved in electron transport, tissue oxidation	Angular stomatitis Glossitis Cheilosis Photophobia Tearing Seborrheic dermatitis (nasolabial fold and scrotum)	FAD-dep red blood cell (RBC) Glutathione reductase activity 24-hour urine riboflavin RBC riboflavin

continued on next page

Table 9-2 continued

VITAMIN DEFICIENCY STATES AND THEIR DETECTION

Vitamin	Role	Deficiency State	Measurement
Pantothenic acid	Precursor of coenzyme A involved in synthesis of fatty acids and steroid hormones	"Burning feet" syndrome Fatigue, leg cramps Paresthesias	
Niacin	Constituent of the coenzymes NAD and NADP involved in hydrogen transport and glycolysis	Pellagra (dementia, diarrhea, dermatitis) Scarlet, raw tongue Fissures of the tongue	Red blood cell (RBC) or urine NAD:NADP ratio
Pyridoxine (B_6)	Coenzyme involved in amino acid metabolism and DNA synthesis Peripheral neuropathy	Convulsions Glossitis Cheilosis Seborrheic dermatitis (eye, nose, and mouth areas)	Plasma pyridoxal phosphate
Biotin	Coenzyme in carboxylation reactions	Dermatitis Alopecia Depression Muscle pain Paresthesias	24-hour urine biotin
Folic acid	Coenzyme in amino acid metabolism and DNA synthesis	Anemia (macrocytic) Stomatitis Diarrhea	RBC folate Homocystine
Cobalamin (B_{12})	Coenzyme in amino acid metabolism and DNA synthesis	Anemia (megaloblastic) Neuropathy Paresthesias Glossitis	Serum B_{12} Methylmalonic acid

continued on next page

Table 9-2 continued

VITAMIN DEFICIENCY STATES
AND THEIR DETECTION

Vitamin	Role	Deficiency State	Measurement
C	Oxidation/reduction reactions	Delayed wound healing Petechia Scurvy	Plasma or white blood cell count Vitamin C
Fat Soluble			
A	Retinal pigment formation Epithelial integrity	Xerophthalmia Keratomalacia Night blindness Delayed wound healing Sterility (males)	Serum vitamin A
D	Calcium and phosphate homeostasis	Osteomalacia (rickets)	Serum 25-OH vitamin D_3
E	Antioxidant	Neuropathy (paresis of gaze, gait disturbance, decreased proprioception)	Serum vitamin E/ total lipid ratio
K	Synthesis of prothrombin factors II, VII, IX, and X	Hemorrhage	Prothrombin time

FMN = flavin mononucleotide
FAD = flavin adenine dinucleotide
NAD = nicotinamide adenine dinucleotide
NADP = nicotinamide adenine dinucleotide phosphate

Table 9-3

TRACE METAL DEFICIENCY STATES

Trace Element	*Signs and Symptoms of Deficiency*
Zinc	Anorexia, growth retardation, dermatitis, hypoguesia, alopecia, diarrhea, impaired wound healing, immune suppression, night blindness, hypogonadism
Copper	Microcytic anemia, leukopenia, neutropenia, osteoporosis, neuropathy, testicular failure, hair and skin depigmentation, poor connective tissue
Manganese	Growth retardation, bone deformities, B cell degeneration, transient dermatitis in animals
Chromium	Impaired glucose tolerance, elevated serum lipids, peripheral neuropathy
Iron	Microcytic anemia
Molybdenum	Growth retardation, impaired methionine and uric acid metabolism in animals
Iodine	Thyroid disease (goiter, hypothyroidism, cretinism)
Selenium	Cardiomyopathy, neuropathy, pseudoalbinism, macrocytosis, myositis, cancer, infection
Silicon	Growth retardation, skeletal deformities, and defective connective tissue formation in animals
Fluoride	Caries, osteoporosis
Cobalt	Pernicious anemia
Nickel	Growth retardation and impaired lipid metabolism in animals
Vanadium	Growth depression, impaired reproduction and lipid metabolism in animals

Other Nutrients	*Nutrient Deficiency State*
Choline	Visual and verbal memory abnormalities, hemorrhagic nephritis (animals), growth retardation (animals)
Carnitine	Cardiomyopathy, myopathy
Taurine	Retinal abnormalities, liver disease

Vitamin D is the most common fat-soluble vitamin (ie, vitamins A, D, E, K) deficiency reported in IBD. Fat-soluble vitamin deficiency results from malabsorption secondary to a reduced bile salt pool resulting from terminal ileal disease or resection. The combination of both vitamin D and calcium malabsorption and corticosteroid use can result in significant metabolic bone disease. Corticosteroids cause both decreased intestinal absorption and increased urinary excretion of calcium. Patients at risk should receive 1500 mg of elemental calcium daily. Measurement of bone density using dual-energy x-ray absorptiometry (DEXA) should be performed early after the diagnosis of IBD. Supplementation with 1000 IU of daily vitamin D has been reported to prevent bone loss in patients with Crohn's disease.[5] Sixteen percent of patients with IBD may also have low serum vitamin A and E concentrations.[6] One study reported a consistent relationship between low vitamin A and E concentrations and disease activity.[6]

Iron deficiency is common in both active Crohn's disease and ulcerative colitis. Iron deficiency has been reported in 20% to 40% of IBD patients, usually resulting from blood loss from the gastrointestinal tract. Iron deficiency is more common in patients whose disease is limited to the colon. Low serum ferritin concentration is the most reliable marker of reduced iron stores, although serum ferritin as an acute phase reactant may be elevated in the presence of systemic inflammation. Anemia in IBD, however, is usually the result of the chronic disease rather than iron deficiency. Zinc deficiency may also occur, especially in patients with significant diarrhea and intestinal fistulas. Zinc deficiency has been reported in about 40% of patients with Crohn's disease.[7] A combination of low serum and urinary zinc concentrations is highly suggestive of zinc deficiency. Zinc can be replaced using 220 mg twice daily of oral zinc sulfate. Magnesium and potassium are electrolytes that may need to be replaced, especially in those patients who have had partial small bowel resections or have significant diarrhea. Intramuscular or intravenous replacement is often necessary because oral magnesium supplements can worsen diarrhea.

GENERAL DIETARY MEASURES

For most nonhospitalized patients, the most important advice is for patients to consume a diet liberal in protein, with sufficient calories to maintain weight. Oral intake of 25 to 35 kcal of ideal body weight per day (40 kcal/kg/day for weight gain) and 1.0 to 1.5 grams per kilogram of protein will meet the requirements of most adults who are normally nourished at the beginning. In regard to the specifics of a diet, controlled studies have not shown benefit of low-residue diets except in those patients with intestinal obstruction. There is some, but limited, data to support the use of high-fiber diets to maintain remission in patients with ulcerative colitis.[8] Soluble fiber is metabolized by colonic bacteria to short-chain fatty acids. One of these, butyrate, is the preferred fuel for the colonocyte and may be useful in the healing process.

Lactose intolerance is not a problem in all patients with IBD as lactase is present in the proximal intestine, uncommonly involved with Crohn's disease. Dietary lactose should only be restricted if patients have symptoms associated with dairy intake and in patients in whom lactose intolerance can be demonstrated by breath hydrogen testing; many patients with symptoms of lactose intolerance are not really lactose intolerant.[9] Lactose-containing foods are an excellent source of dietary calcium. Furthermore, there is no consistent epidemiological data supporting the role of milk as a cause of IBD.

A low oxalate diet may be required in those patients who have had their terminal ileum resected or have significant fat malabsorption and still have part of their colon remaining. These patients have a propensity for oxalate kidney stones.

Liquid dietary supplements may help some patients that are otherwise unable to consume sufficient energy. Most supplements are lactose free and well tolerated.

Initial studies with fish oil supplements (n-3 fatty acids) in ulcerative colitis showed decreased disease activity in patients that received these formulas, but randomized trials in Crohn's disease have failed to show consistent results.[10,11] Fish oil may have anti-inflammatory activity because n-3 fatty acids are thought to compete in the substrate pool of the lipoxygenase pathway, thus reducing the production of inflammatory leukotrienes.[12] A study by Belluzzi et al found that 2.7 grams of n-3 fatty acids administered as an enteric-coated fish oil preparation maintained 59% of Crohn's patients in remission after 1 year compared to 26% in the placebo group, p <0.05.[10] Another study by Lorenz-Meyer et al failed to show a difference in remission rates compared to placebo.[11] In each study, large amounts, which are unpalatable for most people, were given. Studies have not shown any benefit of glutamine supplementation in either patients with Crohn's disease or ulcerative colitis.

WHEN IS NUTRITIONAL SUPPORT NECESSARY?

Nutritional support refers to the use of either intravenous (total parenteral nutrition [TPN]) or enteral tube feeding and is usually administered to hospitalized patients. Nutritional support of the hospitalized patient should be instituted promptly when it has been determined from daily calorie counts that a patient is not taking sufficient oral intake of food for 7 or more days. After approximately 7 to 10 days of nil per os (ie, nothing by mouth [npo]), negative nitrogen balance occurs, which increases the risk of infection and interferes with wound healing. Nutritional support may also be considered an adjunctive therapy in malnourished patients in whom sufficient oral intake to promote nutritional repletion is not immediately achievable. For both active Crohn's disease and ulcerative colitis, nutritional therapy therefore has a significant supportive role. The role of nutritional support as *primary therapy* for IBD is limited, as discussed later. The use of preoperative TPN has been suggested to improve surgical outcome and limit bowel resection in Crohn's patients undergoing small bowel resections but not in large bowel resections.[13] Most of the reports are retrospective and uncontrolled. The analysis of the data showed positive changes in nutritional parameters that were not accompanied by reduced postoperative complications. Therefore, it is our opinion, that 7 to 10 days of preoperative TPN in Crohn's disease should be restricted to seriously malnourished patients (SGA "C") who are not candidates for enteral feeding because of bowel obstruction. For patients who are significantly nutritionally depleted, long-term nutritional support may be required in order to improve postoperative morbidity. It should therefore be pointed out that surgery should not be delayed on account of administration of nutritional support in the majority of patients. Delaying surgery often leads to a further decline in the nutritional reserve of a patient. Nutritional support should be continued or started postoperatively if the patient is considered moderately (SGA "B") or severely malnourished (SGA "C") preoperatively. Patients are usually unable to take sufficient oral nutrition for at least 5 days following intestinal resection as a result of postoperative ileus.

PARENTERAL NUTRITION

Once nutritional support is deemed necessary, which route—parenteral or enteral—should be used? Indications for parenteral feeding usually include small bowel obstruction, which may develop in Crohn's disease because of adhesions related to prior surgery, severe edema with luminal compromise during an acute flare, or chronic, fibrotic scar tissue; severe diarrhea and malabsorption during active disease; small bowel ileus; gastrointestinal hemorrhage; treatment for enterocutaneous or enteroenteric fistulae; and supportive care in patients that are severely malnourished (SGA "C") or who have active disease with compromised absorptive surface. TPN may also be indicated in a patient with ulcerative colitis and toxic megacolon in which enteral nutrition is not possible. TPN is not generally indicated in patients that have a nonobstructive gastrointestinal tract or when the duration of nutritional support is expected to be less than 7 days.

It is thought that the gut "atrophies" in the absence of enteral nutrition. While this may be the case in animal studies, the data in humans fail to support this concept. It is commonly thought that in the absence of enteral nutrition, bacteria will translocate across the intestinal epithelium to the mesenteric lymph nodes and into the systemic circulation, resulting in sepsis and multiorgan failure. Although this has been reported in the rat model, it rarely occurs in humans.[14] When bacterial translocation does occur in humans, it is usually in the setting of small bowel obstruction, is unrelated to the route of feeding and is usually clinically inconsequential.[14]

Whether the combination of complete bowel rest and TPN can be used successfully as *primary therapy* in patients with acute IBD with or without the addition of other medical therapy, including diet, is controversial. The consensus of the literature would suggest that patients with Crohn's enteritis might be placed into clinical remission with the combination of bowel rest and parenteral nutrition alone.[15-20] The composite results suggest that npo and TPN for 3 to 6 weeks will achieve a clinical response rate of 64% in patients with acute Crohn's disease.[20] In most studies, however, prednisone was given simultaneously with TPN, which makes it difficult to discern whether the positive effects observed are totally the result of bowel rest and TPN or the combined effects of prednisone and TPN. On the other hand, the consensus of the literature would suggest that patients with Crohn's colitis and idiopathic ulcerative colitis do not respond any better to TPN and bowel rest (with or without prednisone) than patients treated with prednisone and diet.[21-23] Also reported in many of these reports is a 10% risk of complications associated with TPN, including pneumothorax from central catheter placement, catheter sepsis, and various metabolic complications. Therefore, the potential risk of therapy should be considered before administering a therapy with questionable benefit. TPN is generally reserved for supportive therapy to maintain nutritional reserve rather than as primary treatment.

Intestinal fistula is one circumstance is which npo and bowel rest may serve as primary treatment. A 38% fistula closure rate has been reported in Crohn's patients.[24] However, the reported studies lack a non-TPN control group and there generally was no long-term follow-up reported. In our opinion, if closure is not obvious after 3 months, surgery is usually required. For Medicare reimbursement, 3 months or longer of TPN is usually required and distal enteral feeding has to be documented as "not possible." With newer medications, such as infliximab, TPN and bowel rest may serve less of a role in the treatment of fistulas. A randomized study comparing TPN plus bowel rest to infliximab in addition to an oral diet is needed. Octreotide should only be used in patients with high output proximal fistulas. Octreotide is not compatible with TPN; therefore, they should not be mixed. The role of enteral nutrition is discussed in the sections of this chapter that follow.

CHOOSING THE ROUTE FOR PARENTERAL NUTRITION DELIVERY

Once it has been determined parenteral nutrition (PN) is indicated for a particular patient, a route for delivery must be selected. PN can be delivered via a peripheral or central vein. Peripheral PN is generally used when short-term nutritional support is required (eg, <7 to 10 days). The peripheral access can sometimes be used to supply total nutritional needs (30 to 40 kcal/day), especially if a lipid emulsion is used. Lipid emulsions are isotonic. Because of the hypertonicity of the dextrose, thrombophlebitis is a significant risk when concentrations above 10% are used. The amino acid concentration in the TPN solution should also be <3.5% to ensure the solution has <900 mOsm. Heparin (1000 units/L) and hydrocortisone (10 mg/L) will reduce the risk of thrombophlebitis. Central parenteral nutrition (CPN), more typically referred to as TPN, is infused into a large central vein. Large veins such as the superior vena cava (SVC) or the inferior vena cava (IVC) can tolerate a greater solution osmolarity (up to 1800 mOsm, typically 35% dextrose and 5% amino acids). It is important that the catheter tip resides in either the SVC or IVC. Should the tip be located in a smaller vessel, catheter thrombosis could result when the hypertonic TPN solution is infused. Catheter location within the right atrium may increase the risk of cardiac arrhythmia. A catheter useful for TPN may include a percutaneously inserted central catheter (PICC) that is typically inserted via the brachial (although occasionally the antecubital) vein and advanced to the SVC. The risk of a pneumothorax can be avoided with this method and therefore should be the choice of access in the authors' opinion. A triple, double, or single lumen (preferably) catheter inserted into the subclavian, internal jugular, or femoral vein may also be used, provided the catheter tip is located within the SVC or IVC. For longer-term use, it is typical that a single lumen Hickman, Broviac, or Groshong catheter or a subcutaneous infusion port be inserted. Regardless of the catheter type, it is critical that a catheter lumen be reserved for the exclusive use of TPN to minimize infection risk.

WRITING THE TPN PRESCRIPTION: HOW MUCH IS NECESSARY?

A number of studies have investigated energy expenditure and nitrogen excretion in patients with both active and inactive disease.[25] Patients with inactive disease do not differ from normal controls, whereas patients with active disease may require 1.2 to 1.5 times additional calories above resting energy expenditure. Thirty to 40 kcal/kg/day of ideal body weight and 1 to 1.5 grams per kg of ideal body weight of protein is usually sufficient for most adult patients. Most hospitalized patients only require nutritional support for 2 weeks or less.

Ideal body weight (IBW) can be calculated using the following equations: 48 kg + 2.7 x number of inches over 60 inches in height (males) or 45 kg + 2.3 x number of inches over 60 inches in height (females). Caloric measurement using indirect calorimetry is usually not needed. A minimum of 200 g of dextrose is necessary daily to meet the needs of brain metabolism. The carbohydrate used in TPN solutions is dextrose monohydrate, which contains 3.4 kcal/mL.

Intravenous fat emulsion is typically used to supply 20% to 40% of the daily calories. Only 6% of daily calories are needed as lipid emulsion to prevent essential fatty acid deficiency. Fat emulsions supply either 1.1 or 2.0 kcal/mL, depending upon whether a 10% or 20% emulsion is selected. Fluid requirements can usually be met by using 1 mL per kcal or a 1.5 to 2.0 L TPN formula. Patients with cardiac or renal insufficiency may require less, and patients with significant diarrhea or fistula losses may require more.

Depending upon the specific order form used, one can order TPN either in terms of absolute amounts of macromolecules (ie, dextrose, lipid, and protein) or by indicating a total volume and final concentration of these TPN constituents. Electrolytes, minerals, trace elements, and vitamins can be requested using "standard" amounts (ie, multitrace metals and multiple vitamin solutions) unless the addition of a specific nutrient is required to correct or prevent a deficiency or withholding of a specific ingredient is necessary in order to avoid potential toxicity. For example, a 70 kg man that requires 25 kcal/kg/day and 1.0 g/kg/day of protein for maintenance might receive the following formula: 2 liters of 20% dextrose (400 g, providing 1360 kcal) + 200 mL of 20% lipid emulsion (400 kcal) with 3.5% amino acids (700 g). Again, depending upon the formulation capabilities of the hospital pharmacy, the complete solution can be provided as a 3-in-1 emulsion (ie, dextrose, lipid, and amino acids) or as a 2-in-1 solution (ie, dextrose and amino acids) with the lipid emulsion hung in a "piggybacked" fashion. Initially, the TPN rate should be relatively slow (eg, 40 mL/hr) and even slower in the malnourished patient (see refeeding syndrome on p. 155). The rate can be advanced as rapidly as every 8 hrs in a normally nourished individual without diabetes as long as the blood glucose is <160 mg/dL. During continuous central TPN the blood glucose should be determined every 6 hrs.

MONITORING PARENTERAL NUTRITION

Safety

If used inappropriately or not monitored appropriately, TPN will not have any value to the patient and may even become a life-threatening therapy rather than a life-saving one. It is generally recommended to consult the services of a multidisciplinary nutritional support team (NST) in the hospital to assist in writing the TPN prescription, monitoring the therapy, and making adjustments as required. However, it is imperative that the responsible physician understand the importance of appropriate monitoring, especially in the absence of a NST.

Patients should be weighed daily and accurate inputs and outputs should be recorded. If weight gain is planned, anything more than 1 to 2 kg per week indicates fluid retention. This may occur in the first week or two of TPN; decreasing the rate of TPN is usually sufficient, although occasionally diuretic therapy becomes necessary.

In general, electrolytes should be monitored daily the first few days of starting parenteral TPN and then at least twice weekly. Acid base disturbances can often be managed by increasing or decreasing acetate or chloride in the solution. Metabolic acidosis may be caused by diarrhea and can usually be corrected by a slight increase of potassium acetate to the solution. Hypochloremic metabolic alkalosis may result from nasogastric suction in the absence of adequate replacement fluid. Elevated BUN may result because of the provision of insufficient fluid, excessive amino acid infusion, or renal insufficiency.

Mild elevations in the hepatic aminotransferases (ie, alanine aminotransferase [ALT], aspartate aminotransferase [AST]) as well as the alkaline phosphatase are often observed within 2 to 14 days of initiating TPN and should be determined at baseline and subsequently on a weekly basis.[26] These elevations are generally transient. More persistent elevation in ALT and/or AST may result from hepatic steatosis from overfeeding or choline deficiency.[26-28] Persistently elevated alkaline phosphatase may signify the development of biliary sludge, which will occur in virtually 100% of patients on TPN that are npo. It is normal to see a rise in serum bilirubin as a direct result of TPN. A rise in bilirubin is a concern and other causes besides TPN should be evaluated. A low alkaline phosphatase, especially in the Crohn's patient with chronic diarrhea, may be a sign of zinc deficiency.[29]

The serum triglyceride concentration should be monitored twice weekly during the first week and weekly thereafter in order to ascertain adequate clearance of the lipid emulsion. It should be obtained 4 to 6 hours after infusion of the lipid emulsion has been completed. Although there is no clear evidence of the deleterious effects of a serum triglyceride concentration <1000 mg/dL, it is generally recommended to decrease the infusion rate and/or volume of the lipid emulsion if the triglyceride concentration is greater than 400 to 500 mg/dL; a concentration of >1000 mg/dL may be associated with the development of pancreatitis.[30]

The human body adapts to starvation and weight loss by decreasing resting energy expenditure. When massive amounts of carbohydrate are supplied to a malnourished patient in an overzealous attempt to renourish him or her, refeeding syndrome may result.[31] This potentially life-threatening complication of either TPN or enteral nutritional therapy occurs when carbohydrate intake stimulates pancreatic insulin release, which results in the flow of potassium and magnesium to the intercellular space and results in cardiac arrhythmias. In addition, the demand for phosphate to produce adenosine triphosphate (ATP) from the infused carbohydrate may result in hypophosphatemia with subsequent hemolytic anemia, seizures, rhabdomyolysis, and/or respiratory muscle dysfunction. In rare cases, respiratory failure may ensue. Prevention of refeeding syndrome can be prevented by the slow introduction of carbohydrate and the use of proteins (amino acids) and lipids. Small amounts of supplemental potassium phosphate and magnesium may be helpful. Serum potassium, magnesium, and phosphate concentrations should be determined daily or more frequently if necessary until the caloric support goal and a stable electrolyte pattern in the normal range can be achieved.

Infectious complications are also common in TPN-treated patients. There are three types of catheter infections that can occur.[32] The most common is catheter sepsis in which the catheter tip becomes a nidus for bacterial adherence. Bacteria may reach the catheter tip because of catheter contamination from the skin or the catheter hub (used when connecting infusion tubing to the catheter or directly injecting medications). The most common organisms are generally skin flora, including coagulase negative *staphylococci, S. aureus, Klebsiella pneumonia,* and *E. coli.* Such infections can often be treated without the requirement for catheter removal using a 2-week course of systemic antibiotic therapy. Also a highly concentrated solution of vancomycin or amikacin (2 mg/mL) in 2 mL of saline can be instilled into the catheter every 12 hours (antibiotic lock technique).[33] Ten units of heparin may also be mixed in order to avoid clotting. Treatment is for 7 days. Should fungemia be identified, the catheter must be removed. Regardless of whether the catheter is removed because of fungemia or refractory bacterial sepsis (ie, sepsis syndrome or the inability to relieve the febrile response after 48 to 72 hours of antibiotic therapy), the patient should remain completely afebrile and have negative blood cultures prior to insertion of a new central venous catheter.

Infection may develop surrounding the anchoring cuff of a subcutaneous tunneled catheter. This type of infection is rarely associated with fever or leukocytosis but is invariably diagnosed by the presence of purulent drainage from the catheter skin exit site. Often tenderness can be elicited over the catheter cuff. Coagulase negative *staphylococci* and *S. aureus* are the most common organisms involved. Successful treatment of the infection can be achieved with 2 weeks of systemic antibiotic therapy about 50% of the time. If treatment of the catheter *in situ* is ineffective, the catheter should be removed and a new catheter may be placed in a different site without delay in the absence of systemic infection. Systemic antibiotics should, however, be continued for 5 to 7 days following catheter removal.

The subcutaneous catheter tunnel tract may also become infected. Although it is usually difficult to culture an organism, *S. aureus* is most commonly recovered. Because antibiotic penetration of the tunnel is poor, treatment consists of catheter removal in addition to 1 week of appropriate systemic antibiotic therapy. In the absence of systemic evidence of infection, a new catheter can be inserted in a different site without delay. In order to help prevent the risk of infection, it is imperative that those caring for the catheter learn appropriate catheter care technique. Virtually all catheter-related infections relate either to the skin entrance site or the catheter hub. These must be cleaned appropriately before each use with a bactericidal agent such as povidone-iodine or chlorhexidine; ethanol alone is insufficient. In addition, the skin surrounding the catheter should be cleaned appropriately during dressing changes. We recommend the use of small, sterile gauze covering with a semipermeable dressing placed over the gauze to anchor it to the skin. Semi-permeable membranes alone have been associated with increased infection risk in some studies. Dressings should be changed two to three times weekly; more often if the area becomes wet or dirty.

Catheter occlusion can take the form of either thrombotic or nonthrombotic occlusion and is generally manifested in difficulty with TPN or medication infusion. Routine heparin flushes are a useful preventative measure. However, fibrin can still accumulate and block the catheter tip. If used within the first 24 to 48 hours, 2 mg of tissue plasminogen activator (TPA) infused in a 2 mL volume (in order to completely fill the catheter) is often successful in dissolving the thrombosis.[34] Following instillation of the TPA into the catheter, aspiration should be attempted after 30 minutes. It may be necessary to repeat the procedure. In the inpatient setting, the catheter is often simply removed and replaced, although in the outpatient setting, especially in the case of the short bowel patient, every attempt should be made to preserve venous access sites.

Nonthrombotic occlusion may result from calcium-phosphate precipitates or lipid accumulation. Either 0.2 to 0.5 mL of 0.1 N hydrochloric acid or sodium hydroxide may be useful in clearing the obstruction, although occasionally the catheter will require removal and replacement. Care should be made to avoid the addition of too much supplemental calcium and phosphate simultaneously in the TPN solution. Because the solubility of calcium and phosphate in TPN is dependent on a number of factors, knowledgeable pharmacists should always prepare the formula.

Efficacy

There is no gold standard or specific laboratory test to measure the efficacy of nutrition with either TPN or enteral feeding. Weight gain in the hospital during a 1- to 2-week course of nutritional support is usually the result of fluid and not lean body mass. Serum visceral proteins such as prealbumin can be measured and followed during the course of therapy, if desired. The half-life of prealbumin is 2 days, whereas the half-life of albumin at 21 days is too long to be useful in the inpatient setting. It must be recognized that the serum concentrations of all visceral proteins, including prealbumin, may be affected by many non-nutritional factors, including intra- and extravascular fluid shifts in the postoperative patient, or may be depressed because of the protein-losing enteropathy seen in active IBD or because of decreased synthesis as the liver turns toward increased production of acute phase proteins during active disease. Although serum concentration of visceral proteins may guide nutritional therapy, they should be interpreted with the caveats described above. It must also be recognized that normal visceral protein synthesis cannot occur in the absence of sufficient energy intake because skeletal muscle will be catabolized as a fuel source. Serum transferrin will be low in the face of iron-deficient anemia, and as such is often not useful in patients with IBD.

The nitrogen balance can also be determined if one has a laboratory in which to perform accurate measurements. A 24-hour urine collection is required. Total urine nitrogen (TUN) is measured and subtracted from the nitrogen intake from TPN (or enteral nutrition for that matter). An additional 2 grams are subtracted to account for stool, sweat, and other insensible losses. It is assumed that 95% of nitrogen is generally absorbed and that the average amino acid or protein is 16% nitrogen. Therefore, in order to derive the nitrogen intake, the grams of amino acids (or protein in the case of enteral feeding) are divided by 6.25. If the TUN is not readily available, the urine urea nitrogen (UUN) can be measured. If that is the case, 4 grams should be added to the measured nitrogen excretion in order to account for insensible losses and urinary nitrogen losses that are not in the form of urea. Similar to visceral proteins, a positive nitrogen balance requires not only greater nitrogen intake than excretion, but also an energy intake at least equal to energy expenditure. Maintaining a patient in positive nitrogen balance has been associated with better outcome and lower mortality.

HOME PARENTERAL NUTRITION

Patients may require home TPN (HPN) because they have developed short bowel syndrome from multiple bowel resections for Crohn's disease, have chronically draining enteroenteric or enterocutaneous fistulae, or have become severely malnourished in the face of active disease. Such therapy requires assessment of the home environment for appropriateness and safety and proper training of either the patient or a responsible adult, especially in aseptic catheter care.

The patient should be metabolically stable prior to discharge. It is appropriate to cycle the TPN to a 10- to 12-hour nocturnal infusion prior to discharge. Nocturnal infusion gives the patient more freedom during the day to ambulate. Nocturnal infusion may also help prevent TPN associated liver disease and encourage eating during the normal day. During the cycling process, the patient receives his or her prescribed TPN at a gradually increased rate over a progressively shorter period of time. For example, a patient that receives a 3:1 emulsion containing 2 L of 20% dextrose, 3.5% amino acids, and 200 mL of 20% lipid emulsion over 24 hours (91 mL/hr) would have the same total volume infused over 10 hours (220 mL/hr) as a goal. In order to achieve that goal, the infusion time is shortened by 2 to 4 hour increments during each subsequent 24-hour period. For example, the TPN would be infused at 110 mL/hr for 20 hours, then tapered off to over 30 to 60 minutes. A gradual tapering is required in order to prevent hypoglycemia as endogenous insulin secretion increases significantly. This can be done by decreasing the infusion rate by 50% for 15 to 30 minutes and then by another 50% for another 15 to 30 minutes before discontinuing the TPN. Most pumps used in the home environment can be programmed to automatically and gradually decrease the rate to zero over a 30- to 60-minute period. This time period is not included in the overall infusion time calculation.

During cycling of the TPN, the blood glucose should be obtained 2 hours after starting the TPN, just before beginning the taper period (to detect hyperglycemia) and 30 minutes after the TPN has been discontinued (to detect hypoglycemia). The blood glucose should always be obtained from a peripheral vein opposite the side of the infusion in order to minimize the chance of contamination of the sample from residual dextrose, resulting in a falsely elevated concentration, and to avoid contamination of the catheter. If the blood sugar is >180 mg/dL, regular insulin should be administered subcutaneously. The same amount can be added to the TPN solution just prior to beginning the infusion on subsequent nights. Typically, regular insulin is added 1 unit per 10 g of dextrose (eg, 2 L of 20% dextrose would require 20 units per liter or 40 units per bag), if necessary. If post-TPN hypoglycemia is encountered, the patient should be instructed to drink some sugar-fortified juice when the TPN is discontinued, and the taper period should be lengthened. Once the goal infusion rate has been achieved (patients with cardiac or renal disease may not tolerate an infusion over 10 to 12 hours and may require a slower rate), the TPN does not require ramping up on subsequent nights.

It is strongly recommended that the home TPN patient receive his or her TPN through a reputable home care company that has considerable experience in the care of such patients; many home care companies do not have considerable experience, but welcome the care of such a patient anyway because of the financial remuneration. It is also strongly recommended, because of the complexities involved with HPN, that patients requiring this specialized therapy be referred to a center with a physician experienced in the care of such patients. Because the patient at home should be stable, minimal changes in the TPN prescription should be required. If frequent laboratory monitoring and changes in the TPN formulation are necessary, the patient is probably not ready for discharge.

Patients with IBD are the most common group treated with long-term HPN at most centers. Catheter infection is the most common complication associated with HPN use. Catheter infection is no greater in the IBD group compared to other patients receiving HPN. Patients with IBD have a better-estimated 5-year survival rate than other groups of patients treated with HPN.[35]

ENTERAL NUTRITION

In the absence of bowel obstruction, fistula, or toxic megacolon, enteral nutrition is the preferred form of nutritional support provided the patient will consent to having a nasogastric tube placed. Occasionally, patients are too ill and refuse to have a tube placed in their nose. In general, enteral feeding in the patient with IBD will take place via a nasogastric tube. A small bore, 8 to 10 French feeding tube should be used rather than a larger tube used for gastric decompression. Complications (discussed below) are generally fewer with such a tube. The risk of aspiration is not necessarily decreased with postpyloric feeding; hence, such feeding is rarely necessary in this population. However, because of postoperative gastroparesis, jejunal feeding may be preferred in those individuals. Tube placement should be verified radiologically prior to beginning feeding because physical examination, namely auscultatory confirmation, is often inaccurate for determining tube position. In general, feeding is begun at a relatively slow rate (typically 40 mL/hr) and advanced every 8 hours until the goal rate is achieved and if gastric residuals are <200 mL prior to each rate increase. However, if a small bore feeding tube is used or if jejunal feeding is undertaken, it may be difficult to aspirate and to determine an accurate gastric residual volume. In these patients, abdominal pain, distention, and tenderness are used to determine enteral feeding tolerance. The presence or absence of bowel sounds may be helpful but actually indicates nothing more than an air-fluid interface. Feeding can often be undertaken in the absence of bowel sounds. In malnourished patients, the formula infusion rate should be increased more gradually to avoid refeeding syndrome (see previous section). In addition, jejunal feeding in postoperative patients should be started at as little as 10 mL/hr, although this can often be accomplished in the immediate postoperative phase and advanced as tolerated. Most isotonic formulas are 1.0 to 1.5 kcal/mL and include the protein content in this calculation.

The protein content varies among formulas. No formula provides sufficient free water to meet the daily fluid requirement. Therefore, it is important that patients with normal or increased fluid requirements receive at least the equivalent of 25% of the formula's volume as free water. For example, an additional 500 mL of free water should be supplied to the patient that receives 2000 mL of formula daily. This can be provided in two to four divided doses as a bolus. This amount includes water used to flush medications from the tube. Tap water is fine; sterile or distilled water is unnecessary.

The patient's head and shoulders should be elevated to 30 to 45degrees at all times to prevent aspiration. Gastric residuals should also be checked every 4 hours and if less than 200 mL, the aspirated formula should be returned to the tube as a bolus. The tube should be flushed with 30 mL of water after aspiration. Accurate input and outputs should be recorded and the patient should be weighed at least three times weekly.

Occasionally, the nasogastric feeding tube may become clogged despite proper flushing as described. Often this is related to protein precipitates. Sugar-free, decaffeinated soda is often useful for dislodging this type of occlusion. Sometimes, meat tenderizer (ie, papain) is necessary. One teaspoon of nonpotato flake papain meat tenderizer can be mixed in the smallest amount of tap water required to dissolve it and instilled in the catheter. The specific pancreatic enzyme preparations Pancrease (Ortho-McNeil, Raritan, NJ) or Viokase (Axscan Scandipharm, Birmingham, Ala) can be mixed with one crushed 324-mg sodium bicarbonate tablet in 5 mL of tap water and instilled into the feeding tube. It may be necessary to repeat the procedure. Some medications are not compatible with enteral feedings; therefore, compatibility should be determined prior to using the feeding tube for instillation.

Other complications of tube feeding include esophagitis, esophageal and/or gastric erosions or ulceration, or esophageal stricture or mucosal bridge formation. Esophageal or gastric erosions may be evident within a week, although long-term use is generally required before clinically significant disease, including gastrointestinal hemorrhage, may occur. In addition, nasal erosions and nasal cartilage sloughing may result from excessive pressure on the nasal alae and cartilage; therefore, nasogastric feeding should be undertaken via the same nares for a maximum of 4 to 6 weeks.

Regarding which formula to use, a defined formula given either orally or via a feeding tube may have potential benefit as primary treatment in Crohn's patients.[36-39] The composite data suggest that the administration of either an elemental, peptide based, or polymeric diet for 3 to 6 weeks will achieve a remission rate of approximately 68%, which is similar to the remission rate reported with TPN and bowel rest. The reason that patients with active Crohn's disease may respond to polymeric enteral formulas but not an ad-lib regular oral diet is unclear, but it may be related to the lipid composition of the enteral formula. Diets high in long chain triglycerides and polyunsaturated fats may be risk factors for the relapse of Crohn's disease.[40]

REFERENCES

1. Seidman EG. Nutritional management of inflammatory bowel disease. *Gastroenterol Clin North Am.* 1989;18:129-155.

2. Detsky AS, McLaughlin JR, Baker JP, et al. What is subjective global assessment of nutritional status? *Journal of Parenteral and Enteral Nutrition.* 1987;11(1):8-13.

3. Franklin JL, Rosenberg IH. Impaired folic acid absorption in inflammatory bowel disease: effects of salicylazosulfapyridine. *Gastroenterology.* 1973;64:517-525.

4. Behrend C, Jeppesen PB, Mortensen PB. Vitamin B_{12} absorption after ileorectal anastomosis for Crohn's disease: effect of ileal resection and time span after surgery. *Eur J Gastroenterol Hepatol.* 1995;7:397-400.

5. Vogelsang H, Ferenci P, Resch H, et al. Prevention of bone mineral loss in patients with Crohn's disease by long-term oral vitamin D supplementation. *Eur J Gastroenterol Hepatol.* 1995;7:609-614.

6. Bousvaros A, Zurakowski D, Duggan C, et al. Vitamins A and E serum levels in children and young adults with inflammatory bowel disease: effect of disease activity. *J Ped Gastro Nutr.* 1999;26:129-134.

7. Valberg LS, Flanagan PR, Kertesz A, et al. Zinc absorption in inflammatory bowel disease. *Dig Dis Sci.* 1986;31:724-731.

8. Fernandez-Banares F, Hinojosa J, Sanchez-Lombrana JL, et al. Randomized clinical trial of Plantago ovata seeds (dietary fiber) as compared with mesalamine in maintaining remission in ulcerative colitis. *Am J Gastroenterol.* 1999; 94:427-433.

9. Suarez FL, Savaiano DA, Levitt MD. A comparison of symptoms after the consumption of milk or lactose-hydrolyzed milk by people with self-reported severe lactose intolerance. *New Engl J Med.* 1995;333:1-4.

10. Belluzzi A, Brignola C, Campieri M, et al. Effect of enteric coated fish oil preparations on relapses in Crohn's disease. *New Engl J Med.* 1996;334:1557-1560.

11. Lorenz-Meyer H, Nicolay C, Schulz B, et al. Omega 3 fatty acids and low carbohydrate diet for maintenance of remission in Crohn's disease: a randomized controlled multicenter trial. *Scand J Gastroenterol.* 1996;31:778-785.

12. Caughey GE, Mantzioris E, Gibson RA, et al. The effect on human tumor necrosis factor alpha and interleukin 1 beta production of diets enriched in n-3 fatty acids from vegetable oil or fish. *Am J Clin Nutr.* 1996;63:116-122.

13. Lashner BA, Evans AA, Hanauer SB. Preoperative total parenteral nutrition for bowel resection in Crohn's disease. *Dig Dis Sci.* 1989;34:741-746.

14. Sedman PC, MacFie J, Palmer MD, et al. Preoperative total parenteral nutrition is not associated with mucosal atrophy or bacterial translocation in humans. *Br J Surg.* 1995;82:1663-1667.

15. Ostro MJ, Greenberg GR, Jeejeebhoy KN. Total parenteral nutrition and complete bowel rest in the management of Crohn's disease. *Journal of Parenteral and Enteral Nutrition.* 1985;9:280-287.

16. Reilly J, Ryan JA, Stole W, et al. Hyperalimentation in inflammatory bowel disease. *Am J Surg.* 1976;131:192-200.

17. Mullen JL, Hargrove WC, Dudrick SJ, et al. Ten years experience with intravenous hyperalimentation and inflammatory bowel disease. *Ann Surg.* 1978;187:523-529.

18. Greenberg GR, Fleming CR, Jeejeebhoy KN. Controlled trial of bowel rest and nutritional support in the management of Crohn's disease. *Gut.* 1988;29:1309-1315.

19. Lochs SH, Meryn S, Marosi L, et al. Has total bowel rest had a beneficial effect in the treatment of Crohn's disease? *Clin Nutr.* 1983;2:61-64.

20. Greenberg GR. Nutritional management of inflammatory bowel disease. *Semin Gastrointest Dis.* 1993;4:69-86.

21. Dickinson RJ, Ashton MG, Axon AT, et al. Controlled trial of intravenous hyperalimentation and bowel rest as an adjunct to routine therapy of acute colitis. *Gastroenterology.* 1980;79:1199-1204.

22. McIntyre PB, Powell-Tuck J, Wood SR. Controlled trial of bowel rest in the treatment of severe acute colitis. *Gut.* 1986;27:481-485.

23. Sitzmann JV, Converse RL, Bayless TM. Favorable response to parenteral nutrition and medical therapy in Crohn's colitis. *Gastroenterology.* 1990;99:1647-1652.

24. Afonso JJ, Rombeau JL. Nutritional care for patients with Crohn's disease. *Hepatogastroenterology.* 1990;37:32-41.

25. Chan ATH, Fleming CR, O'Fallon WM, et al. Estimated versus measured basal energy requirements in patients with Crohn's disease. *Gastroenterology.* 1986;91:75-78.

26. Buchman AL, Ament ME. Liver disease and total parenteral nutrition. In: Zakim D, Boyer TD, eds. *Textbook of Liver Disease.* 3rd ed. Philadelphia, Pa: WB Saunders; 1996: 1812-1821.

27. Buchman AL. *Handbook of Nutritional Support.* Baltimore, Md: Williams and Wilkins; 1997.

28. Buchman AL, Sohel M, Dubin M, Jenden DJ, Roch M. Choline deficiency causes reversible hepatic abnormalities in patients during parenteral nutrition: proof of a human choline requirement; a placebo-controlled trial. *Journal of Parenteral and Enteral Nutrition.* 2001;25:260-268.

29. Samman S, Soto C, Cooke L, et al. Is erythrocyte alkaline phosphatase activity a marker of serum zinc status in humans? *Biol Trace Elem Res.* 1996;51:285-291.

30. Toskes PP. Hyperlipidemic pancreatitis. *Gastroenterol Clin North Am.* 1990; 19:783-791.

31. Solomon SM, Kirby DF. The refeeding syndrome: a review. *Journal of Parenteral and Enteral Nutrition.* 1990;14:90-97.

32. Buchman AL, Moukarzel A, Goodson B, et al. Catheter-related infections associated with home parenteral nutrition and predictive factors for the need for catheter removal in their treatment. *Journal of Parenteral and Enteral Nutrition.* 1994;18:297-302.

33. Messing B, Peitra-Cohen S, Debure A, et al. Antibiotic-lock technique: a new approach to optimal therapy for catheter-related sepsis in home-parenteral nutrition patients. *Journal of Parenteral and Enteral Nutrition.* 1988;12:185-189.

34. Atkinson JB, Bagnall HA, Gomperts E. Investigational use of tissue plasminogen activator (t-PA) for occluded central venous catheters. *Journal of Parenteral and Enteral Nutrition.* 1990;14:310-311.

35. Scolapio JS, Fleming CR, Kelly DG, et al. Survival of home parenteral nutrition treated patients: 20 year experience at the Mayo Clinic. *Mayo Clinic Proc.* 1999;74:217-222.

36. O'Morain C, Segal AW, Levi AJ, et al. Elemental diet as primary treatment of acute Crohn's disease: a controlled trial. *Br Med J.* 1984;288:1859-1862.

37. Jones VA. Comparison of total parenteral nutrition and elemental diet in induction of remission of Crohn's disease. *Dig Dis Sci.* 1987;32:100-107.

38. Gonzalez-Huix F, de Leon R, Fernandez-Banares F, et al. Polymeric enteral diets as primary treatment of active Crohn's disease: a prospective steroid controlled trial. *Gut.* 1993;34:778-782.

39. Rigaud D, Cosnes J, Le Quintree Y, et al. Controlled trial comparing two types of enteral nutrition in treatment of active Crohn's disease: elemental vs polymeric diet. *Gut.* 1991;32:1492-1497.

40. Miura S, Tsuzuki Y, Hokari R, Ishii H. Modulation of intestinal immune system by dietary fat intake: relevance to Crohn's disease. *J Gastroenterol Hepatol.* 1998;13:1183-1190.

chapter 10

Pregnancy and Fertility With Inflammatory Bowel Disease

Jeffry A. Katz, MD

Inflammatory bowel disease (IBD) often presents before or during child-bearing years, and young women with IBD may become pregnant. Women are naturally concerned about the effects of IBD on fertility, pregnancy, and the fetus. Additionally, patients worry about how pregnancy may affect their disease activity. Major concerns of the gastroenterologist and obstetrician should be the optimal timing of the pregnancy, the potential for symptomatic recurrence of IBD during pregnancy and after delivery, and the safety of and need for treatment during pregnancy.

INHERITANCE

It has been recognized for decades that genetic factors play a role in the pathogenesis of Crohn's disease (CD) and ulcerative colitis (UC), which are, in large part, genetic diseases with complex nonmendelian patterns of inheritance. The most established risk factor for IBD is a positive family history. Many studies have shown a greater risk of CD when a first-degree relative has CD as compared to the familial risk of UC. When the proband has CD, the lifetime risk has been estimated at between 5.2% to 7.8%; when the proband

Table 10-1

GENETIC RISK OF INFLAMMATORY BOWEL DISEASE

	Proband	Risk to First-Degree Relative
Crohn's Disease	Jewish	8%
	Non-Jewish	5%
Ulcerative Colitis	Jewish	4%
	Non-Jewish	1%

has UC, a 1.6% to 4.5% risk has been reported (Table 10-1). These risks appear to be higher among Jews than among non-Jews. Overall, a child of affected parents has a 5% to 10% risk of developing IBD. When both parents have IBD, this risk has been reported to be much higher. The recent discovery of a gene associated with CD makes it likely that we may soon be able to identify persons at high risk of developing CD.

FERTILITY

Some studies have suggested that women with UC have decreased fertility compared to the normal population; however, when adjusted for patient age and desire for children, the fertility rate is normal. In CD fertility appears to be slightly decreased compared to the normal population, although some of this may be voluntary (Table 10-2). Among women with IBD, those whose first pregnancy occurred after disease onset have had fewer pregnancies compared to controls, whereas women whose first pregnancies occurred before the disease onset have the same average number of pregnancies as controls. This suggests that the observed reduced fertility was due in part to the patient's choice and not due to disease-related impairment and that fear of pregnancy may play a role in the reported reduced fertility seen in women with CD. Fertility is also reduced in CD in proportion to the disease activity and can be restored when drug therapy achieves disease remission. Occasionally, the ovaries and the fallopian tubes are affected by the inflammatory process of CD, especially on the right side due to the proximity of the terminal ileum, and this may help explain some reduced fertility in CD. Additionally, CD patients with perianal disease may have secondary dyspareunia and decreased libido contributing to lower fertility rates. Fever, pain, diarrhea, and malnutrition have also been implicated in decreased fertility in IBD.

Table 10-2	
FERTILITY IN PATIENTS WITH **INFLAMMATORY BOWEL DISEASE**	
Patient Population	*Fertility*
Women with ulcerative colitis	Normal
Women with Crohn's disease	Decreased slightly
Men with ulcerative colitis	Normal
Men with Crohn's disease	Normal

Infertility in male patients with IBD caused by sulfasalazine has been well documented. Within 2 months of starting therapy, the density of the patient's semen decreases, abnormal forms of spermatozoa increase, and sperm motility reduces. These events are dose related and do not respond to supplemental folate. Two to 3 months after withdrawal of sulfasalazine, semen quality returns to normal. A male patient whose partner is trying to conceive should be switched to an oral mesalamine preparation. The overall reproductive capacity of men with IBD is not markedly diminished, although male patients with CD have been noted to have small families.

EFFECT OF ULCERATIVE COLITIS ON FETAL OUTCOME

Retrospective studies have suggested no significant impact of UC on pregnancy outcome. Rates of healthy offspring between 76% to 97%, spontaneous abortions of 5% to 13%, stillbirths of 1% to 3%, and congenital abnormalities of 1% to 3% do not differ significantly from those expected in the normal population (Figure 10-1). However, some population-based investigations have shown an increased risk of preterm birth, low birth weight, and small for gestational age. The risk of preterm birth appears to be particularly increased when the first hospitalization for UC occurred during pregnancy. The presence of UC has not influenced the mode of delivery or the incidence of eclampsia or preeclampsia.

EFFECT OF CROHN'S DISEASE ON FETAL OUTCOME

As with UC, retrospective studies suggest that the rates of prematurity, fetal loss, and congenital anomalies in CD approximate the incidence of these findings in the normal population (see Figure 10-1). However, the majority of

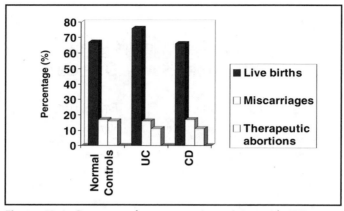

Figure 10-1. Outcome of pregnancy in patients with IBD compared to a normal population (data from Nielsen OH, Andreasson B, Bondesen S, Jarnum S. Pregnancy in ulcerative colitis. *Scand J Gastroenterol.* 1983;18:735-742; Ventura SJ, Mosher WD, Curtin SC, Abma JC, Henshaw S. Trends in pregnancies and pregnancy rates by outcome: estimates for the United States, 1976-96. *National Center for Health Statistics Vital Health Stat.* 2000;21:1-59; and Hudson M, Flett G, Sinclair TS, Brunt PW, Templeton A, Mowat NA. Fertility and pregnancy in inflammatory bowel disease. *Int J Gynaecol Obstet.* 1997;58:229-237).

female IBD patients who experience stillbirths, spontaneous abortions, or children with birth defects have CD. Recent population-based studies from Scandinavia have found children born to mothers with CD have lower birth weights and are small for gestational age. Patients who have ileal disease or have undergone previous surgery may be particularly at risk for these events.

INFLUENCE OF PREGNANCY ON INFLAMMATORY BOWEL DISEASE

The course of UC during pregnancy correlates with disease activity at the time of conception (Figure 10-2A). Among pregnancies occurring in patients with inactive UC, approximately 34% will relapse during gestation and puerperium, similar to the relapse rate in nonpregnant UC patients. Most relapses occur during the first trimester; this may partially be related to patients stopping maintenance medications. Approximately two-thirds of pregnant UC patients will have quiescent disease throughout the pregnancy.

Without drug therapy, active UC at conception is at risk of worsening during pregnancy. In women with active UC at the time of conception, the dis-

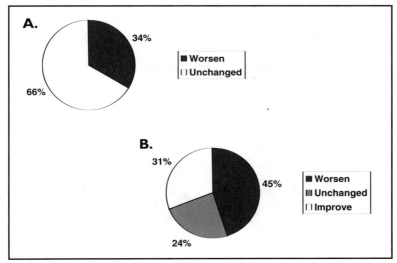

Figure 10-2. The effect of pregnancy on the activity of ulcerative colitis. A. Ulcerative colitis *inactive* at the time of conception. B. Ulcerative colitis *active* at the time of conception.

ease activity worsens in 45%, remains unchanged in 24%, and improves in 31% (Figure 10-2B). Occasionally, pregnancy will induce an improvement in disease activity or clinical remission, usually in the first trimester. Not infrequently, the first presentation of UC will coincide with pregnancy. Additionally, some patients will have symptomatic disease only when pregnant, with quiescence between pregnancies and exacerbations during subsequent pregnancies.

The course of CD during pregnancy is similar to that of UC. Patients with quiescent disease at conception will typically remain in remission, whereas active disease at conception is likely to remain active (Figures 10-3A and 10-3B). Women who have active disease at conception remain active one third of the time and worsen one third of the time. No data exist on the optimal duration of remission before conception that will insure a good outcome for both mother and fetus; however, in general, the longer the remission, the better the outcome.

The clinical course or outcome of previous pregnancies can predict neither the clinical course of IBD nor the outcome of pregnancy. The activity of IBD remains the primary predictor of the course of pregnancy.

ROLE OF THE MODE OF DELIVERY

Retrospective analysis of pregnancy outcomes in IBD has documented a higher rate of cesarean section versus controls, and population studies have

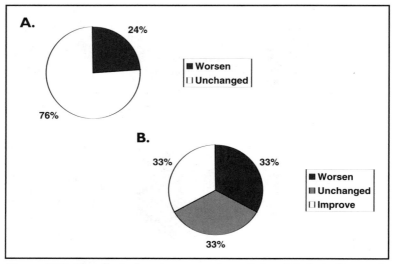

Figure 10-3. The effect of pregnancy on the activity of Crohn's disease. A. Crohn's disease *inactive* at the time of conception. B. Crohn's disease *active* at the time of conception.

confirmed these findings. The explanation for this finding is uncertain, although it may relate to concerns over the potential risk of perineal trauma causing postpartum complications. Although data are limited, in patients with CD and no pre-existing perineal involvement the overall rate of developing perineal disease after vaginal delivery ranges between 5% to 18%, with most studies reporting perianal complications in less than 10% of patients. Few CD patients with inactive perianal disease who have an episiotomy at delivery progress to develop recurrent perineal disease during follow-up. Thus, women with CD and either no perianal disease or inactive perianal disease at term do not require a cesarean section solely because of a concern about the integrity of the perineum. If an episiotomy is needed, a mediolateral episiotomy should be done to avoid trauma to the rectal sphincter.

ASSESSING DISEASE ACTIVITY DURING PREGNANCY

An accurate assessment of disease activity in the pregnant patient is often difficult. Many pregnant women will have intermittent abdominal discomfort related to changes in bowel habits or gastroesophageal reflux. In addition, it is important to remember that abdominal pain in the pregnant IBD patient could be related to cholelithiasis, pancreatitis, toxemia, or a problem with the pregnancy itself, rather than CD. Clinically, these processes can be distinguished from a flare of IBD by careful history, examination, and laboratory evaluation.

During pregnancy a number of changes occur in routine laboratory parameters that are considered physiologically normal and should not be attributed to worsening disease activity. These include a normal 1 g/dL fall in the hemoglobin due to dilution and reduced iron stores, a two to three fold increase in the erythrocyte sedimentation rate, a 1 g/dL fall in the serum albumin, and a 1.5-fold rise in the serum alkaline phosphatase.

Flexible sigmoidoscopy can be used safely during pregnancy to evaluate disease activity. Although colonoscopy has been reported to be safe in pregnancy, its use should probably be restricted to those patients in which the information gained is critical to the patient care. During colonoscopy, close fetal monitoring is indicated.

Both ultrasound and magnetic resonance imaging can be used safely in pregnancy. It is best to avoid exposure of the fetus to radiation from abdominal x-rays, especially early in the pregnancy; however, the absolute risk to the fetus during abdominal radiography is minimal, and clinical necessity should guide decision making.

MEDICAL THERAPY DURING PREGNANCY

Two important questions surround the medical therapy of IBD in the pregnant patient. First, does the outcome of the pregnancy differ among pregnant IBD patients on drug therapy when compared to those not on treatment, and second, are medications used to treat the pregnant IBD patient safe and effective? Although some studies suggest an increase in the frequency of prematurity, spontaneous abortion, and fetal malformations among mothers with IBD undergoing medical treatment, most investigations show that medical therapy, when analyzed as an independent variable, has no effect on pregnancy outcome. As discussed above, it is quite evident that disease activity, not medication, most strongly affects pregnancy outcome, and there is little evidence that drug therapy increases the risk of pregnancy-related complications in the IBD patient.

Most pregnant women are concerned about the risks of drugs to the fetus. Decisions surrounding continued medical therapy during pregnancy might be particularly difficult for the woman with IBD who must balance concerns for the developing fetus against fears of increased disease activity. Although controlled, prospective studies are lacking, much information exists on the safety of medical therapy for IBD during pregnancy, allowing for thorough and thoughtful counseling of the patient and family (Table 10-3).

SYMPTOMATIC THERAPY

There are little data on the use of antidiarrheal and antispasmodic agents during pregnancy. Bulking agents, such as psyllium and methylcellulose, are

Table 10-3

SAFETY OF DRUG THERAPY IN INFLAMMATORY BOWEL DISEASE DURING PREGNANCY

Safe	Probably Safe	Not Safe
Loperamide	Azathioprine	Diphenoxylate
Sulfasalazine	6-mercaptopurine	Methotrexate
Mesalamine	Ciprofloxacin	Thalidomide
Corticosteroids	Metronidazole	
Total parenteral nutrition	Cyclosporine	

safe during pregnancy, as is kaolin and pectin. Codeine has been used for many years during pregnancy without report of associated fetal abnormalities. Drug dependence and withdrawal in the newborn can occur but are rare. Loperamide has been found to be safe in pregnancy, but diphenoxylate with atropine is teratogenic in animals and fetal malformations have been observed in infants exposed to diphenoxylate during the first trimester. Both loperamide and diphenoxylate are excreted in breast milk, and their safety during breast feeding is unknown. Bismuth subsalicylate should also not be used during pregnancy because salicylate absorption can occur and has been associated with prolonged labor, decreased birth weight, and increased perinatal mortality. Anticholinergics and antispasmodics have been associated with nonlife-threatening fetal malformations and are best avoided during pregnancy.

5-AMINOSALICYLIC ACID

Sulfasalazine

Sulfasalazine interferes with normal folate metabolism through competitive inhibition of the enzyme folate conjugase. Folate is critical to normal fetal development and folate supplementation in early pregnancy prevents neural tube defects. Pregnant women are recommended to take 0.4 mg of supplemental folate daily; pregnant IBD patients on sulfasalazine should receive 2 mg of supplemental folate daily.

Both sulfasalazine and sulfapyridine cross the placenta with fetal serum levels equivalent to maternal levels. Although sulfasalazine and sulfapyridine are excreted in breast milk, the levels are lower than in serum, and sulfasalazine is only occasionally detected in the serum of breast fed infants whose mothers were taking the drug. Because sulfa drugs can displace bilirubin bound to albumin, there has been concern that circulating fetal sulfasalazine and sulfapyridine could put newborns at risk for jaundice and kernicterus. However, multiple studies have shown that in the term infant there is no increased incidence of neonatal jaundice or kernicterus associated with the use of sulfasalazine by pregnant women.

Sulfasalazine has been used for the treatment of IBD for over 60 years and has been used safely in many pregnant patients. Although there are occasional case reports of congenital abnormalities in babies born to women who took sulfasalazine during pregnancy, larger studies have proved sulfasalazine to be safe throughout pregnancy.

MESALAMINE

5-aminosalicylic acid (5-ASA) and its metabolite acetyl-5-aminosalicylic acid (Ac-5-ASA) are found in both maternal and fetal plasma in women taking mesalamine, and the concentrations are comparable to those found in women taking equivalent doses of sulfasalazine. Mesalamine and its metabolites are also present at low levels in the breast milk of lactating women. Although these drugs have only been used for little over a decade, information on their safe use during pregnancy is gradually increasing. A single case report exists of an infant exposed to mesalamine between the third and fifth month of gestation who developed renal insufficiency characterized by interstitial fibrosis and tubular atrophy. Most studies, however, suggest that mesalamine is safe during pregnancy.

Recently, a prospective controlled cohort study of 165 women exposed to mesalamine during pregnancy has been conducted; 146 women had first trimester exposure. Pregnancy outcome was compared to a matched control group counseled for nonteratogenic exposure. There was no increase in major malformations for the mesalamine-treated women compared to controls, and no significant differences in rates of live births, miscarriages, pregnancy termination, delivery method, or fetal distress were detected between the two groups. A statistically significant increase in preterm deliveries (13% vs. 5%), decrease in mean maternal weight gain (13 kg vs. 15 kg), and decrease in mean birth weight (3253 g vs. 3461 g) was reported. However, it was the women with active IBD during pregnancy who had significantly lower birth weights babies compared to women with inactive disease. Likewise, women treated with polytherapy had significantly lower birth weight and lower gestational age babies compared to those women on monotherapy. This data again support a significant effect of disease activity on pregnancy outcome rather than an effect of mesalamine.

ANTIBIOTICS

For the treatment of IBD, metronidazole and ciprofloxacin are the most widely used antibiotics. Animal studies have not shown evidence of teratogenicity or increased fetal loss with metronidazole. Although there have been case reports of fetal malformation, particularly cleft lip, with use of metronidazole early in pregnancy, two meta-analyses have found no relationship between metronidazole exposure during pregnancy and birth defects.

In animal studies, no teratogenicity has been observed with ciprofloxacin, although arthropathy has been identified in immature animals. This has led to restricted use of ciprofloxacin during pregnancy, although these problems have not been identified in pregnant women taking ciprofloxacin. However, a higher rate of therapeutic abortions has been observed in quinolone-exposed pregnant women compared to controls (ie, women treated with nonembryotoxic antimicrobials for similar indications). The reasons for this observation are uncertain.

Review of the non-IBD literature suggests it is safe to use short courses of both metronidazole and ciprofloxacin during pregnancy. However, these agents are more commonly used for longer duration in IBD, and there currently exists no direct safety data on prolonged therapeutic use of these agents during pregnancy. Alternative agents, while probably safe, are at least as efficacious as metronidazole and ciprofloxacin with more long-term safety data, and so the use of these two antibiotics during pregnancy should currently be restricted to short courses of treatment.

CORTICOSTEROIDS

Corticosteroids have been used to treat a variety of illnesses during pregnancy. Case series examining corticosteroid therapy in asthma and rheumatoid arthritis have not revealed an increased risk of fetal malformation. However, older animal studies in pregnant mice have shown an increase in cleft palate, and similar concerns have been raised for the human fetus. Corticosteroids cross the placenta and are transferred into breast milk, but the ratio of maternal-to-fetal serum concentration depends upon the corticosteroid used. Prednisolone is more efficiently metabolized compared to dexamethasone, and fetal levels are only approximately 10% of maternal levels. Although there is a concern regarding possible adrenal suppression among the neonates of mothers taking corticosteroids, in practice this has rarely occurred. If steroids must be used during pregnancy, it makes sense to use one more extensively metabolized by the placenta, such as prednisone or prednisolone.

Among patients with IBD, corticosteroid therapy has not been found to be harmful to the fetus. No increased incidence of prematurity, spontaneous abortion, stillbirth, or developmental defects has been reported for pregnant women with IBD treated with corticosteroids. When necessary corticosteroids can be safely used to control active disease during pregnancy.

IMMUNOSUPPRESSANTS

As more and more patients with IBD are treated with immunosuppressant therapy, there is a growing need for information on the effects of these therapies on the pregnant patient and fetus. Unfortunately, little direct study of immunosuppressant use in the pregnant woman with IBD has been performed. However, there is a large volume of literature on the use of azathioprine/6-mercaptopurine (AZA/6-MP), cyclosporine (CsA), and methotrexate

(MTX) among pregnant transplant recipients and patients with autoimmune diseases. This information can be used to help guide the rational and safe use of immunosuppressant therapy for the woman with IBD who is or wishes to become pregnant.

Azathioprine/6-mercaptopurine

AZA/6-MP has been shown to be teratogenic in mice and rabbits but not in rats. These differences among species suggest that variable metabolism may play a role in potential drug toxicity and make extrapolation of animal data to pregnant humans difficult. In addition, genetic variance for AZA/6-MP metabolism may make some people more susceptible than others to adverse drug effects. AZA crosses the placenta, but the fetal liver lacks the enzyme inosinate pyrophosphorylase, which converts AZA to its active metabolite, and, as expected, only trace amounts of its metabolites are detected in fetal serum. Both AZA/6-MP are excreted in low amounts in the breast milk and can have immunosuppressant effects on the fetus.

The available published literature among IBD patients, though limited, suggests that AZA/6-MP is safe and well tolerated during pregnancy. A retrospective analysis of 16 pregnancies among 14 women with IBD being treated with AZA found no increase in spontaneous abortion, fetal abnormalities, prematurity, or low birth weight. Seven women continued AZA throughout the pregnancy; five stopped before week 16 and two had elective termination of pregnancy. One mother did contract hepatitis B infection during pregnancy. All pregnancies went to term, except for the voluntary terminations and an elective cesarean section at 32 weeks gestation. No congenital anomalies or subsequent health problems occurred among 15 children. All neonates weighed 2.5 kg or greater. The authors recommended continuing AZA therapy throughout pregnancy if the drug is considered to play an important part in the control of the disease.

Most of the concern surrounding the use of AZA/6-MP has focused on the pregnant woman; however, concerns have been raised recently regarding the risk of pregnancy related complications when the father is or has taken 6-MP. Retrospective analysis of pregnancy outcome among fathers treated with 6-MP compared to fathers who had never been treated with 6-MP suggests an increased incidence of pregnancy-related complications when fathers used 6-MP within 3 months of conception. Specifically, there were two spontaneous abortions (first trimester) and two congenital anomalies among 13 pregnancies in which the father took 6-MP within 3 months of conception. However, the true impact of this observation is limited by the retrospective nature of the evaluation, the small sample size, the lack of a true normal control group, and the lack of information regarding disease activity in the fathers and comorbid conditions in the mother.

With regard to AZA/6MP, when are they to be used during pregnancy? The days of recommending voluntary termination following any fetal exposure to AZA/6-MP have passed. All IBD couples considering conception should be carefully counseled regarding the limits of our knowledge regarding the safety of these therapies during pregnancy but also reassured that most data support their safe use. Remembering that active disease represents the greatest difficulty to conception and pregnancy for the IBD patient, if AZA/6MP is important to maintaining the health of the mother, then therapy with these drugs should be continued during pregnancy. For a couple who feels strongly that they do not wish to conceive while continuing AZA/6-MP, the drug should be stopped for at least 3 months before proceeding with attempts at conception. It must be emphasized to this group that corticosteroid therapy would likely be recommended should the disease flare during pregnancy. At present there is no information or rationale supporting the initiation of AZA/6-MP in the mother after conception occurs.

Methotrexate

MTX is increasingly used for the therapy of resistant CD. MTX inhibits the enzyme dihydrofolate reductase and interferes with purine biosynthesis. Adequate folic acid is critical to early neural tube development, and supplemental folic acid is recommended for all pregnant women. In a variety of animals, including chickens, rats, and mice, embryonic exposure to MTX has been associated with fetal loss and congenital anomalies, including neural tube and craniofacial defects. In humans, high dose MTX is an abortifacient. Spontaneous abortions as high as 40% have been reported after MTX exposure, as have frequent neural tube defects, such as spina bifida.

It is not surprising, therefore, that MTX is contraindicated before conception and during pregnancy. However, with increasing use among IBD patients, inadvertent pregnancies are bound to occur. What advice should be given to a couple in this situation? Clearly, the risk of fetal loss and congenital malformation is high. Although some congenital abnormalities, such as spina bifida, can be screened for with blood tests and ultrasound, others are undetectable. Weighing against this increased risk is the fact that not all infants will be adversely affected by MTX exposure. In this difficult situation, it is probably best to carefully discuss the issue of pregnancy termination with each couple individually. It is best, however, to avoid this situation through careful counseling and effective contraception prior to initiation of MTX therapy.

Cyclosporine

CsA is useful for the treatment of refractory UC unresponsive to high-dose intravenous corticosteroid therapy. In this role, its safety is of particular interest given the occasional presentation of fulminant UC during pregnancy in which delaying surgery for even just a few weeks to allow fetal maturation may profoundly affect fetal viability. Unlike AZA/6-MP or MTX, CsA does not interfere with cell proliferation and turnover. Rather, it blocks IL-2 signaling in T cells. This may possibly make CsA safer than other immunosuppressants during pregnancy. CsA at 10mg/kg/day showed no fetal toxicity in rats; however, renal tubular damage was noted at higher doses, as is seen in adult humans. It is likely that this effect relates directly to the general nephrotoxicity of CsA rather than any specific effects on the fetus. CsA crosses the placenta, but the concentration of the drug in the newborn falls rapidly within days.

As with AZA/6-MP, most of our knowledge about CsA and pregnancy comes from the transplantation literature. Growth retardation and prematurity have occurred in up to 40% of neonates, and babies have had minor laboratory abnormalities, including thrombocytopenia, leukopenia, hypoglycemia, and low grade disseminated intravascular coagulation. Transplant patients treated with CsA-based immunosuppressive regimens have increased rates of low birth weight and prematurity. Despite these results, pregnant transplant patients treated with CsA have been reported to have lower neonatal complications and congenital malformations than pregnant transplant patients not treated with CsA. Follow-up studies have found no persistent nephrotoxicity among the children of mothers treated with CsA.

There are only case reports and small case series of CsA use during pregnancy in patients with IBD. No congenital abnormalities were observed and no renal toxicity was noted in the neonates, although two of four infants were premature (<37 weeks) and weighed less than 2500 g. These results were deemed favorable when compared to the results of surgery in the pregnant patient with severe colitis. In pregnancy, properly used and monitored CsA is probably as safe as AZA/6-MP. Use of CsA should be considered in cases of severe colitis as a means of avoiding urgent surgery and reaching a gestational age when the fetus can be safely delivered.

TOTAL PARENTERAL AND ENTERAL NUTRITION

Undernutrition during gestation is accompanied by a significant increase in perinatal morbidity and mortality. Given the poor nutrition that often accompanies IBD, it is not at all surprising that both total parenteral (TPN) and enteral supplementation have been used to support the pregnant IBD patient. Pregnant women with IBD have been safely treated with TPN from conception to delivery. Despite concerns about possible fat embolization to the placenta, pregnant patients receiving TPN with intravenous lipids have done well. The infants born to these mothers have been healthy, and examination of the placenta has shown no signs of fat. Elemental diets have also been used safely during pregnancy both as primary therapy for active CD and as a source of supplemental nutrition. Obviously, the nutritional needs of the pregnant IBD patient are quite different from the nonpregnant IBD patient, and close monitoring with a nutritional expert is necessary.

OTHER MEDICAL THERAPIES

Recently, a variety of other therapies have begun to be used to treat IBD. Thalidomide has been found to have a variety of beneficial anti-inflammatory and immunomodulatory effects, including effects on tumor necrosis factor (TNF-a), and has been used to treat refractory CD. Thalidomide, however, is a potent teratogen and should not be given to women of child-bearing age, except after the most careful counseling and strict adherence to contraceptive use.

Infliximab (Centocor, Inc., Malvern, Pa) is a chimeric monoclonal antibody to TNF-a used for the treatment of active CD and fistulizing CD. Although it is not recommended for use during pregnancy, some patients have been exposed to infliximab early in pregnancy without obvious harm; however, more information is clearly needed.

SURGICAL THERAPY DURING PREGNANCY

Planned nonobstetric surgical procedures performed in the second trimester in the pregnant patient without IBD do not carry a significant increase in perinatal mortality. In the pregnant IBD patient, however, elective surgical intervention is uncommon. When the need for surgery is obvious, as in the patient with fulminant colitis, toxic megacolon, or perforation, a decision to proceed with surgery is relatively easy. By contrast, in a pregnant patient with a disease flare who is incompletely responsive to medical therapy, the natural tendency is to push continued medical therapy in the hope that the patient may eventually respond. However, this approach only further increases the risk to both mother and fetus; the greater risk to the fetus is continued maternal illness rather than surgical intervention. Doing what is best for the mother generally ends up being what is best for the fetus.

What operation to perform in the pregnant IBD patient depends on the disease and the specific indication for surgery. A variety of procedures have been performed, including panproctocolectomy, subtotal colectomy with ileostomy, hemicolectomy or segmental colectomy with primary anastomosis or ileostomy, and combined subtotal colectomy and cesarean section. Two general points bear noting: first, primary anastomosis carries a greater risk of postoperative complications and a temporary ileostomy is generally preferred, and second, if the fetus is sufficiently mature, cesarean section along with bowel resection is indicated.

Total proctocolectomy followed by ileal pouch-anal anastomosis (IPAA) is the preferred surgical procedure for UC. In women with an IPAA, fertility and sexual functioning have been maintained and successful pregnancy and delivery have been possible. There is debate about whether women who have had IPAA should be allowed to deliver vaginally or whether a cesarean section should be planned. Studies suggest that women who have had an IPAA tolerate pregnancy well and have a lower complication rate lower than in women who have had an ileostomy. Follow-up of women with an IPAA who delivered vaginally showed no adverse long-term effects on pouch function. Women with IPAA may note increases in stool frequency, incontinence, and pad usage while pregnant; these symptoms improve to baseline after delivery. Obstetric considerations should dictate the type of delivery in patients with an IPAA.

CONCLUSION

Since UC and CD typically present in the second, third, and fourth decades, discussions of fertility and pregnancy should be part of the routine education of the IBD patient. If IBD is inactive at the time of conception and remains inactive during the pregnancy, most patients with IBD can expect to conceive, carry to term, and deliver a healthy baby, similar to the non-IBD population. However, if the disease is active, then conception will be difficult and the risk of fetal loss and premature delivery greatly increased. It is wise to discuss plans for dealing with disease flares during pregnancy before conception occurs. The potential benefits of folate supplementation should be reinforced.

Disease activity during pregnancy will improve in roughly one third of patients, stay the same in one-third, and worsen in the remaining third. Fortunately, clinical experience shows that most medications used to treat IBD can be used safely during pregnancy, and active disease is a far greater risk to the fetus than medical therapy. Symptoms of increasing disease activity should be aggressively evaluated and treated. Sigmoidoscopy, ultrasonography, and magnetic resonance imaging are all safe during pregnancy. Data support the overall safety of sulfasalazine, mesalamine, and corticosteroids throughout pregnancy. Short courses of metronidazole and ciprofloxacin are likely safe but should be avoided if possible. Little direct data suggest a significant risk from AZA/6-MP and cyclosporine therapy before or during pregnancy, but individual case should be discussed in detail with each couple. When IBD does not respond to medical therapy, then surgical intervention may be necessary. Decisions regarding surgery for the pregnant IBD patient are often difficult, but worsening disease in the mother is a greater risk to the fetus than surgery. Surgical procedures should be delayed only if this delay would allow critical maturation of the fetus to occur. Although the pregnant IBD patient requires particularly rigorous care, the basic principles of caring for such patients do not change. A close interaction between the patient, treating gastroenterologist or internist, and obstetrician should allow for a successful pregnancy and healthy infant.

BIBLIOGRAPHY

Alstead EM, Ritchie JK, Lennard-Jones JE, Farthing MJ, Clark ML. Safety of azathioprine in pregnancy in inflammatory bowel disease. *Gastroenterology.* 1990;99:443-446.

Baird DD, Narendranathan M, Sandler RS. Increased risk of preterm birth for women with inflammatory bowel disease. *Gastroenterology.* 1990;99:987-994.

Diav-Citrin O, Park YH, Veerasuntharam G, et al. The safety of mesalamine in human pregnancy: a prospective controlled cohort study. *Gastroenterology.* 1998;114:23-28.

Donnenfield AE, Pastuszak A, Noah JS, Schick B, Rose NC, Koren G. Methotrexate exposure prior to and during pregnancy. *Teratology.* 1994;49:79-81.

Fedorkow DM, Persaud D, Nimrod CA. Inflammatory bowel disease: a controlled study of late pregnancy outcome. *Am J Obstet Gynecol.* 1989;160:998-1001.

Fonager K, Sorensen HT, Olsen J, Dahlerup JF, Rasmussen SN. Pregnancy outcome for women with Crohn's disease: a follow-up study based on linkage between national registries. *Am J Gastroenterol.* 1998;93:2426-2430.

Habel FM, Hui G, Greenberg G. Oral 5-aminosalicylic acid for inflammatory bowel disease in pregnancy: safety and clinical course. *Gastroenterology.* 1993;105:1057-1060.

Hudson M, Flett G, Sinclair TS, Brunt PW, Templeton A, Mowat NA. Fertility and pregnancy in inflammatory bowel disease. *Int J Gynaecol Obstet.* 1997;58:229-237.

Hugot JP, Chamaillard M, Zouali H, et al. Associations of NOD2 leucine-rich repeat variants with susceptibility to Crohn's disease. *Nature.* 2001;411:599-603.

Juhasz ES, Fozard B, Dozois RR, Ilstrup DM, Nelson H. Ileal pouch-anal anastomosis function following childbirth. An extended evaluation. *Dis Colon Rectum.* 1995;38:159-165.

Katz JA, Pore G. Inflammatory bowel disease and pregnancy. *Inflamm Bowel Dis.* 2001;7:146-157.

Kornfeld D, Cnattingius S, Ekbom A. Pregnancy outcomes in women with inflammatory bowel disease—a population-based cohort study. *Am J Obstet Gynecol.* 1997;177:942-946.

Marion JF, Rubin PH, Lichtiger S, Chapman M, Hanauer S, Present DH. Cyclosporine is safe for severe colitis complicating pregnancy [abstract]. *Am J Gastroenterol.* 1996;91:1975.

Miller JP. Inflammatory bowel disease in pregnancy: a review. *J R Soc Med.* 1986;79:221-225.

Moser MA, Okun NB, Mayes DC, Bailey RJ. Crohn's disease, pregnancy, and birth weight. *Am J Gastroenterol.* 2000;95:1021-1026.

Nielsen OH, Andreasson B, Bondesen S, Jarnum S. Pregnancy in ulcerative colitis. *Scand J Gastroenterol.* 1983;18:735-742.

Norgard B, Fonager K, Sorensen HT, Olsen J. Birth outcomes of women with ulcerative colitis: a nationwide Danish cohort study. *Am J Gastroenterol.* 2000;95:3165-3170.

Nugent FW, Rajala M, O'Shea RA, et al. Total parenteral nutrition in pregnancy: conception to delivery. *Journal of Parenteral and Enteral Nutrition.* 1987;11:424-427.

Ogura Y, Bonen DK, Inohara N, et al. A frameshift mutation in NOD2 associated with susceptibility to Crohn's disease. *Nature.* 2001;411:603-606.

Rajapaske RO, Korelitz BI, Zlatanic J, Baiocco PJ, Gleim GW. Outcome of pregnancies when fathers are treated with 6-mercaptopurine for inflammatory bowel disease. *Am J Gastroenterol.* 2000;95:684-688.

Ramsey-Goldman R, Schilling E. Immunosuppressive drug use during pregnancy. *Rheum Clin North Am.* 1997;23:149-167.

Subhani JM, Hamilton MI. Review article: the management of inflammatory bowel disease during pregnancy. *Aliment Pharmacol Ther.* 1998;12:1039-1053.

Ventura SJ, Mosher WD, Curtin SC, Abma JC, Henshaw S. Trends in pregnancies and pregnancy rates by outcome: estimates for the United States, 1976-96. *National Center for Health Statistics Vital Health Stat.* 2000;21:1-59.

Yang H, Rotter J. Genetics of inflammatory bowel disease. In: Targan S, Shanahan F, eds. *Inflammatory Bowel Disease: From Bench to Bedside.* Baltimore, Md: Williams and Wilkins; 1994: 32-64.

chapter 11

Indications for Surgery in Inflammatory Bowel Disease

David Black, MD and Alain Bitton, MD, FRCPC

INTRODUCTION

Surgery in inflammatory bowel disease (IBD) is undertaken when medical therapy has failed or when serious complications occur. For some indications, such as unrelenting hemorrhage, perforation, abdominal abscess, or colorectal cancer the need for surgery is unequivocal. However, for other indications, the decision to undergo surgery is arrived at after careful planning between the patient, gastroenterologist or internist, and surgeon with consideration of the patient's quality of life, the presence of disease- or medication-related complications, and the type of surgery. This chapter provides an overview of the urgent and nonurgent indications for surgery in ulcerative colitis (UC) and Crohn's disease (CD) (Tables 11-1 and 11-2).

Table 11-1

SURGICAL INDICATIONS FOR ULCERATIVE COLITIS

Urgent[a]	*Nonurgent*[b]
Severe/fulminant colitis[c]	Medically refractory disease[d]
Toxic megacolon[c]	Unacceptable medication-related toxicity
Perforation	Dysplasia, DALM, or suspected cancer
Massive hemorrhage	Selected extraintestinal manifestations
Acute colonic obstruction	Growth failure in children
Colon cancer	

DALM = dysplasia-associated lesion or mass
[a]Immediate surgery warranted
[b]Prompt but not immediate surgery warranted
[c]Refractory to medical therapy
[d]Refractory to 5-aminosalicylic acid, corticosteroids, and immunomodulators

Table 11-2

SURGICAL INDICATIONS FOR CROHN'S DISEASE

Urgent[a]	*Nonurgent*[b]
Severe/fulminant colitis	Medically refractory disease[d]
Toxic megacolon[c]	Unacceptable medication-related toxicity
Perforation	Colonic dysplasia or suspected cancer
Massive hemorrhage	Chronic low-grade obstruction
Acute gastrointestinal obstruction	Fistulizing disease (enteric and perianal)[c]
Intra-abdominal abscess[e]	Inflammatory mass with or without obstructive uropathy
Perianal abscess	Selected extraintestinal manifestations
Small bowel or colon cancer	Growth failure in children

[a]Immediate surgery warranted
[b]Prompt but not immediate surgery warranted
[c]Refractory to medical therapy
[d]Refractory to antibiotics, corticosteroids, and immunomodulators
[e]Not amenable to percutaneous drainage

ULCERATIVE COLITIS

CHRONIC ACTIVE DISEASE (STEROID-DEPENDENT OR STEROID-REFRACTORY)

UC is a chronic illness characterized by exacerbations and remissions of disease activity. A subset of patients evolve into a chronically active state that can be characterized based on response to corticosteroid therapy. Patients are said to be *steroid-dependent* if they have achieved satisfactory control of their symptoms but are unable to eliminate corticosteroid use without experiencing recurrent symptoms. Patients are deemed *steroid-refractory* if they remain symptomatic despite maximal doses of corticosteroids. Therapeutic options in both types of patients include surgery or steroid-sparing immunomodulating therapy such as 6-mercaptopurine (6-MP) or azathioprine. The choice of treatment is based on various considerations; all of which must be discussed carefully and decided upon by the patient and physician. These include personal and psychosocial issues, disease-related complications, and corticosteroid-related toxicity. Major corticosteroid side effects, such as osteoporosis, avascular necrosis, diabetes, and myopathy as well as effects on psychological well-being and physical appearance will influence the decision for surgery. Issues relating to surgical outcome must also be considered in the therapeutic equation. Patients should be informed that surgery for UC is curative but should be made aware that the ileal pouch-anal procedure, which preserves continence, may occasionally fail or be complicated by pouchitis. In patients who decide on a trial of 6-MP or azathioprine, optimal dosage and duration of these agents must be ensured prior to considering surgery. Surgical intervention in steroid-dependent cases is semi-elective but is more pressing in steroid-refractory cases given the attendant risks of disease-related complications.

SEVERE COLITIS

It is important to be able to assess the severity of disease in a patient who presents with an exacerbation of UC. Truelove and Witts' criteria have traditionally been used for this purpose (Table 11-3). Severe colitis can be defined as greater than six bloody bowel movements per day with volume depletion, anemia, and hypoalbuminemia. Patients with severe colitis should be evaluated and followed by experienced medical (gastroenterologist or internist) and surgical personnel from the day of admission. Bowel rest, volume repletion, and parenteral corticosteroids are the mainstays of therapy. Clinical response is gauged by daily monitoring of symptoms and physical exam findings as well as the interpretation of laboratory tests and periodic abdominal x-rays. Full colonoscopy is not recommended in patients with severe colitis. However, in the patient with new-onset colitis, a gentle limited sigmoidoscopy with no air insufflation may be helpful to distinguish the type of colitis (ie, pseudomembranous colitis versus UC versus CD). Stool cultures may rule out infectious

---

Table 11-3

CRITERIA FOR DISEASE ACTIVITY
IN ULCERATIVE COLITIS

	Mild	*Moderate*	*Severe*
Number of bowel movements/day	<4 Minimal blood	4 to 6 Bloody	>6 Bloody
Fever (°F)	None	±	>99.5°
Heart rate (beats/min)	<90	>90 but <100	>100
Hemoglobin (g/dL)	12 to 14	10 to 12	<10
Sedimentation rate (mm/hour)	<10	>10 but <30	>30
Albumin (g/dL)*	>3.5	3.0 to 3.5	<3.0

*Albumin was not part of Truelove and Witts' initial criteria.

Data from Truelove SC, Witts LJ. Cortisone in ulcerative colitis. *Br Med J*. 1955;2:1041-1048.

---

colitides. Several investigators have attempted to identify clinical, laboratory, or endoscopic parameters that predict a poor response to medical treatment. Low serum albumin (<3.0 g/dL), persistently elevated C-reactive protein, and extensive ulceration at colonoscopy early in the hospitalization have been reported as predictors of a surgical outcome in severe UC. Likewise, the presence of increased small bowel gas may be a sign of impending toxic megacolon. These predictors can help guide clinicians during the first few days of admission but are not a substitute for good clinical judgement.

For patients with severe colitis who do not respond to a 7- to 10-day course of parenteral corticosteroids, therapeutic options include surgery or cyclosporine A (CsA) (Figure 11-1). CsA should be reserved for patients without systemic toxicity. Patients should be apprised of the risks and benefits of each therapy (Table 11-4). The patient who has had long-standing UC, multiple exacerbations, and been on prolonged medical therapy may opt for a surgical intervention. The young patient with new-onset severe UC, who may not be psychologically prepared for colectomy, may be more suitable for CsA treatment.

FULMINANT COLITIS AND TOXIC MEGACOLON

Fulminant colitis is defined as severe colitis with indications of systemic toxicity, such as fever, leukocytosis (elevated bands), tachycardia, orthostasis,

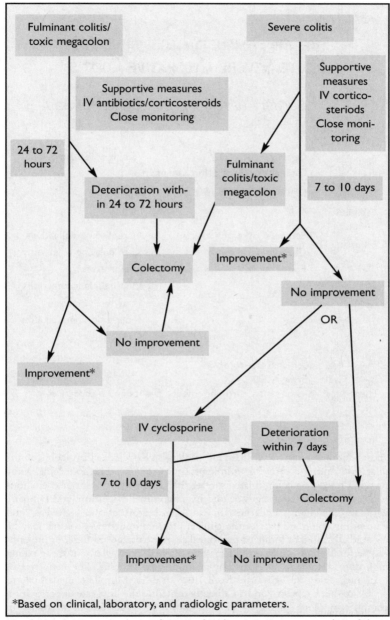

Figure 11-1. Management and surgical indications in severe colitis, fulminant colitis, and toxic megacolon.

Table 11-4

SURGERY VERSUS CYCLOSPORINE A IN
ACUTE SEVERE ULCERATIVE COLITIS

	Surgery (IPAA)	*Cyclosporine A*
Benefits		
	Curative	Avoids colectomy
	Eliminates risk of colon cancer	
	Avoids permanent ileostomy	
Risks		
	Standard risks of surgery	Increased complications
	Chronic pouchitis	from delaying colectomy[*]
	Pouch failure	Nephrotoxicity
		Opportunistic infections
		Long-term immuno-suppression needed after CsA

IPAA = Ileal pouch-anal anastomosis
CsA = Cyclosporine A
[*]Theoretical risks of sepsis, thromboembolic events, and perforation

---

and abdominal tenderness. Toxic megacolon is characterized by acute colonic dilatation during a severe or fulminant attack of UC. The abdominal x-ray reveals a transverse colon dilated greater than 6 cm with absent or edematous haustral folds. Systemic signs of toxicity, abdominal distension, and tympany with accompanying tenderness in the distribution of the transverse and descending colon are part of the clinical presentation. Bowel sounds may be reduced. Diffused or localized peritoneal signs are present in frank or impending perforation of the colon but may be masked, particularly in those taking high dose steroids or in elderly or malnourished patients. The incidence of toxic megacolon in UC ranges from 1.6% to 22%. Mortality rates of 0% to 45% have been reported and are directly related to the high rate of perforation complicating this condition. The significant improvement in mortality in more recent series is attributable to the earlier recognition of the condition and the vigorous medical and surgical treatment offered to these patients.

Patients presenting with fulminant colitis or toxic megacolon should be managed intensively. Diligent monitoring of vital signs, physical examination findings, laboratory tests, and daily abdominal series is the rule. Supportive measures include peripheral parenteral nutrition, correction of hypovolemia and electrolyte abnormalities, and blood transfusions as needed. Precipitants of megacolon should be avoided and include anticholinergic drugs, opiates, hypokalemia, and full colonoscopy or barium enema. Medical therapy includes parenteral corticosteroids and broad-spectrum antibiotics. In the patient with toxic megacolon and small bowel ileus, placement of a nasogastric tube and adoption of a prone or "knee-elbow" position will enhance the evacuation of gas from the gastrointestinal tract. A 24- to 72-hour trial of medical treatment is often undertaken with the proviso that the patient will undergo urgent colectomy if signs of deterioration develop (see Figure 11-1). About half of the patients presenting with toxic megacolon respond to aggressive medical treatment. Patients who progress to fulminant colitis or toxic megacolon during an admission for severe UC should undergo urgent colectomy.

PERFORATION

Colonic perforation in UC is uncommon. Its occurrence is often a function of the extent and severity of the colitis and does not require the presence of colonic dilatation. A free perforation entails spillage of intestinal contents into the general peritoneal cavity with resulting diffuse peritonitis. A sealed perforation is contained by an adherent mass of omentum and adjacent structures causing localized peritonitis. Abrupt changes in the patient's condition should raise concerns that a perforation has occurred. The clinician should watch for fever, tachycardia, sudden increase in abdominal pain and distension, a precipitous drop in the frequency of bowel movements, loss of the hepatic dullness on percussion, and peritoneal signs. Malnourished patients on high-dose corticosteroids may initially be lacking signs of peritonitis. Patients who deteriorate and do not have overt peritoneal signs should have an abdominal x-ray and a computerized tomography (CT) scan to assess for free air or an inflammatory mass, suggesting a sealed perforation. Perforation is associated with a high mortality rate and is an absolute indication for urgent surgery.

MASSIVE HEMORRHAGE

Massive, incessant hemorrhage requiring emergent surgery occurs rarely in UC patients. It is important that clinicians recognize the point at which further medical and supportive therapy is futile and when surgery is required. The principles used for the diagnosis and management of acute lower gastrointestinal bleeding of any cause should be applied. Hemodynamic stability should be ensured. Supportive therapy includes blood transfusions and correction of coagulation abnormalities in addition to the standard medical treatment for UC. If the origin of bleeding is unclear, an upper endoscopy can rule out a gastroduodenal source. In certain clinical settings, such as the elderly UC patient with no overt signs of active colitis, other causes of massive lower gastrointestinal bleeding should be considered (eg, angiodysplasia, diverticula, ischemic colitis, or carcinoma). In general, the requirement of 6 to 8 units of packed red blood cells over 24 to 48 hours is an indication for urgent surgical intervention. Because bleeding is usually the result of diffuse mucosal ulceration, it is not amenable to angiographic or endoscopic therapy. Subtotal colectomy is the procedure of choice, leaving the rectal remnant for future ileal pouch-anal anastomosis. One must be aware, however, that the rectal remnant itself may be the source of ongoing bleeding.

OBSTRUCTION

Colonic obstruction in UC is rare and usually occurs in the setting of a colorectal stricture. Stricture formation results from submucosal fibrosis and hypertrophy. Although most strictures are benign, a high index of suspicion for malignancy must be maintained. Factors favoring malignancy in a stricture include location in the proximal colon, development in the face of long-standing UC, and the presence of obstructive symptoms. Acute or low-grade obstruction resulting from a stricture is an indication for surgery. Strictures should be biopsied, but results that are negative for neoplasia do not rule out malignancy and may provide a false sense of security. It is prudent to recommend surgery in all patients with long-standing UC diagnosed with a colorectal stricture, even if asymptomatic, because of the possibility that there may be an underlying malignancy.

DYSPLASIA AND COLORECTAL CARCINOMA

The risk of colon cancer in UC depends on the extent and duration of the disease. Greater than average risk of colon cancer begins after 7 to 8 years of extensive colitis and increases yearly thereafter. Dysplasia is a neoplastic transformation of the colonic epithelium without extension into the lamina propria. Dysplasia is categorized as negative, indefinite, low grade, and high grade. The finding of dysplasia on colonoscopic biopsies poses a therapeutic challenge (Figure 11-2). Prior to any decision to perform colectomy histologic specimens must be reviewed by at least two pathologists to confirm the diagnosis of dysplasia and exclude reactive inflammatory atypia.

High-grade dysplasia (HGD) is a marker for synchronous colorectal cancer and is therefore an indication for surgery. Low-grade dysplasia (LGD) has been associated with concurrent cancer or progression to HGD or cancer. In patients with LGD, clinicians should consider either colectomy or close colonoscopic surveillance with repeat biopsies in 3 months. The decision to perform colectomy may be more compelling in the patient with long-standing UC who continues to have multiple flares and is on prolonged medical therapy. In patients who understand the risk of foregoing colectomy and choose rigorous colonoscopic monitoring, the persistence of LGD during surveillance is an indication for surgery. Patients who have mucosal biopsies showing indefinite dysplasia should undergo close periodic endoscopic monitoring.

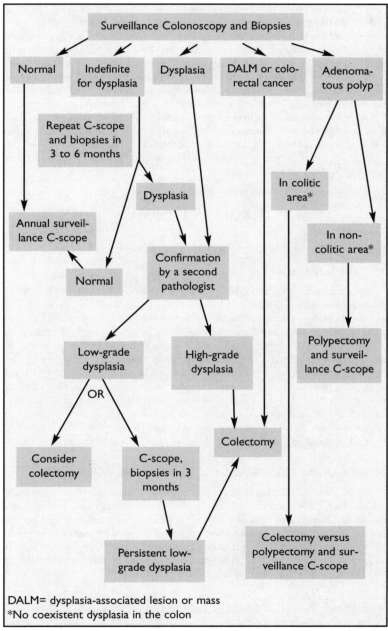

Figure 11-2. Dysplasia and colon cancer in ulcerative colitis. Indication for surgery based on findings at surveillance colonoscopy.

The management of colonic polyps in UC is still not precisely defined. Pedunculated or sessile colonic polyps proximal to areas of colitis with no associated dysplasia elsewhere in the colon can be treated like sporadic adenomas with endoscopic polypectomy and follow-up. Management of patients with diminutive, sessile, or pedunculated polyps in areas of colitis that resemble sporadic adenomas is somewhat controversial. A diminutive polyp may represent raised dysplastic epithelium and warrant colectomy; however, in the absence of concurrent dysplasia elsewhere in the colon, complete removal of such polyps followed by vigorous surveillance may be suitable. The finding of raised, irregular, and broad-based mucosa that harbors dysplasia (ie, dysplasia associated lesion or mass [DALM]) is an absolute indication for surgery because of the high incidence of coexistent carcinoma. The diagnosis of colorectal cancer, of course, mandates prompt surgery.

CROHN'S DISEASE

CHRONIC ACTIVE DISEASE (STEROID-DEPENDENT OR STEROID-REFRACTORY)

Approximately 20% to 30% of patients with CD can become either steroid-dependent or steroid-refractory. Decision-making regarding surgery in chronic active disease differs from that of UC for two reasons: first, surgery in CD is not curative and second, certain operations, such as a permanent ileostomy or extensive bowel resection, may have a significant effect on a patient's quality of life, psychosocial functioning, and nutritional status. Consequently, if the patient is not acutely ill, there may be an attempt to avoid or delay surgery until all medical therapies have been explored. Patients who are steroid-dependent or steroid-refractory may opt for immunomodulator therapy, such as methotrexate, 6-MP (or azathioprine), or infliximab (chimeric monoclonal antibody to tumor necrosis factor) to induce and maintain a symptom-free remission. Patients resistant to or intolerant of these agents will invariably require surgery.

SEVERE COLITIS, FULMINANT COLITIS, AND TOXIC MEGACOLON

Severe colitis, fulminant colitis, and toxic megacolon can complicate colonic CD. Toxic megacolon is less common in CD than UC, and its presence is not required to cause a perforation. Although the etiology and pathogenesis of toxic megacolon may differ between these two diseases, similar management principles and surgical indications apply to both (see Figure 11-1). If surgery is required, the ileal pouch-anal anastomosis is not recommended in CD because of the high rate of subsequent pouch failure.

OBSTRUCTION

Obstruction in CD is secondary to inflammation, fibrotic strictures, adhesions, or carcinoma and can occur at any site in the gastrointestinal tract.

Gastroduodenal CD

Gastroduodenal involvement occurs in less than 4% of patients with CD and is usually associated with concurrent intestinal disease. Symptoms may mimic peptic ulcer disease. Patients may describe worsening postprandial epigastric pain, nausea and vomiting, and significant weight loss. Rarely, hematemesis or melena may occur. Patients may also present more acutely with symptoms of frank gastroduodenal obstruction. Medical therapy is initiated in this situation with bowel rest, total parenteral nutrition, nasogastric suctioning, fluid repletion, and parenteral corticosteroids. Upper endoscopy and biopsies should be performed to exclude malignancy. Endoscopic balloon dilatation of the gastroduodenal stricture may be beneficial. Failure of medical therapy mandates surgery.

Small Bowel CD

The small bowel is the most common site of obstruction in CD. Patients with acute obstruction present with abdominal pain and distention, nausea and vomiting, and obstipation. Abdominal x-rays show distended loops of small bowel with air-fluid levels. CT scan may at times identify the site and cause of small bowel occlusion. Small bowel obstruction occurs secondary to fibrotic strictures with superimposed spasm, edema, and inflammation. Most episodes of obstruction are partial and respond well to nasogastric suctioning and parenteral corticosteroids. Food boluses that become acutely impacted in a stenosed area or small bowel adhesions can also cause obstruction. These usually respond well to conservative measures. Patients with acute obstruction who do not improve with medical therapy as gauged by radiologic imaging, persistent symptoms, and inability to progress their diet should be referred for surgery. Other indications for surgery include recurrent bouts of acute bowel obstruction and multiple small bowel strictures resulting in chronic low-grade obstruction, bacterial overgrowth, and malnutrition. In the latter situation, strictureplasty, which is a bowel-conserving measure, is the surgical treatment of choice.

Colonic CD

Surgery for obstructive colonic CD is not as common as it is for intractable inflammatory disease. Obstruction is usually secondary to a colorectal stricture that may be benign or neoplastic. Such strictures in CD are probably less likely to harbor malignancy than in UC. Patients presenting acutely with a high-grade colonic obstruction should be surgically treated. Low-grade obstructive symptoms should prompt clinicians to consider surgery, both to alleviate symptoms and to rule out underlying cancer. At times a short stricture may be amenable to endoscopic balloon dilatation. Strictures arising in long-standing CD are associated with a higher risk of malignancy. A stricture that cannot be adequately traversed and biopsied for surveillance, particularly in long-standing CD, should be managed with surgery.

MASSIVE HEMORRHAGE

Massive lower gastrointestinal hemorrhage in CD occurs in less than 2% of patients and is more frequent with colonic or ileocolonic disease. The management guidelines outlined for massive hemorrhage in UC should be followed. Lower gastrointestinal bleeding spontaneously stops in 50% of patients, but the rate of rebleeding is high. Unrelenting hemorrhage is an urgent indication for resection of the involved bowel segment. Rarely, gastroduodenal CD presents with massive upper gastrointestinal bleeding, requiring surgery.

PERFORATION

Intestinal perforation is an uncommon complication of CD. Free intestinal perforation may occur spontaneously or secondary to a ruptured abscess in the peritoneal cavity. Patients present acutely with signs of systemic toxicity and generalized peritonitis. The presentation may be less acute in elderly individuals or those on corticosteroids. Immediate surgery is warranted. A bowel microperforation with localized peritonitis can also occur and may be managed with parenteral antibiotics with or without surgical resection, depending on the patient's course. The individual who presents with an appendicitis-like problem deserves particular mention. Such patients often undergo laparotomy at which time ileitis, not appendicitis, is discovered. In the absence of a perforation ileal resection is not recommended for two reasons: an adequate course of medical treatment for CD has not yet been attempted or the ileitis may be due to a self-limited infection such as *Yersinia*. If the cecum is normal, appendectomy should be performed so that future symptomatic episodes will not be attributed to appendicitis. If the cecum is involved, the appendix should not be removed because of the increased risk of postoperative enterocutaneous fistula.

ENTEROENTERIC, ENTEROVESICAL, AND ENTEROCUTANEOUS FISTULAS

Enteroenteric fistulas occur between a diseased segment of bowel and adjacent involved or uninvolved bowel. Ileocecal, ileo-right colon, and ileosigmoid are the most common types of fistulas and rarely cause significant symptoms. Fistulas can also occur between the colon and stomach or duodenum. Fistulas originating from the small bowel can be visualized with a small bowel series or enteroclysis. Large bowel fistulas can be identified by barium enema or colonoscopy. Cologastric or coloduodenal fistulas can be detected by upper gastrointestinal barium studies or upper endoscopy. Abdominal CT scanning is also useful in diagnosing fistulas. Enteroenteric fistulas as such are not an indication for surgery unless they are symptomatic. Medical therapy with antibiotics or immunomodulators, including the purine analogues, cyclosporine, or infliximab, may be beneficial. Indications for surgery include significant diarrhea resulting from the fistula bypassing a long segment of bowel (eg, cologastric or coloduodenal fistula) or complicated internal fistulas with concomitant sepsis and obstruction not manageable by medical therapy alone medical therapy (Table 11-5).

Enterovesical fistula occur in less than 10% of patients with CD. The most common intestinal site of origin is the ileum. Presenting symptoms include

Table 11-5

INDICATIONS FOR SURGERY IN FISTULIZING CROHN'S DISEASE

Type of Fistula	Surgical Indications
Perianal	Simple low-lying fistula[a]
	Complex fistula[b]
Enteroenteric	High output fistula
	Complex fistulas with sepsis and obstruction
Enterocutaneous[b]	High output fistula
	Difficulty in maintaining hygiene[c]
Enterovesical	Repeated urosepsis
Ano- or rectovaginal[b]	Difficulty in maintaining hygiene[c]

[a]Refractory to antibiotics
[b]Refractory to antibiotics and immunomodulators
[c]At times, disabling and distressing for the patient

pneumaturia, fecaluria, and urinary tract infection. A trial of medical therapy can be initiated in patients with minimal symptoms. Repeated episodes of urinary sepsis are an indication for surgery.

Enterocutaneous fistulas originate from a diseased intestinal segment fistulizing through the skin, usually at the site of a surgical scar or at the opening of a percutaneously or spontaneously drained abscess. An initial trial of medical therapy may be offered. Surgery is warranted in patients who fail medical treatment, develop copious fistula drainage, or who encounter great difficulty in maintaining hygiene.

INTRA-ABDOMINAL ABSCESS AND INFLAMMATORY MASS

Patients with intra-abdominal abscesses may present with increasing abdominal pain, fever, leukocytosis, and a palpable abdominal mass. An ileopsoas abscess may be characterized by right-sided flank, hip, or thigh pain with a positive psoas sign. Abscess drainage and antibiotics followed by medical or surgical treatment of the underlying bowel disease are the mainstays of therapy. Percutaneous drainage under CT scan guidance may be a successful, albeit temporary, measure prior to surgery.

Inflammatory masses most commonly complicate ileal or ileocolonic CD. An abdominal CT scan should be performed to rule out a frank abscess, although interloop or small abscesses may escape detection. In the absence of an abscess, medical treatment is undertaken. Failure to respond to medical therapy mandates surgery. Ureteral obstruction with hydronephrosis can complicate an inflammatory mass and is often an indication for surgery.

DYSPLASIA AND SMALL AND LARGE BOWEL CANCER

CD is associated with an increased risk of small and large bowel carcinoma. The low incidence of carcinoma and the difficulty of thoroughly surveying the small intestine make it difficult to establish surveillance programs for small bowel cancer. Extensive colonic CD is associated with an increased risk of colon cancer that may approach that of UC. High-grade dysplasia can be found in areas adjacent to or distant from a CD cancer. Dysplasia in CD appears to have similar significance as in UC as an indicator of concurrent cancer so that endoscopic surveillance programs are recommended. There are no firm recommendations regarding surgical indications when dysplasia is detected in CD, although following the guidelines for UC seems reasonable. The type of surgery (ie, segmental colectomy versus total colectomy) also remains controversial and will depend on various factors, such as extent of colonic involvement, presence of coexistent dysplasia, and concerns of the patient.

PERIANAL DISEASE

Anal Fissure

Symptomatic anal fissures in CD often respond to measures such as normalization of bowel movements, local hygiene, topical steroids, and metronidazole. Fissures that remain painful may require surgery. An exam under general anesthesia is indicated to rule out an occult abscess. Treatment with a limited internal sphincterotomy can be successful without inducing damage to the anal sphincter mechanism.

Fistula

Perianal fistulas are more common with colonic and ileocolonic CD than with disease limited to the small bowel. Fistulas can precede intestinal symptoms by years. Symptoms secondary to fistulas include anal pain, painful defecation, and purulent discharge from the perianal opening. Perianal fistulas can be classified as simple or complex according to anatomic extent and relation to the anal sphincter.

The initial treatment of choice for a fistula is antibiotic therapy. Concomitant rectal CD should be treated with appropriate systemic or topical medical therapy. Patients who remain symptomatic despite optimal antibiotic therapy are candidates for immunomodulators or surgery. In the case of a simple low-lying fistula a surgical approach with fistulotomy is the preferred option. Fistulotomy for this indication is highly successful with a low recurrence rate and preservation of fecal continence. In addition, it avoids long-term immunosuppression. Complex fistulas (multiple or high) resistant to antibiotics can be treated with immunomodulators including 6-MP (or azathioprine), cyclosporine A, or infliximab. Immunomodulators may also be beneficial for coexistent intestinal disease that is chronically active. Complex fistulas often will not respond to medical therapy alone and will need surgery. Probing under general anesthesia to define the anatomy of these fistulas is necessary. Biopsy and curettage of refractory fistulous tracts should be considered to rule out the remote possibility of anal cancer. Rarely, patients with intractable perianal fistulas or sepsis and severe rectal disease will require proctocolectomy with ileostomy.

Anovaginal or rectovaginal fistulas occur in <10% of females with perianal CD. In general, these fistulas are difficult to treat—medically or surgically. Patients may present with dyspareunia, incontinence of air and/or foul smelling discharge from the vagina, and recurrent yeast infections. The inability to maintain hygiene may be very disabling for the patient. Asymptomatic patients do not require treatment. Medical therapy similar to that for perianal disease may be tried in symptomatic cases. Recalcitrant symptoms that are distressing to the patient warrant surgery. The type and the success of surgery will depend on the presence or absence of disease in the rectum.

Perianal Abscess

A perianal abscess is a surgical emergency requiring immediate drainage in order to avoid consequent sepsis. Perianal abscesses can occur in up to 50% of patients with perianal CD. Clinical presentation often includes severe anal pain with a tender, erythematous or fluctuant area on perianal exam with or without systemic symptoms of fever and malaise. Patients may occasionally present with painful defecation and no overt signs on physical exam. In this situation, a digital rectal exam and radiologic imaging, such as pelvic CT, pelvic MRI, or endoanal ultrasound, are helpful in making a diagnosis.

OTHER INDICATIONS FOR SURGERY IN IBD

EXTRAINTESTINAL MANIFESTATIONS

Extraintestinal manifestations are rarely the sole indication for surgery in IBD. Patients can be considered for surgery at times when symptoms are incapacitating and refractory to medical therapy. Peripheral arthritis, pyoderma gangrenosum, and uveitis are most often associated with colonic disease and tend to respond the most to colectomy. CsA and more recently infliximab should be considered in refractory cases of pyoderma gangrenosum prior to the decision to perform surgery. Proctocolectomy does not stop or change the course of primary sclerosing cholangitis, ankylosing spondylitis, or sacroiliitis—all of which follow a course independent from the intestinal disease. Rarely, hypercoagulable states associated with IBD may not be controlled with measures such as anticoagulation, venous filters, and avoidance of prothrombotic factors (eg, dehydration, immobilization, sepsis, smoking, and estrogens). Life-saving colectomy has been reported in this situation. Autoimmune hemolytic anemia is also rare and may be life threatening. Cases that do not respond to medical treatment may be cured by colectomy with concomitant splenectomy.

ILEAL POUCH-ANAL ANASTOMOSIS

The ileal pouch-anal anastomosis (IPAA) is the procedure of choice in patients who have undergone colectomy for UC. It avoids the need for a permanent ileostomy while preserving fecal continence. The pouch will have to be excised and replaced with a permanent abdominal ileostomy in approximately 5% to 12% of patients. Indications for pouch removal include debilitating fecal incontinence, unremitting chronic pouchitis, pouch-vaginal fistula in women, complex perineal-pouch fistulas, and pelvic sepsis. These situations should raise the possibility of previously unsuspected CD. Rarely, cancer may arise in the pouch mucosa and require pouch removal.

GROWTH FAILURE IN CHILDREN

Growth in children is most accurately reflected by height velocity. Growth failure is defined as height velocity in the third percentile or lower. Fifteen percent to 30% of children with CD and 5% to 10% of those with UC meet this definition. Delayed puberty frequently accompanies delayed skeletal maturation, both of which can have serious psychosocial effects on children and their parents. With an appropriately-timed intervention, patients can experience a compensatory increase in growth and achieve their maximal growth potential.

Growth failure is thought to be a result of three main factors: malnutrition, inflammation, and the growth hormone-blunting effects of corticosteroids. The latter two factors may be addressed by surgery, which serves to eliminate foci of inflammation in the bowel and obviates the need for corticosteroids for variable periods of time. Indications for surgery include failure of medical therapy to induce remission, steroid-dependence, and the inability to adhere to medical treatment. The timing of surgery is critical. Surgery performed prior to the adolescent growth spurt is more likely to have the greatest benefit. Children in early stages of puberty (Tanner stages 1 to 3) show significantly increased height velocities after surgery. However, for patients in stages 4 and 5, the benefits are marginal (Table 11-6).

Children with CD should have the extent of their disease well defined prior to surgery, as resection of all involved areas carries the best prognosis. In widespread disease, surgery is not always feasible and patients are better served with nutritional therapy with or without limited resection.

CONCLUSION

Surgery in IBD is reserved for medically refractory disease or to treat complications inherent to the disease. It is important for the clinician to recognize the potentially life-threatening complications that require immediate surgery

Table 11-6

HEIGHT VELOCITY BEFORE AND AFTER
INTESTINAL RESECTION FOR CD IN 42 CHILDREN

Stages	Male		Female	
	HV Before Resection (cm/yr)	HV After Resection (cm/yr)	HV Before Resection (cm/yr)	HV After Resection (cm/yr)
Pubertal stage 1 (n = 18)	1.85	7.40	1.64	9.08
Pubertal stage 2 and 3 (n = 14)	2.81	8.20	2.23	7.14
Pubertal stage 4 and 5 (n = 10)	3.32	4.50	2.87	3.09

*Mean annual HV; children grouped according to pubertal stage
HV=height velocity
Adapted from Walker-Smith JA. Management of growth failure in Crohn's disease. *Arch Dis Child.* 1996;75:351-354.

versus those that could be addressed on a more elective basis. For nonurgent indications, the decision for surgery will depend on a host of factors, including personal issues and the type of surgery involved. Surgery in UC is curative, and the IPAA most often precludes the need for a permanent ileostomy. In CD, the benefits of surgery must be weighed against the tendency for CD to recur and the risk of adverse effects of surgery on psychosocial functioning and nutrition. A therapeutic strategy incorporating both medical and surgical therapy must be clearly delineated for each IBD patient. Whether urgent or nonurgent, the decision to proceed to surgery should result from the close collaboration between the patient, gastroenterologist or internist, and surgeon.

BIBLIOGRAPHY

Becker JM. Surgical therapy for ulcerative colitis and Crohn's disease. *Gastroenterol Clin North Am.* 1999;28:371-390.

Bitton A, Belliveau P. Perianal complications of Crohn's disease. *Uptodate.* 1999;7:3.

Bitton A, Peppercorn MA. Emergencies in inflammatory bowel disease. *Crit Care Clin.* 1995;11:513-529.

Blomberg B, Jarnerot G. Clinical evaluation and management of acute severe colitis. *Inflamm Bowel Dis.* 2000;6:21-27.

Glotzer DJ. Surgical therapy for Crohn's disease. *Gastroenterol Clin North Am.* 1995;24:577-596.

Gumaste V, Sachar DB, Greenstein AJ. Benign and malignant colorectal strictures in ulcerative colitis. *Gut.* 1992;33:938-941.

Jewell DP, Caprilli R, Mortensen N, et al. Indications and timing of surgery for severe ulcerative colitis. *Gastroenterol Int.* 1991;4:161-164.

Kornbluth A, Sachar DB. Ulcerative colitis practice guidelines in adults. *Am J Gastroenterol.* 1997;92:204-211.

Lewis JD, Deren JL, Lichtenstein GR. Cancer risk in patients with inflammatory bowel disease. *Gastroenterol Clin North Am.* 1999;28,459-477.

Lichtenstein GR. Treatment of fistulizing Crohn's disease. *Gastroenterology.* 2000;119:1132-1147.

Lichtiger S, Present DH, Kornbluth A, et al. Cyclosporine in severe ulcerative colitis refractory to steroid therapy. *N Engl J Med.* 1994;330:1841-1845.

McClane SJ, Rombeau JL. Anorectal Crohn's disease. *Surg Clin North Am.* 2001;81:169-183.

Present DH. Toxic megacolon. *Med Clin North Am.* 1993;77:1129-1148.

Steinhart AS, Mcleod RS. Clinical review: medical and surgical management in perianal Crohn's disease. *Inflamm Bowel Dis.* 1996;2:200-210.

Walker-Smith JA. Management of growth failure in Crohn's disease. *Arch Dis Child.* 1996;75:351-354.

Yamazaki Y, Ribiero MD, Sachar DB, Aufses AH Jr, Greenstein AJ. Malignant colorectal strictures in Crohn's disease. *Am J Gastroenterol.* 1991;86:882-885.

chapter 12

Surgical Therapy for Inflammatory Bowel Disease

Lisa Poritz, MD and Walter A. Koltun, MD

ULCERATIVE COLITIS

Chronic ulcerative colitis (CUC) is an idiopathic inflammatory disease that affects only the mucosa of the colon and rectum. The cause is unknown, and the only cure is the surgical removal of the entire colon and rectum. Indications for surgery include complications of CUC, such as toxic megacolon or perforation, failure of medical management, development of cancer or prophylaxis for an increased risk of cancer, intolerance to or complications from medications, and patient preference.

CUC starts in the rectum, and the disease moves proximally to the cecum usually without skip lesions. How far the disease proximally extends varies from patient to patient. Surgery for CUC should remove the entire colon and rectum regardless of how far the disease proximally extends. Procedures that remove only part of the colon, such as partial colectomy, are inappropriate, as the disease will recur in the remaining colon.

There are four surgical procedures for the treatment of CUC that will be discussed in this part of the chapter: total proctocolectomy with permanent ileostomy (TPC), total proctocolectomy with Kock pouch (KP), total abdominal proctocolectomy with ileal pouch-anal anastomosis (IPAA), and subtotal

Figure 12-1. Total proctocolectomy and ileostomy.

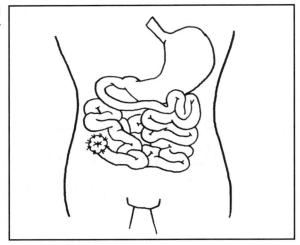

colectomy with ileorectal anastomosis (IR). All of the procedures except for the subtotal colectomy with IR involve the removal of the entire colon and rectum with cure of consequential CUC.

TOTAL PROCTOCOLECTOMY WITH PERMANENT ILEOSTOMY

Total proctocolectomy with permanent ileostomy (TPC) is the gold standard for CUC to which all other operations are compared. The entire colon, rectum, and anus are removed, and a permanent ileostomy is formed from the terminal ileum. This procedure is generally done in the older age group because they are more likely to have difficulties with the number of bowel movements and incontinence after IPAA. This is also the appropriate procedure for a patient who has had a sphincter injury in the past or already has problems with fecal incontinence, as they are likely to worsen after IPAA or IRA.

Technical Aspects (Figures 12-1 and 12-2)

The entire colon is mobilized and the terminal ileum is transected at the ileocecal junction to preserve as much small bowel as possible. The blood supply to the colon is then sequentially divided. Rectal dissection is then completed as low in the pelvis as possible. Dissection is carried out close to the rectum to prevent injury to the sympathetic and parasympathetic nerves. Final dissection of the anus is carried out from the perineal approach using an intersphincteric dissection. The remaining soft tissues in the perineum are then closed after the colon and rectum are removed. The ileostomy is then created from the terminal ileum in a previously marked position. It is important to

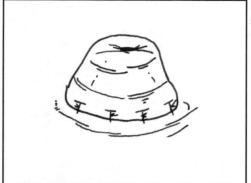

Figure 12-2. Brooke ileostomy.

place the ileostomy well so that the patient does not have problems maintaining it and keeping an ostomy appliance on the site. The ileostomy should be created in a Brooked manner so that it forms a spout to help keep the caustic enteric contents off of the skin.

Advantages

The main advantage of TPC is that it removes all of the colonic and rectal mucosa; therefore, the risk of subsequent development of cancer is essentially nonexistent.

Disadvantages

The main disadvantage to a TPC is that it results in the formation of a permanent ileostomy because the anus and anal sphincter muscles are removed. This type of ileostomy requires a stoma appliance at all times because the effluent from the stoma is liquid and there is no sphincter mechanism to control the flow.

Early Complications

Commonly seen complications in the immediate postoperative period include wound infection (of either the abdominal wound or the perineal wound), urinary tract infection, and bowel obstruction. Infected wounds should be opened and packed. Antibiotics are only necessary if there is cellulitis associated with the wound or if the patient is immunosuppressed. Most bowel obstructions in the immediate postoperative period will resolve with bowel rest and nasogastric decompression. They are often due to edema in the bowel wall and partial kinking of the small intestine.

Less commonly seen complications include bladder dysfunction, sexual dysfunction, enterocutaneous fistula development, wound dehiscence, ureteral injury, and necrosis of the ileostomy. Bladder and sexual dysfunction can develop when the nerves are disturbed during rectal dissection. The sympathetic nerves run near the sacrum and are responsible for ejaculation. Injury to those nerves can result in retrograde ejaculation. The parasympathetic nerves which arise from the second through fourth sacral root deliver impulses through the nervi erigentes. The nervi erigentes run deeper in the pelvis and lateral to the rectum near the seminal vesicles and lateral ligaments. They are responsible for erection, and injury can result in impotence. Dissection in the proper planes near the rectum should avoid injury to these nerves. The incidence of sexual dysfunction should be only 2% to 3% with the majority of difficulties occurring in older men who may already have some degree of underlying bladder and sexual dysfunction. Bladder dysfunction after a TPC is rare and usually results in a flaccid bladder and sometimes overflow incontinence. This usually resolves with time with either an indwelling Foley or intermittent catheterization. The incidence of both these complications also rises significantly if there is also an associated rectal cancer, necessitating a wider dissection to include all the draining lymph nodes and putting the nerves at greater risk.

Both the right and left ureters are subject to injury during dissection during TPC; however, the left is more vulnerable than the right, especially during sigmoid mobilization. Injuries that are recognized at the time of the initial procedure should be immediately repaired and can usually be done primarily. Unfortunately, most ureteral injuries are not recognized at the time of surgery and require more extensive reconstruction at a later date.

Enterocutaneous fistula development is a rare but potentially catastrophic complication. The cause, site, and size of the fistula help determine whether or not the fistula will close nonoperatively. Initial treatment includes fluid resuscitation, correction of sepsis, and control of the effluent. If these goals can be accomplished, then nonoperative treatment is often employed. If the fistula fails to close after several months, surgery is then undertaken.

Wound dehiscence (ie, separation of the fascia so that the intestine is exposed) is also a rare complication but can be seen, especially if fascial healing is compromised by longstanding steroid use. Repair of this requires an immediate return to the operating room for reclosure of the fascia.

Necrosis of the ileostomy is also a rare complication. It can occur from compromise of the blood supply during thinning of the mesentery to help make the small bowel reach the abdominal wall. Necrotic stomas must be resected and revised with a laparotomy. Mucosal ischemia usually do not require revision, and congestion due to edema or obstruction to venous outflow in the mesentery due to a "tight" ileostomy will usually resolve and should not be confused with full thickness necrosis.

Late Complications

Complications other than an abdominal wall hernia after the immediate postoperative period usually involve either the ileostomy or the perineal wound. Complications from an ileostomy include hernia, prolapse, retraction, stenosis, bleeding and pouching problems. Most ileostomy problems can be repaired with a local procedure at the site of the ileostomy. Large peristomal hernias, however, usually require moving the ileostomy to a new site.

Another, more unusual complication is the development of a perineal hernia. This occurs rarely and less commonly than after an APR because in the TPC the sphincter muscles are left in place and they help support the pelvic floor. If a perineal hernia does occur, surgical correction is required.

An unhealed perineal wound or a persistent perineal sinus can occur in up to 10% to 15% of patients who undergo TPC for CUC. They tend to occur more frequently in the older population. Initial treatment includes multiple trips to the operating room for debridement and curettage of the wound. If this fails to heal the wound, then various muscle grafts/flaps can be used to cover the defect.

Long-Term Results and Follow-Up

Long-term results are good with a normal life expectancy and a zero risk of developing colon and rectal cancer. Follow-up past the immediate postoperative period is usually on an as needed basis.

TOTAL PROCTOCOLECTOMY WITH KOCK POUCH

Although the TPC is the gold standard operation for CUC, both curing the disease and preventing the development of colorectal cancer, many patients are reluctant to undergo the surgery because of the requirement for a permanent ileostomy. In 1969 Niles G. Kock[1] developed a method of making the ileostomy continent so that the flow of the effluent could be controlled and that the patient would not have to wear a stoma appliance. A reservoir of small intestine is made from the terminal ileum to store the enteric contents, and a nipple valve is constructed to prevent spontaneous leakage of the fluid from the reservoir. The pouch is emptied by intubation through a small stoma with a special catheter several times a day. A bandage is worn over the stoma, and a stoma appliance is not necessary. The concept is a novel one, but unfortunately the nipple valve is difficult to create and not very durable. Up to 50% of patients require further surgery for problems with their Kock pouch, almost all of them related to the nipple valve. Many of these patients ultimately end up with a permanent ileostomy. Because of this and the availability of an IPAA, few people undergo this operation today. It is usually reserved for patients who have already undergone a TPC but now desire a continent ileostomy and patients who have been denied an IPAA because of fecal incontinence.

Technical Aspects (Figure 12-3)

The colon, rectum, and anus are removed as in the TPC (as discussed). The pouch is created from the terminal ileum by folding it over into an S shape and suturing the folds in place. The most distal 18 to 20 cm of terminal ileum is used to create the nipple valve by intussuscepting it on itself. The valve is then sutured flush to the skin through a small aperture in the abdominal wall so that the pouch can be emptied. This nipple valve prevents the enteric contents from leaking out of the pouch. The catheter is left in the pouch for several weeks to facilitate drainage and also to allow the pouch and valve to heal. After this period the patient then empties the pouch four to six times a day with a special

Figure 12-3. Kock pouch.

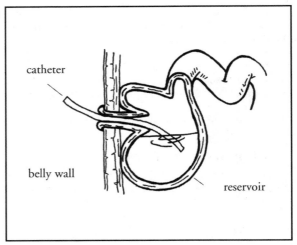

catheter. The stoma site is small and flush to the skin so it can be covered with a bandage.

Advantages

The main advantage to this procedure is that in addition to removing all of the colonic and rectal mucosa, thereby eliminating the possibility of cancer development the patient has a continent ileostomy and does not have to wear a stoma appliance.

Disadvantages

The main disadvantage is the lack of durability of the nipple valve. Approximately 50% of patients will require further surgery for problems with the nipple valve, including slippage of the valve, which causes leakage and pouch intubation difficulty, and stenosis of the valve, which also makes intubation of the pouch difficult.

Early Complications

Early complications include all those listed under TPC except necrosis of the ileostomy. Additionally, because the Kock pouch is hand sewn and there is not a diverting stoma, the risk of leakage from one of the suture lines is a real and serious complication that requires operative revision.

Ischemia of the nipple valve is also a potential early complication analogous to necrosis of the ileostomy. In order to form the intussusception, the mesentery to the nipple valve is often stripped of its fat and injury to the vasculature can occur during this process leading to ischemia.

Late Complications

The majority of late complications of this procedure involve the pouch and the nipple valve. Perineal hernia and an unhealed perineal wound can also occur as seen in TPC.

When the nipple valve slips or reduces itself this leads to both incontinence and difficulty in intubating the pouch. Incontinence results because a properly functioning valve is necessary to keep the liquid contents of the pouch from leaking. The patient also has difficulty intubating the pouch because the slipped valve often takes on an acute angle, leading to obstruction and incomplete emptying of the pouch. Surgical revision is often required in this situation. Many of the pouches are not salvageable, and conversion to a permanent Brooke ileostomy is required.

Pouchitis is characterized by abdominal pain, fever, diarrhea, and bleeding from the pouch. It occurs in 7% to 43% of patients with a continent ileostomy. The specific etiology is unknown, but it is thought to occur from overgrowth of anaerobic organisms due to stasis in the pouch. It usually responds to oral Flagyl with resolution of symptoms. Recurrence is common.

Long-Term Results and Follow-Up

Up to 50% of patients require further surgery and revision of their Kock pouch, almost always for problems with the nipple valve. A significant portion of these patients will eventually have a permanent ileostomy. Those patients who are unhappy with their conventional ileostomy and successfully undergo conversion to a Kock pouch have an improved quality of life. Follow-up after the immediate postoperative period is usually on an as needed basis.

ILEAL POUCH-ANAL ANASTOMOSIS

Because of the difficulties with construction of the nipple valve and frequent requirement for revision, Parks and Nicholls[2] placed the ileal pouch in the pelvis and used the anal sphincter mechanism as the valve to maintain continence. The procedure has many names, including restorative proctocolectomy; J, S, or W pouch; and pelvic pouch, but is most commonly referred to as an IPAA. In this operation the entire colon and rectum are removed and a pouch is fashioned out of the terminal ileum, placed into the pelvis, and attached to the anal canal. This operation is extensive and can be done in one, two, or three stages, depending on the patient's health and the surgeon's experience. IPAA cures the patient of CUC, decreases the risk of colorectal cancer to near zero, and allows patients to defecate through their anus. Because there is no colon to absorb the water, the stool has a pasty consistency. The average patient defecates four to seven times per day and has good continence. Some patients will get up one to two times per night for a bowel movement and a few will have nighttime soiling. The urgency that the patients had with their CUC is gone, and they can often defer a bowel movement for 30 minutes after they feel the urge to defecate. This is the operation of choice for most patients with CUC today.

Figure 12-4. Ileal pouch-anal anastomosis.

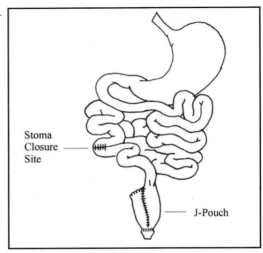

Technical Aspects (Figure 12-4)

The entire colon is mobilized, and the terminal ileum is transected at the ileocecal junction to preserve as much small bowel as possible. The blood supply to the colon is then sequentially divided. Rectal dissection is then completed to the top of the anal canal. Dissection is carried out close to the rectum to prevent injury to the sympathetic and parasympathetic nerves. The rectum is then transected at the anorectal junction. The distal 30 cm of the terminal ileum is then made into a pouch. The most common configuration for this pouch is a J shape. The distal 30 cm is folded and the apex of the fold is opened. Endomechanical staples are then used to create the pouch. The anastomosis is then created between the apex of the pouch and the top of the anal canal with either sutures or endomechanical staples. If the pouch is hand sewn, a mucosectomy is usually included to remove any remaining rectal or columnar epithelium. A mucosectomy is not performed with a stapled anastomosis. A diverting loop ileostomy is then usually created proximal to the pouch to allow the sutures or staple lines to heal. The ileostomy is closed 2 to 3 months later after a Gastrografin enema has ensured proper healing of the pouch.

The sickest patients usually undergo the operation in three stages. The first stage is a total abdominal colectomy with an end ileostomy. The rectum is left in place. The removal of the colon allows the patient to become and feel well again, to be weaned off of steroids (and recover from some of the effects of chronic steroids), and to regain a healthy weight and nutritional status. The second stage of the operation is performed 6 months later. This stage consists of removal of the remaining rectum and construction of the pouch with a diverting loop ileostomy. The ileostomy is then closed 2 to 3 months later after the pouch has healed.

Healthier patients usually have the operation in two stages. The entire colon and rectum are removed at the first stage and the ileal pouch is constructed with a diverting loop ileostomy. After radiographic demonstration that the pouch has healed, the loop ileostomy can be closed 2 to 3 months later. The majority of patients have the operation done this way.

Some surgeons will perform the entire operation at one time (ie, removing the entire colon and rectum and then constructing the ileal pouch without a loop ileostomy). This is only done in the healthiest of patients who are not on steroids. The benefit of doing the operation in one stage is still debated. Although these patients only undergo one operation, the complication rate is slightly higher and the length of stay in the hospital is longer.

After closure of the loop ileostomy, patients usually have multiple loose bowel movements often numbering about 10 a day. As the pouch adapts it will absorb more water, the stool will become thicker, and the number of bowel movements should decrease. Dietary manipulations such as the addition of bananas, peanut butter, rice, and fiber supplements will also help to thicken the stool. Antimotility agents are often added to the regimen to slow the stool transit time and decrease the number of bowel movements. Over the ensuing months, the number of bowel movements should decrease to a stable number—somewhere between four to seven per day.

Advantages

The main advantages of this operation compared to the others is that the pouch is internal in the pelvis and patients defecate through their anus. In addition, all but about 1% of the colonic and rectal mucosa is removed, nearly eliminating the risk of subsequent cancer development.

Disadvantages

The main disadvantage to an IPAA is that construction usually requires two or more surgical procedures.

Early Complications

Early complications are similar to those for TPC and the Kock pouch. Intestinal obstruction is one of the most frequent complications of this procedure and occurs in 15% to 22% of patients, with half requiring subsequent surgery. Anastomotic leak rate is approximately 10%; however, most patients are protected with a covering loop ileostomy so small leaks usually heal without sequelae.

Late Complications

These complications tend to occur after the ileostomy has been closed and include pouchitis, fecal incontinence, anal stricture and pouch anal or pouch vaginal fistulae. Pouchitis is characterized by abdominal pain, fever, diarrhea, and bleeding from the pouch. It is the most common late complication of IPAA and occurs in 18% to 51% of patients. The specific etiology is unknown but it is thought to occur from overgrowth of anaerobic organisms due to stasis in the pouch. It usually responds to oral Flagyl with resolution of symptoms. Recurrence is common.

Long-Term Results and Follow-Up

The success rate of IPAA is 90% to 95%. Approximately 5% of patients will need to have their pouches removed and converted to a permanent ileostomy. Another 1% to 5% of patients will retain their pouch but the function will not be perfect. Eighty percent of patients will have perfect fecal control and the remainder will have occasional nighttime soiling. Within 6 months of surgery, the majority of patients will be have five to seven bowel movements a day.

Patients are followed closely in the immediate postoperative period and then on a yearly basis to inspect the remaining rectal mucosa for signs of dysplasia.

TOTAL COLECTOMY WITH ILEORECTAL ANASTOMOSIS

This is the fourth and least used option for the surgical management of CUC. Very few patients will develop CUC with rectal sparing, and in these patients it is sometimes appropriate to manage them with colectomy and ileorectal anastomosis. This procedure can also be used if the diagnosis of CUC versus Crohn's disease (CD) is in doubt. If performed for CUC of the colon, the patient has the risk of later development of CUC in the rectal remnant and, more seriously, the development of cancer in the remaining rectum. The advantage of this procedure for the few patients for which it is appropriate is that there is no dissection in the pelvis; therefore, the possible complications of alteration of bladder and sexual function are avoided. The risks of this procedure in the development of CUC and cancer in the remaining rectum often outweigh the benefits of avoiding the rectal dissection, and the procedure should be only rarely used in specific cases.

Technical Aspects (Figure 12-5)

The entire colon is mobilized and the terminal ileum is transected at the ileocecal junction to preserve as much small bowel as possible. The blood supply to the colon is then sequentially divided. The colon is then transected at the top of the rectum, and an anastomosis is performed between the terminal ileum and the proximal rectum. The anastomosis can either be hand sewn or fashioned with endomechanical staples.

Advantages

The main advantage to the procedure is the avoidance of rectal dissection and subsequent risk (although small) to bladder and sexual function. Also by leaving the rectum in place the patient retains a natural reservoir for fecal, material decreasing the number of bowel movements per day compared with IPAA and lowering the risk of fecal incontinence or nighttime soiling.

Disadvantages

The obvious disadvantage is that the rectum is left in place and it can subsequently develop CUC or cancer. Twenty-nine percent to 55% of patients require subsequent proctectomy for either intractable symptoms or for neoplasia.

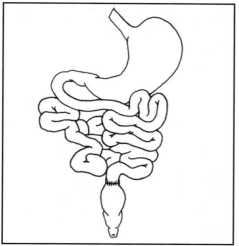

Figure 12-5. Sub-total colectomy/ileorectal anastomosis.

Early Complications

Early complications are similar to those of TPC, although bladder and sexual dysfunction should not be seen nor is there an ileostomy.

Anastomotic leak is the most feared complication with this procedure but should occur less than 5% of the time. Leak usually requires surgical revision, often with a diverting loop ileostomy.

Late Complications

Late complications are the development of cancer of the rectum and progression of the CUC to involve the rectum.

Long-Term Results and Follow-Up

Long-term results for about one-half the patients are excellent with a manageable number of bowel movements. They do, however, require frequent endoscopic evaluation of the rectum to watch for recurrence of the disease and development of cancer. Unfortunately, about half of the patients that undergo this operation will need subsequent proctectomy with either IPAA or permanent ileostomy for progression of CUC to involve the rectum or development of cancer in the rectum. The success of this operation depends on careful selection of patients.

SUMMARY

CUC patients can be weaned off of steroids while other inflammatory bowel medications, such as 5-ASA products, can be stopped after surgery. They generally feel better and can resume a less restricted diet and lifestyle. Although patients with IPAA may still have frequent bowel movements (five to seven per day), they no longer have urgency and the restrictions imposed by needing to be near a toilet are gone. Many patients feel that they have their life back.

CROHN'S DISEASE

There are some common principles of surgical management of any patient with Crohn's disease. The first is to operate on the complications of CD (such as fistula, obstruction, or hemorrhage) rather than the disease itself, since it is not surgically curable. Having said that, overall, approximately 25% to 30% of CD patients after resection will have negligible recurrence of their disease, acting as if they have been cured, thus definitive resection is still a goal at the time of surgery. Second, only the bowel that needs to be removed based on gross inspection should be resected, accepting microscopic involvement of surgical margins. Preservation of bowel length to avoid short gut syndrome should also be a priority, since recurrence and repeat resection are common. Nearly all incisions should be midline so as to not interfere with possible future stoma siting. Incidental appendectomy should be performed to remove appendicitis from the differential in future bouts of abdominal pain. Finally, in the critically ill patient with sepsis, malnutrition, and immune suppression, resection of the site of sepsis with the placement of a diversionary stoma is the safest choice with reconstitution of the digestive tract preserved for a second operation.

Crohn's disease can affect the colon, ileocolonic area, small bowel, and perineal area and surgery of each region will be discussed in turn.

COLONIC DISEASE

Operations for Crohn's disease of the colon are generally of three sorts: segmental colectomy with colocolonic anastomosis, proctectomy with colostomy (also known as abdominoperineal resection [APR]), and total proctocolectomy with end ileostomy. Another variation, which will be discussed under ileocolonic Crohn's disease, is the subtotal colectomy with ileorectal anastomosis. The choice of operation largely depends on the site of colonic disease, the amount of remaining bowel, and the anticipated disease recurrence.

Segmental Colectomy (Figure 12-6)

Crohn's disease is known to manifest with "skip" lesions, but isolated areas of colonic involvement amenable to segmental resection with colocolonic anastomosis are relatively uncommon, representing only about 20% of patients with colonic CD. This is because such disease is frequently in continuity with the right colon (thus necessitating an ileocolectomy for ileocolonic disease [see below]) or is associated with perineal disease (thus precipitating a total proctocolectomy). In addition, recurrence rates after segmental colonic resection and anastomosis are relatively high, on the order of 40% to 50% at 5 years. Such segmental colonic resections are done, therefore, more in patients with short

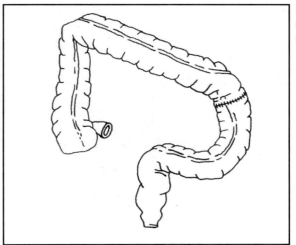

Figure 12-6. Segmental colectomy.

areas of disease, without anal or ileal involvement, especially if the resorptive surface area of the gastrointestinal (GI) tract needs to be preserved due to previous intestinal resection

Proctectomy With Colostomy (Figure 12-7)

Isolated Crohn's proctitis with or without anal disease is the usual indication for proctectomy and colostomy. The remaining portions of the colon should be without disease and even then recurrence in the colon and involving the colostomy are on the order of 25% to 35% which makes some surgeons recommend a total proctocolectomy with ileostomy over the APR for any colonic disease. The technical considerations are significant, since a nonhealing perineal wound is one complication of APR in CD. This can be minimized by an intersphincteric dissection (facilitated by lack of perineal disease), placement of abdominal drains, and omental flaps to fill the dead space left by the removal of the rectum. Sometimes gracilis muscle flaps from the legs are necessary to prophylax against or correct a nonhealing perineal wound. Sexual and urologic dysfunction in the male is avoided by keeping the dissection very close to the rectal tissues themselves and should be less than 5%.

Total Proctocolectomy With Ileostomy

Pancolonic involvement, including the rectum and anus, requires total proctocolectomy and ileostomy (see Figure 12-1). This is a relatively straight-forward operation and in the patient without small bowel disease has a low recurrence rate of disease, generally less than 20%. The sexual and urologic considerations in the male are the same as for the APR. Ileostomy siting must be done preoperatively to take into account skin folds, bony prominences, and clothing preferences. The function of the stoma, including appliance adhesion,

Figure 12-7. Proctectomy/colostomy.

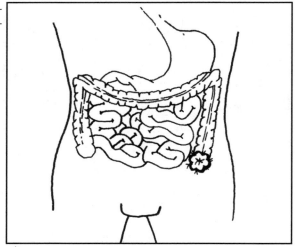

is the feature that correlates most with patient satisfaction with this operation, since ileal effluent can be quite irritating to the skin and disabling for the patient if leakage occurs. The continent ileostomy (also know as the Kock pouch) and the IPAA (see surgery for UC) are not presently recommended in the patient with known CD due to the high recurrence rate of CD in the reservoir (greater than 50%) and the resultant need for pouch removal.

ILEOCOLONIC DISEASE

Ileocolonic involvement is the most common form of Crohn's disease and the one most successfully treated by simple surgical resection and anastomosis (Figure 12-8). Indications for surgery are more commonly abscess/fistula (30%) or obstruction (30%), with a shift toward the latter in this age of TNF antagonist therapy. Recurrence rates are variable, depending on technique of assessment. By endoscopy, inflammation can be seen at the anastomosis as soon as 1 year after resection, but repeat ileocolic resection for recurrence is probably less than 50% at 10 years. There is data that suggest the efficacy of Asacol is increased in the patient with an ileocolic resection and that use of this medication in the patient without an ileocolic valve prolongs the "disease-free" interval.

Typically, the technique of resection is very straight forward, with most patients undergoing a ileocecal resection with less than 15 cm of small bowel and only the cecal pole being resected and then primarily anastomosed. Cholestyramine is frequently prescribed to minimize bile-salt induced diarrhea postoperatively. The operation is commonly performed using laparoscopic techniques that facilitate early hospital discharge, unless complicated fistulous disease or sepsis is encountered. Not uncommonly, however, there is an associ-

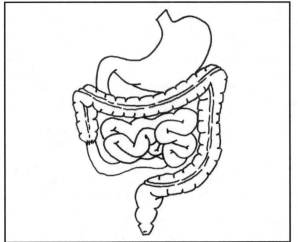

Figure 12-8. Ileocolectomy.

ated ileal fistula to an otherwise healthy appearing rectum that requires simple division and oversewing on the rectal side. Preoperative preparation is the same as for any patient undergoing colonic surgery (ie, oral laxative preparation and antibiotics) but should also include either a CT or IVP to exclude a urinary-enteric fistula. If the bladder is involved with an ileal fistula analogous to the undiseased rectum, the fistula is simply divided and the bladder oversewn while removing the inciting ileum.

Another typical presentation of ileocolic disease is that of obstruction and abscess. Under these circumstances, percutaneous CT-guided drainage and then 7 days of intravenous steroids and broad spectrum antibiotics are administered. The patient can then safely undergo resection and anastomosis with rarely the need for a diverting stoma.

When there is extensive right-sided colonic involvement with Crohn's disease, a total abdominal colectomy (also know as a subtotal colectomy) preserving the rectum, with an ileorectal anastomosis may be performed (see Figure 12-5). The recurrence rate after such an operation is on the order of 50% to 70% after 5 years but can provide the patient with a prolonged period of "stoma-free" life in spite of initially extensive disease. Bowel movement frequency is relatively unpredictable, however, and depends on the severity or recurrence of disease in the remaining rectum.

SMALL BOWEL DISEASE

CD of the small bowel is found either proximally in the duodenum or distally in the jejunum or ileum. It can be addressed with resection and anastomosis, strictureplasty, or bypass. Primary resection and anastomosis is usually done for discrete, short areas of disease in the jejunum or ileum. This has the advantage of removing diseased intestine and maintaining GI continuity with a minimum of intestinal foreshortening. The duodenum, with its proximity to the pancreas and other retroperitoneal structures, does not lend itself well to resection and anastomosis. Duodenal disease, therefore, is most commonly treated with either bypass (such as gastrojejunostomy) or strictureplasty. Most commonly, strictureplasty is done for multiple areas of jejunal or ileal disease in which multiple resections would risk the consequences of short gut, either immediately or upon subsequent operation.

Jejunoileal disease represents about 30% of patients with Crohn's disease and indications for surgery are most commonly obstruction and intractability, including persistent need for steroids. Fistulous disease as an indication is most commonly associated with the terminal ileum and requires ileocolectomy (see above). Preoperative preparation of the patient with small bowel Crohn's disease usually includes nutritional assessment/supplementation and the use of oral antibiotics due to the propensity for bacterial overgrowth in the semi-obstructed intestine. Steroids and ASA derivatives are maintained, but 6-MP and its analogs are discontinued a week before surgery.

In the patient with one or two relatively short areas of small bowel stricturing, resection of grossly affected bowel and anastomosis of normal intestine are done. About 25% of such patients will never again require surgery, providing rationale for the removal of all gross disease whenever possible. However, extensive or multiple areas of disease will probably risk short gut if entirely removed, thus strictureplasty has become increasingly the operative choice. Strictureplasty (Figure 12-9) involves a full-thickness linear incision through the stricture, which is then closed in a transverse fashion with either staples or sutures. It is important to note that such a procedure should be performed in relatively rigid, fibrotic bowel, not edematous, acutely inflamed intestine. Though intuition may suggest poor healing, in fact, strictureplasty leak rates are no higher than that found for conventional anastomosis, about 1% to 3%. Long-term studies of strictureplasty patients have shown that recurrent disease requiring operation (about 30% at 5 years) is rarely at the site of previous strictureplasty, but most commonly due to disease at a new site in the small bowel. At the time of strictureplasty, the surgeon must remember to be wary of the possibility of small bowel adenocarcinoma and biopsy any suspicious tissue because resection will not be performed.

Duodenal Crohn's disease is a relatively rare entity but represents a very difficult surgical problem. Obstruction is the most common indication, with gastroduodenal fistula to adjacent bowel accounting for the remaining patients. There is ongoing debate as to the preferred surgical treatment—bypass or strictureplasty. If the disease is extensive, strictureplasty will be impossible. Gastrojejunostomy (Figure 12-10), however, is associated with a relatively high disease recurrence rate (70% to 80% at 10 years) and marginal ulceration in the small bowel at the anastomosis due to acid (30% to 80%). Though vagotomy probably should be performed at the time of gastrojejunostomy, this too is controversial because the procedure can worsen the already present predisposition to diarrhea in these patients. Therefore, some suggest that a highly selective vagotomy should be performed, but there is no objective data that

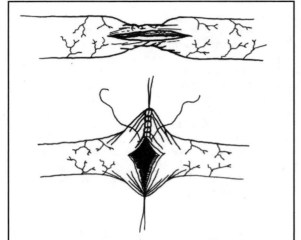

Figure 12-9. Strictureplasty.

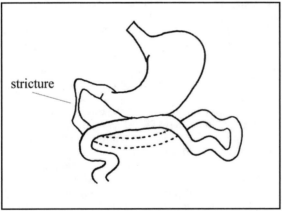

Figure 12-10. Gastroenterostomy.

stricture

confirm its value in decreasing marginal ulceration or diarrhea in the Crohn's patient. If the duodenal disease is short, direct strictureplasty or duodenojejunostomy is possible and avoids the peptic ulceration problem. However, this technique is associated with a relatively high incidence of perioperative complications such as persistent obstructive symptoms, anastomotic leak, or postoperative fistula.

PERINEAL DISEASE

The management of the affected perineum of the Crohn's disease patient is a complicated and difficult problem, frequently relying on simultaneous medical and surgical management. Surgery of the perineum should be viewed as attempting to control the local septic complications of a systemic illness. Thus, disease activity in the perineum mirrors that of the patient in general. Of paramount importance is the goal of minimizing injuries that result in incontinence. These injuries can be due to either the disease itself (abscess, fistula) or surgical intervention (sphincter injury from drainage procedures). It is also important to note that the management of a fistula or skin tag in the CD patient is much more difficult in the presence of a diseased anorectal canal with proctitis than in the patient without such low rectal disease. The approach to management of the patient with perineal CD can be separated into "benign" versus "aggressive" perineal complications of CD.

Benign Perineal Complications

Benign perineal complications of Crohn's disease include skin tags, fissures, hemorrhoids, and strictures. Generally speaking, such nonseptic complications are not an indication for surgery. In fact, hemorrhoidectomy in the CD patient is associated with a high incidence of nonhealing with eventual proctectomy and colostomy. Thus, the mainstay of therapy is stool modifying agents and salves or hygienic maneuvers to minimize discomfort and skin irritation. A discussion of such medical management is found elsewhere in this text but includes topical steroid creams or suppositories, metronidazole containing compounds and stool modifying agents (ie, fiber, cholestyramine, Lomotil). Fissures can be treated as they are in non-CD patients with botulinum toxin injections or diluted nitroglycerine ointment (0.2% three times a day), although there are no studies to date objectively evaluating these therapies in CD patients. We have never had to perform a sphincterotomy in a CD patient for a fissure that has failed to heal, but this was sometimes due to the diffuse severity of the anorectal disease present, recognizing it would accomplish little.

Rarely, we have operated on patients with dramatically large skin tags that presented with significant hygiene problems. This is always done in the context of quiescent intestinal disease (ie, not during a flare) and while on metronidazole. A single skin tag was excised as a trial. After successful healing, the remaining tags were removed 4 weeks later with similarly successful healing.

Lastly, the occasional patient with anorectal stricturing can be helped by an anal dilatation under anesthesia if obstructive symptoms are present. Such stricturing is increasingly being found as a consequence of successful TNF antagonist therapy. It needs to be recognized that such a stricture, however, may be partially responsible for the patient's continence. Therefore, no more than a single digit is used, even if recurrence occurs a few months later, since repetitive dilatations are preferable to incontinence from an overly aggressive dilatation.

Aggressive Perineal Complications

These include abscesses and the consequential fistula, including rectovaginal fistula. The Crohn's disease patient presenting with increasing perineal pain mandates examination, even in the operating room if necessary. This is because most of the benign complications of perineal CD, as well as long standing fistulae, are amazingly well tolerated by the CD patient. Thus, pain bespeaks abscess.

The surgical treatment of an abscess is incision, usually excising a small skin divot to facilitate drainage. At times, the abscess cavity can be very large and packing is anatomically difficult for the patient. A mushroom tip catheter placed within the cavity through which the patient can irrigate saline while sitting on the toilet greatly facilitates care. The catheter can be removed several days later or changed over to one of smaller caliber, as the cavity collapses. A consequential fistula is usually guaranteed and frequently such fistulae are complex with numerous tracts and several external openings, but usually only one common internal opening at the dentate line. After the acute process has calmed with drainage, irrigation, and antibiotics, an examination in the operating room under anesthesia can locate the internal opening and allow the placement of a seton drain. This is simply a soft piece of rubber the size of a conventional rubber band that is passed through the main fistula tract. Such a drain is very well tolerated by the patient and effectively eliminates the ability of the tissues to reaccumulate purulence, so obviating the usual recrudescing course of recurrent abscess formation. Sometimes patients will require several setons for several fistulae. Not infrequently, patients will live with their setons for months or even years, satisfied with the elimination of the painful abscesses they had suffered before.

Alternatively, repair of the fistula can be undertaken. This is most successful in the nondiseased rectum and anorectal canal. The choices for surgical correction are fistulotomy (usually done for very low, shallow, intersphincteric fistulae), advancement flap repair (in the patient with a soft, nondiseased anorectal canal, which allows surgical mobilization of the rectal mucosa to close the fistula), or debridement and fibrin glue instillation. More recently, the coordinated efforts of the gastroenterologist administering anti-TNF medication and the surgeon placing and then timing the removal of the seton has become successful. This involves the placement of the seton by the surgeon with the subsequent administration of TNF antagonist (infliximab) for three doses (5 mg/kg at 0, 2, and 6 weeks). The seton is removed between the second and third dose, as the effects of the medication promote fistula closure. This is usually reflected in a tightening of the tissues around the seton, causing it to feel snug. Such a protocol has resulted in a perineal fistula healing rate of approximately 45%.

Fecal diversion in the form of a temporary stoma can provide the patient with much relief from the septic complications of CD. However, such diversion treats the sepsis secondary to the anatomic abnormalities present (ie, fistulae) but does not treat the primary CD. As such, reversal of the stoma most frequently results in recrudescence of disease. In fact, the vast majority of such "temporary" diversionary stomas become permanent. Some suggest that when done for perineal CD, a loop ileostomy is preferable to a colostomy. Certainly, a stoma should not be created in an area of disease, whether it be in the colon or terminal ileum.

Finally, in the patient with severe perineal disease, proctectomy can be performed to good effect and is discussed above. Some suggest that due to recurrence of disease at the colostomy or in the remaining colon, a total proctocolectomy and ileostomy is preferred. Overall, the patient with significant perineal CD has about a 10% chance of proctectomy at 10 years of disease, with rectovaginal fistula and proctitis increasing the chances of eventual permanent stoma.

REFERENCES

1. Kock NG. Intra-abdominal "reservoir" in patients with permanent ileostomy: preliminary observations on a procedure resulting in fecal "continence" in five ileostomy patients. *Arch Surg.* 1969;99:223.
2. Parks AG, Nicholls RJ. Proctocolectomy without ileostomy for ulcerative colitis. *Br Med J.* 1978;2:85.

BIBLIOGRAPHY

Corman ML, Veidenheimer MC, Collar JA, Ross VH. Perineal wound healing after proctectomy for inflammatory bowel disease. *Dis Colon Rectum.* 1978;21:155.

Fazio VW. Complications and function of the continent ileostomy at the Cleveland Clinic. *World J Surg.* 1988;12:148.

Fazio VW, Ziv Y, Church JM, et al. Ileal pouch-anal anastomoses: complications and function in 1005 patients. *Ann Surg.* 1995;222:120.

Hawley PR. Ileorectal anastomosis. *Br J Surg.* 1985;72(Suppl):S75.

Hughes LE. Clinical classification of perianal Crohn's disease. *Dis Colon Rectum.* 1992;35:928-932.

Lyttle JA, Parks AG. Intersphincteric excision of the rectum. *Br J Surg.* 1977;64:413.

Murray JJ, Schoetz DJ Jr, Nugent FW, et al. Surgical management of Crohn's disease involving the duodenum. *Am J Surg.* 1984;147:58-65.

Ozuner G, Fazio VW, Lavery IC, et al. How safe is strictureplasty in the management of Crohn's disease? *Am J Surg.* 1996;171:57-60.

Peck DA. Stapled ileal reservoir to anal anastomosis. *Surg Gynecol Obstet.* 1988;166:562.

Poritz LS, Rowe WA, Koltun WA. Remicade does not abolish the need for surgery in fistulizing Crohn's disease. *Dis Colon Rectum.* 2002;45(6):771-775.

Sangwan YP, Schoetz DJ, Murray JJ, et al. Perianal Crohn's disease: results of local surgical treatment. *Dis Colon Rectum.* 1996;39:529-535.

Scammell BE, Andrews H, Allan RN, Alexander-Williams J, Keighly MR. Results of proctocolectomy for Crohn's disease. *Br J Surg.* 1987;74:671-674.

Stern HS, Goldberg SM. Rothenberger DA, et al. Segmental versus total colectomy for large bowel Crohn's disease. *World J Surg.* 1984;8:118-122.

Utsunomiya J, Iwana T, Imajo M, et al. Total colectomy, mucosal proctectomy, and ileoanal anastomosis. *Dis Colon Rectum.* 1980;23:459.

Wolff BG, Culp CE, Beart RW Jr, et al. Anorectal Crohn's disease: a long-term perspective. *Dis Colon Rectum.* 1985;28:709-711.

Worsey MJ, Hull T, Ryland L, Fazio V. Strictureplasty is an effective option in the operative management of duodenal Crohn's disease. *Dis Colon Rectum.* 1999;42:596-600.

Yamamoto T, Bain IM, Connoly AB, et al. Outcome of strictureplasty for duodenal Crohn's disease. *Br J Surg.* 1999;86:259-262.

Yeager ES, van Heerden JA. Sexual dysfunction following proctocolectomy and abdominal perineal resection. *Ann Surg,* 1980;191:169.

chapter **13**

Medical Therapy
for Crohn's Disease

Radhika Srinivasan, MD; Chinyu G. Su, MD; and
Gary R. Lichtenstein, MD

Introduction

Inflammatory bowel disease is a chronic, relapsing, remitting disease that poses several therapeutic challenges. Ulcerative colitis (UC) affects the colon alone while Crohn's disease (CD) can affect any part of the gastrointestinal (GI) tract. CD involves the ileocecal area in 40% to 50% of patients, small bowel only in 30% to 40%, and the colon only in 20% of patients. In addition, both diseases are frequently associated with the presence of extra-intestinal manifestations. This chapter will focus on medical management of CD and Chapter 14 will address medical management of UC.

Goals of Medical Therapy

Proper management of patients with CD depends on assessing both the location and severity of the disease. In general, medical therapies can be broadly classified based on the disease activity for which the medications are targeted. In patients with active CD, medical therapies are administered to induce remission. Standardized instruments have been developed to assess disease activity in patients with CD; however, most of these are inconvenient for daily practice and are best reserved for clinical trials. An example of this is the Crohn's disease activity index (CDAI). This is an index derived from eight weighted subjective and objective components. The index requires the patient to keep a diary for 1 week prior to the office visit. The maximum attainable score is 600 points. A patient is considered to have mild to moderate disease activity if the score is 200 to 450 and severe disease activity if the score is >450. Remission is defined as <150 points. From a practical standpoint, patients are generally considered to have mildly to moderately active disease when they are ambulatory; are able to tolerate an oral diet; and manifest no signs of dehydration, toxicities, abdominal tenderness, painful mass or obstruction. Moderate to severe disease refers to patients refractory to treatment for mild to moderate disease or those with prominent symptoms of fever, significant weight loss, abdominal pain and tenderness, nausea and vomiting (without obstruction), or significant anemia. Severe or fulminant disease applies to patients with persistent symptoms despite corticosteroid therapy or those exhibiting high fever, persistent vomiting, evidence of intestinal obstruction, rebound tenderness, cachexia, or evidence of an abscess.

Once remission is achieved via either medications or surgery, maintenance therapies may be provided to prevent recurrent disease. This is not necessarily appropriate in all patients. Based on the CDAI, a patient is considered to be in remission if the score is less than 150. In general, patients who are asymptomatic or have no inflammatory sequelae are considered in remission. As remission can be achieved via medical or surgical therapy (such as by surgical resection of the ileocecal region), appropriate maintenance agents may be different based on available data. The decision to use maintenance therapy should be based on the frequency and severity of active disease and the potential consequence of additional flare and therapy in an individual. In general, patients who have experienced frequent and/or severe recurrences or have had multiple surgeries with potential short gut syndrome should be placed on maintenance therapy once remission is achieved.

Given the chronic, relapsing nature of the disease, medical therapies for CD should ideally possess all of the following features: efficacy in relieving symptoms, modifying disease process, and maintaining remission; efficacy in improving quality of life; low toxicity profile; and easy administration. This chapter will review medical therapies for induction of remission followed by therapies for maintenance of remission. The use of these various agents for the induction and maintenance of remission in patients with CD is summarized in Table 13-1. In addition, recommended guidelines for management of specific clinical scenarios based on disease severity are also outlined in Figures 13-1 to 13-5.

AMINOSALICYLATES

Mechanism of Action and Pharmacology

Sulfasalazine was initially utilized in patients to treat rheumatoid arthritis in the 1930s. It was initially used by Dr. Nana Svartz of the Karolinska

Table 13-1

THERAPEUTIC INDICATIONS OF MEDICATIONS FOR CROHN'S DISEASE

Sulfasalazine

- Induction of remission for mildly to moderately active disease
- More effective in ileocolonic and colonic disease
- Maintenance of remission

Mesalamine

- Induction of remission for mildly to moderately active disease
- Induction of remission for active disease on concurrent corticosteroids (reducing steroid dependency)
- More effective in ileal disease
- Maintenance of remission (most effective in surgically induced remission)

Corticosteroids

- Induction of remission for moderately to severely active disease (intravenous for more severe disease)

Budesonide

- Induction of remission for mildly to moderately active disease (involving ileum and right-sided colon)

Metronidazole and/or Ciprofloxacin

- Induction of remission for active Crohn's colitis
- Induction of remission for active perianal CD (closure of fistula)
- Maintenance of remission for surgically induced remission

Azathioprine/6-mercaptopurine

- Induction of remission for active CD
- Induction of remission for steroid-dependent CD (allowing steroid withdrawal)
- Fistulous CD
- Maintenance of medically induced and possibly surgically induced remission

Methotrexate

- Induction of remission for active CD

continued on next page

Table 13-1 (Continued)

THERAPEUTIC INDICATIONS OF MEDICATIONS FOR CROHN'S DISEASE

- Induction of remission for steroid-dependent CD (allowing steroid-withdrawal)
- Maintenance of remission

Cyclosporine
- Fistulous CD refractory to other medical therapies (antibiotics, AZA/6-MP, anti-TNF therapies)

Infliximab
- Induction of remission for moderately to severely active CD
- Induction of remission for active fistulous disease
- Maintenance of remission for quiescent CD induced by infliximab

TPN or Elemental Diet
- Induction of remission for severely active small bowel CD

Institute. It was noted that the use of sulfasalazine to treat patients with presumed rheumatoid arthritis serendipitously led to a reduction in diarrhea in patients with coexistent UC. Sulfasalazine is comprised of sulfapyridine linked to a 5-aminosalicylic acid group (5-ASA) by an azobond. Upon reaching the colon, sulfasalazine is cleaved by bacterial azo-reductases, which release the 5-ASA molecules. Studies support the notion that the 5-ASA constituent serves as the active ingredient, while the sulfapyridine moiety primarily acts as a carrier, preventing proximal bowel absorption. The exact mechanism of action of the aminosalicylates remains unclear. Sulfasalazine appears to inhibit nuclear factor (NF) kappa B, which is a potent proinflammatory cytokine. Furthermore, sulfasalazine and the newer 5-ASA agents have important effects on prostaglandin synthesis, oxygen free radical production, lymphocyte and monocyte activity, the production of other proinflammatory cytokines such as interleukin-1 (IL-1), and tumor necrosis factor-alpha.

With the use of sulfasalazine, approximately 90% of the compound is delivered to the colon. The newer mesalamine derivatives (Table 13-2) are designed to deliver 5-ASA to specific sites of the gastrointestinal tract without the sulfapyridine moiety, which is thought to be responsible for many of the side effects of sulfasalazine (Table 13-3). Pentasa uses ethylcellulose-coated microgranules that release mesalamine from the duodenum throughout the remainder of the small bowel and the colon. Asacol is an Eudragit-S-coated

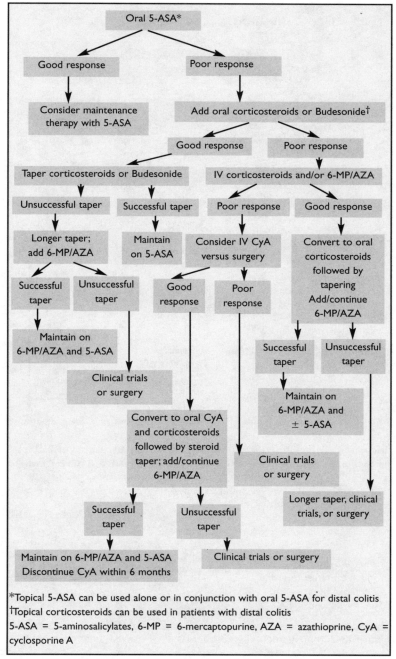

*Topical 5-ASA can be used alone or in conjunction with oral 5-ASA for distal colitis
†Topical corticosteroids can be used in patients with distal colitis
5-ASA = 5-aminosalicylates, 6-MP = 6-mercaptopurine, AZA = azathioprine, CyA = cyclosporine A

Figure 13-1. Management algorithm for mildly to moderately active ulcerative colitis.

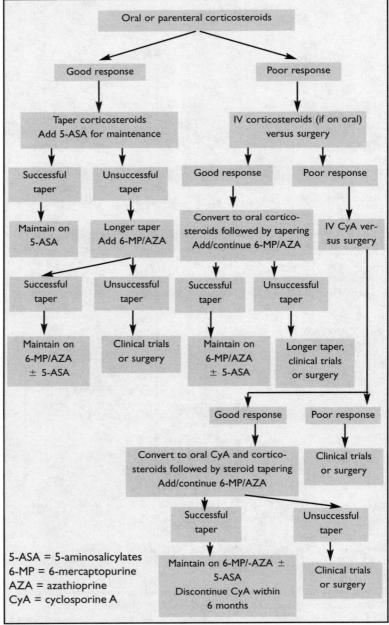

Figure 13-2. Management algorithm for severely active ulcerative colitis.

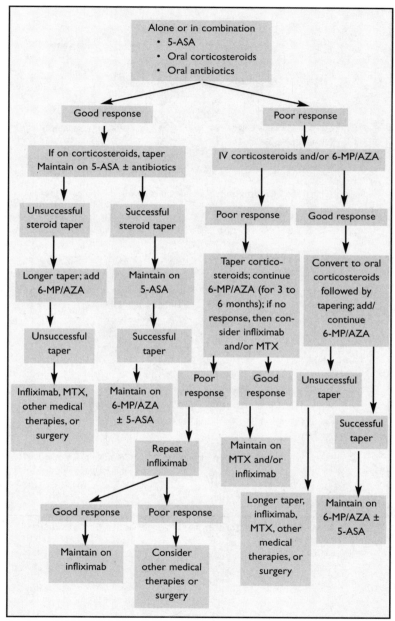

Figure 13-3. Management algorithm for mildly to moderately active Crohn's disease.

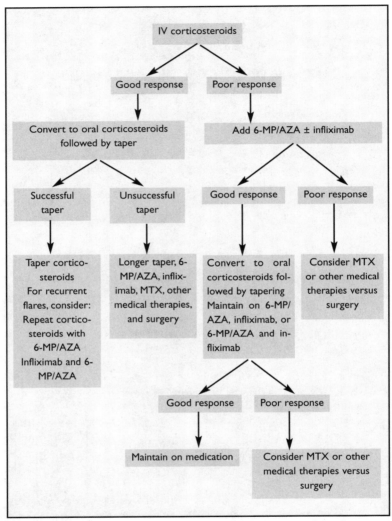

Figure 13-4. Management algorithm for severely active Crohn's disease.

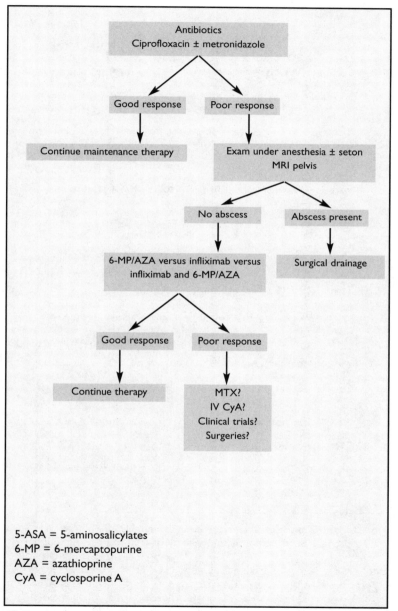

Figure 13-5. Management algorithm for fistulous and perianal Crohn's disease.

Table 13-2

5-AMINOSALICYLATE (5-ASA) PREPARATIONS

Drug	Constituents	Site of Release	Formulation	Dosages
Oral				
Sulfasalazine	Sulfapyridine, 5-ASA	Colon	500 mg tablet	4 to 6 g/day[a] 2 to 4 g/day[b]
Olsalazine (Dipentum [Pharmacia, Peapack, NJ])	5-ASA dimer	Distal ileum, colon	250 mg gelatin capsule	1.5 to 3 g/day
Balsalazide (Colozal [Salix, Raleigh, NC])	5-ASA + 4-aminobenzoyl + β-alanine	Colon	750 mg capsule	2 to 6 g/day
Mesalamine derivatives Asacol (Proctor & Gamble, Mason, Ohio)	5-ASA	Distal ileum, colon	400 mg pH-sensitive, resin-coated tablet	2 to 4.8 g/day

[a]Treatment of active disease
[b]Maintenance dose

continued on next page

Table 13-2 (Continued)

5-AMINOSALICYLATE (5-ASA) PREPARATIONS

Drug	Constituents	Site of Release	Formulation	Dosages
Pentasa (Shire, Florence, Ky)	5-ASA	Duodenum, jejunum, ileum, colon	200 or 500 mg ethyl-cellulose-coated micro-granules in a capsule	2 to 4.8 g/day
Topical				
Mesalamine suppository (Canasa [Axcan Scandi-pharm, Birmingham, Ala])	5-ASA	Rectum	500 mg suppository	500 mg to 1 g/day
Mesalamine enema (Rowasa [Solvay, Marietta, Ga])	5-ASA	Distal colon	4 g enema	2 to 4 g/day

Table 13-3

DOSING AND ADVERSE EFFECTS OF DRUGS
COMMONLY USED IN IBD

Agent	Route	Dose	Adverse Effects
Sulfasalazine	PO	See Table 13-2	Nausea, headache, rash, fever, hypersensitivity reactions, folate malabsorption, sperm abnormalities
5-ASA	PO, topical	See Table 13-2	Nausea, dyspepsia, headache, rare hypersensitivity reactions*
Corticosteroids	IV, PO, topical	See Table 13-4	Fat redistribution (47%), acne (30%), weight gain, striae (6%), mood changes, myopathy, hyperglycemia, cataracts[†] (22%), osteoporosis, osteonecrosis,[†] growth failure in children[†]
Metronidazole	PO	10 to 20 mg/kg/d	Nausea, abdominal pain, metallic taste, disulfuram-like reaction with alcohol, peripheral neuropathy
Ciprofloxacin	PO	1 mg/d	Dyspepsia, diarrhea, headache, rash, abnormal liver chemistry, Achilles' tendon ruptures
AZA/6-MP	PO	AZA: 2.0 to 2.5 mg/kg/d 6-MP: 1.0 to 1.5 mg/kg/d	Nausea, fever, rash, pancreatitis (3% to 15%), infection (7%), bone marrow suppression[‡] (2% to 11%), increased LFTs (<1%)

continued on next page

Table 13-3 (Continued)

DOSING AND ADVERSE EFFECTS OF DRUGS
COMMONLY USED IN IBD

Agent	Route	Dose	Adverse Effects
Cyclosporine	IV, PO	4 mg/kg/d	Hypertension (11%), headache (5%), electrolyte abnormalities, tremor (7%), paresthesia (26%), increaed LFTs, gingival hyperplasia (2%), nephrotoxicity (6%), seizure (rare), opportunistic infections (rare)
Methotrexate	PO, IM, SC	25 mg/wk§	Nausea, vomiting, diarrhea, leukopenia (10% to 24%), hepatic fibrosis (rare), pneumonitis (rare)
Infliximab	IV	5 mg/kg	Nausea, abdominal pain, upper respiratory infection, myalgias, infusion reactions (0.5%), possible delayed hypersensitivity-like reactions, CHF exacerbation, tuberculosis

*5-ASA is usually well tolerated. Eighty percent of patients intolerant to sulfasalazine are able to tolerate 5-ASA.

†Subcapsular cataracts, osteonecrosis, and growth failure in children are usually associated with prolonged exposure to corticosteroids.

‡Bone marrow suppression with AZA or 6-MP may be delayed.

§MTX 15 mg/wk SC can be used for maintenance of remission.

PO = by mouth, 5-ASA = 5-aminosalicylate, AZA = azathioprine, 6-MP = 6-mercaptopurine, IV = intravenous, IM = intramuscular, SC = subcutaneous, LFTs = liver function tests, CHF = congestive heart failure mesalamine tablet that is released at a pH-dependent fashion in the distal ileum and the colon. Approximately 70% to 85% of Asacol reaches the colon. In contrast, balsalazide (eg, Colazal), which consists of a 5-ASA molecule azo bonded to a 4-aminobenzoic acid derivative, delivers 99% of the intact drug to the colon.

CLINICAL EFFICACY

Sulfasalazine appears to provide benefit (based upon data from over 500 patients from the National Crohn's Cooperative Study and the European Crohn's Cooperative Study) in patients with ileocolonic and colonic CD but not in those with isolated small bowel disease. Sulfasalazine in the presence of small bowel disease alone is no more beneficial than a placebo. The dose that is required to have clinical efficacy is 3 to 5 g daily. However, those with jejunal and ileal disease may benefit from newer mesalamine preparations that deliver 5-ASA to the small bowel (see Table 13-2). Two placebo-controlled, double-blind trials have shown the efficacy of mesalamine in induction of remission in mild to moderate CD. In one study involving 310 patients, a 43% remission rate was seen in patients taking 4 g/day of mesalamine at week 16 versus 18% in those receiving placebo. In another smaller study using 3.2 g/day of oral mesalamine (ie, Asacol), a similar efficacy was shown for inducing a clinical response (not remission). When assessing two unpublished studies and combining them with the large study of 310 patients, the data for efficacy of 4 g of Pentasa to induce remission is more effective than placebo (p = 0.04); however, the difference in the CDAI (18 points) is of uncertain clinical significance because the variation of patients CDAI for an individual in remission with CD is 55 points (based upon the initial derivation/validation of the CDAI). It should be pointed out, however, perhaps higher doses of mesalamine (more than 4 g daily) will be effective for induction of remission in patients with CD. There also may be subsets of patients who respond well and are easily induced into remission with doses of 4 g of mesalamine daily (such as patients with ileal disease alone). Recent data also suggest that 4 g/day Asacol may be as effective as 40 mg/day of oral methylprednisolone for the treatment of active Crohn's ileitis. Additionally, based on data from a large controlled trial the use of mesalamine at a dose of 4 g daily in addition to prednisone was shown to be effective in the reduction of the percent of patients who become steroid dependent compared to a group that received prednisone alone (in the absence of concurrent use of mesalamine).

Although there has been no randomized-controlled trials evaluating its efficacy, topical mesalamine (see Table 13-2) can be used in patients with colonic CD. In patients with left-sided Crohn's colitis, mesalamine enemas can be used alone or in conjunction with oral agents.

Results of a recently published meta-analysis indicate that oral mesalamine preparations are beneficial in maintaining remission of CD, although the benefit was mainly observed in patients with surgically induced remission, ileitis, and/or prolonged disease duration. Mesalamine seems to have a somewhat limited role in facilitating withdrawal from steroid therapy once remission has been achieved.

INDICATIONS, DOSING, AND TOXICITY

The indications and dosing for using aminosalicylates in patients with CD are listed in Tables 13-1 and 13-2. In general, sulfasalazine and mesalamine are not effective as primary therapies for severely active CD. Side effects associated with aminosalicylate therapy are listed in Table 13-3. One of the most common side effects is headache. This side effect usually responds to a decrease in dose and improves with time and administration of medications with food. Folate malabsorption can occur, and patients should be given folate supplements. Sperm abnormalities are a common reversible side effect that has been reported with sulfasalazine. Male patients should be informed of this potential toxicity prior to initiating sulfasalazine and be advised for possible sperm banking if it should be desired.

CORTICOSTEROIDS

MECHANISM OF ACTION AND PHARMACOLOGY

Corticosteroids have a multitude of effects on the immunoinflammatory cascade. They decrease eicosanoid production, inhibit the release of proinflammatory cytokines such as IL-1 and IL-2, and down-regulate NF-kappa B production. They also interfere with phagocytic activity and decrease chemotaxis of monocytes, eosinophils, and neutrophils.

Prednisone is the most commonly used glucocorticoid and owes its activity to its metabolite, prednisolone. The conversion of prednisone to prednisolone occurs in the liver. Due to their intracellular location of action, the activity of glucocorticoids cannot be correlated to plasma level. Wide variations in the absorption of prednisolone have been found in patients with CD. The systemic availability of prednisolone is approximately 80%. The site of action of topically administered steroids is thought to be primarily local. However, systemic absorption occurs through the rectal mucosa with most topical agents, and approximately 50% of administered hydrocortisone reaches the systemic circulation.

Newer corticosteroid preparations (eg, budesonide) may provide certain advantages over traditional corticosteroids by achieving clinical efficacy associated with fewer systemic side effects and less adrenal suppression. The improved toxicity profile of these agents relates to their low systemic bioavailability (10%), which is achieved via their extensive first pass metabolism in the liver and erythrocytes. Oral budesonide is the best studied of these newer corticosteroids. It is structurally related to 16a-hydroxyprednisolone. The budesonide capsule contains 1 mm acid stable microcapsules. There is an outer resin coating that dissolves at a pH of 5.5 or higher (Eudragit-L) and another coating (ethylcellulose). Commonly used glucocorticoids are listed in Table 13-4.

CLINICAL EFFICACY

Corticosteroids have traditionally been one of the mainstays of therapy for active CD. Corticosteroids, given orally or parentally, are efficacious for the treatment of active luminal CD, regardless of disease distribution. In moderate to severe flares of inflammatory bowel disease, corticosteroids in doses equivalent to 40 to 60 mg/day of prednisone are effective first-line therapy for the induction of remission. The use of higher doses is associated with increased side effects without appreciable clinical benefit. In moderately to severely active Crohn's colitis, adding sulfasalazine to corticosteroids does not result in better efficacy compared with corticosteroids alone. Although no controlled studies have directly compared oral versus intravenous corticosteroids, patients with severe or fulminant disease or small bowel obstruction should be hospitalized and receive intravenous corticosteroid therapy. Additionally, it is important to use defined tapering regimens in the treatment of patients with CD. A standard tapering regimen that might be considered is tapering 5 mg per week then at a dose of 20 mg one might consider a slower rate (if deemed appropriate) at a rate of 2.5 mg weekly. In general, it should be stressed that prior to tapering an individual who is on corticosteroids it is appropriate to be certain that they have inactive disease. The rate of tapering has also been advocated to be more rapid by some individuals; however, it has not been tested in a formal controlled fashion. The use of topical steroids for patients with CD has not been evaluated in controlled studies. In general, topical corticosteroids can be used alone or in combination with oral agents in patients with CD involving the distal colon.

Studies have demonstrated that budesonide is superior to placebo in the treatment of active CD, with the optimal dose being 9 mg/d (taken as three 3 mg capsules once daily). Subsequent studies have also shown budesonide to have comparable efficacy as traditional corticosteroids (equivalent to prednisolone 40 mg/d) for patients with mildly to moderately active CD. Individuals with severely active CD apparently have not benefited as much as those with mild to moderate CD; hence, its use in severe disease is not currently advocated. Importantly, budesonide is associated with significantly fewer side effects and less adrenal suppression compared to the traditional corticosteroids. When compared to mesalamine 4 g/d, budesonide in the form of controlled-ileal release (CIR) preparation at 9 mg/d is superior in inducing remission in CD patients with active ileal and right-sided colonic disease. Based upon its release pattern, approximately 30% of all individuals with CD will not be appropriate candidates to receive therapy with budesonide (ie, those individuals who have colonic disease alone).

In contrast to the traditional corticosteroids, budesonide was initially thought to have a maintenance benefit. An initial study suggests that budesonide might prolong time to relapse in patients with CD. Additional placebo-

Table 13-4

COMMONLY USED CORTICOSTEROIDS

Oral

	Glucocorticoid Potency	Equivalent Glucocorticoid Dose (mg)	Mineralocorticoid Activity
Hydrocortisone	1	20	Yes
Cortisone	0.8	25	Yes
Prednisone	4	5	No
Prednisolone	4	5	No
Methylprednisolone	5	4	No
Budesonide	60	1.1	No

Topical

	Trade Name	Dose	Route
Hydrocortisone	Cortenema (Solvay, Marietta, Ga)	100 mg	Enema
Hydrocortisone	Cortifoam (Schwarz Pharma, Mequon, Wis)	80 mg	Foam
Hydrocortisone	Proctocort (Monarch, Bristol, Tenn)	30 mg	Suppository

controlled trials have also demonstrated benefit of oral budesonide as mainte-nance therapy in CD; however, sustained benefit is not observed at 1 year of follow-up. Budesonide has also been shown in another short-term study to reduce endoscopic recurrence in patients who had surgery for active disease but not in those who had fibrostenotic disease as the indication for surgery.

INDICATIONS, DOSING, AND TOXICITY

Traditional corticosteroids are indicated only in moderately or severely active disease and are not indicated for maintenance of remission (see Table 13-1). The dose for the treatment of active disease and the tapering regimen are reviewed in the previous section. Corticosteroids are potentially associated with multiple and possibly serious side effects (see Table 13-3). The toxicities are usually related to the dose and duration of therapy. Although topical steroids are associated with less systemic absorption compared to oral agents, prolonged treatment with topical corticosteroids may still be associated with steroid-related side effects. In fact, as the inflammation subsides in the intestinal mucosa, the uptake of steroids increases and the number of individuals experiencing side effects increases as this occurs. Several well-known adverse events may occur in patients with CD while on corticosteroids. Important considerations in these patients with CD include promoting intestinal perforation with the use of corticosteroids or the masking of its presence, osteonecrosis, promoting the formation of posterior sublenticular cataracts, and metabolic bone disease (osteopenia and osteoporosis). Another significant irreversible side effect includes striae. The presence of striae may only be reversed with surgical intervention. In addition to minimizing corticosteroid use and close monitoring of potential side effects, patients with CD receiving corticosteroids should receive daily calcium (1200 to 1500 mg/d) and vitamin D (400 to 800 IU/d). Patients with CD should undergo baseline and follow-up bone densitometry studies. Hormone replacement and biphosphonates may be beneficial in preventing bone loss, and their use should be considered in appropriate patients.

ANTIBIOTICS

MECHANISM OF ACTION AND PHARMACOLOGY

Experimental and clinical evidence suggests that bacterial flora may play a role in the pathogenesis of inflammatory bowel disease. Patients with CD have been shown to have abnormal intestinal flora, and intestinal bacteria have been demonstrated in the bowel wall and mesenteric lymph nodes of patients with CD. In addition, diversion of the fecal stream has been shown to delay post-operative recurrence of CD and lessen the severity of CD while healing the inflammatory response. Based on these observations, various antimicrobial agents have been used for CD, although no specific causative bacterial agents have been identified.

The two most commonly used antibiotics for the treatment of CD are metronidazole and ciprofloxacin. Oral metronidazole is well absorbed. The primary metabolic site is the liver. Urinary excretion accounts for 60% to 80% of the administered dose. A reddish-brown discoloration of the urine may be noted due to the metabolites, but this is of no clinical significance. Ciprofloxacin has a bioavailability of approximately 70%. Urinary and fecal excretion account for up to two thirds of the administered dose.

CLINICAL EFFICACY

Treatment with metronidazole at doses of 10 to 20 mg/kg/day as primary therapy for active Crohn's colitis has demonstrated efficacy equal to sulfasalazine at 3 mg/d. Ciprofloxacin 1g/day may have immunomodulatory properties as well as antimicrobial activity, and one preliminary report demonstrated equal efficacy of ciprofloxacin and 5-ASA for the induction of remission of active CD. However, there have been no large controlled studies to date demonstrating antibiotic effectiveness over placebo in CD. Adding ciprofloxacin to metronidazole has also been shown to be beneficial in some patients, but it is unknown if the combination therapy is superior to single agent therapy.

Ciprofloxacin and metronidazole are the most widely used antibiotics to treat patients with active CD. Other antibiotics have been used and tested in clinical trials. Clarithromycin has been used in an open label study of 25 patients with active CD. Patients were maintained on other agents like 5-ASA, steroids, or azathioprine (AZA). Within 4 weeks after initiation of therapy with clarithromycin, 48% of patients entered remission. Eleven of the 25 patients continued the antibiotic for a median of 28 weeks, 73% remained in remission. After the antibiotic treatment was withdrawn, three remained in remission, while five relapsed after a median of 5 months.

Antibiotics may be particularly useful in the management of perineal disease. In an open label trial of 24 patients with perianal fistulas, metronidazole at 20 mg/kg reduced drainage, erythema, and induration, with a complete healing rate of 48%. Advanced healing was achieved in 24% of patients. Four additional open label studies support the observation that treatment with metronidazole may result in closure of perianal fistulas in approximately 34% to 50% of patients. There is now an ongoing multicenter, randomized controlled trial comparing metronidazole to ciprofloxacin to placebo. Ciprofloxacin similarly may be beneficial in treating fistulae and perianal symptoms in CD.

Metronidazole may also be beneficial in preventing postoperative recurrence in CD. A preliminary study found that the use of metronidazole for 3 months postoperatively decreased the severity of endoscopic recurrence after ileal resection for CD. Nitroimidazole, a compound similar to metronidazole but with less intolerance, has demonstrated similar efficacy in preventing postoperative recurrence. No randomized, controlled studies have evaluated the efficacy of metronidazole for the maintenance of remission in nonoperative CD.

INDICATIONS, DOSING, AND TOXICITIES

Antibiotics can be used for the treatment of active Crohn's colitis, active perineal CD, and prevention of postoperative recurrence (see Table 13-1). The dosage and side effects of metronidazole and ciprofloxacin are listed in Table 13-3. The most common side effects of metronidazole are gastrointestinal. Up to 90% of patients receiving metronidazole report a metallic taste. Peripheral neuropathy is common with prolonged use. It is associated with higher doses and longer duration of therapy, occurring in >50% of patients receiving 1 g/day of metronidazole for over 6 months and is reversible if recognized early and the dose decreased or stopped. Ciprofloxacin is generally better tolerated; however, Achilles' tendon rupture and secondary fungal infection have been reported with ciprofloxacin therapy. In patients intolerant of metronidazole, ciprofloxacin constitutes an important alternative.

IMMUNOMODULATORS

AZATHIOPRINE AND 6-MERCAPTOPURINE

Mechanisms of Action and Pharmacology

Since the initial report of 6-mercaptopurine (6-MP) for the treatment of UC in 1962, immunomodulatory therapy has gained an important role in the management of CD. Azathioprine (AZA) and 6-MP are thiopurine analogues that modulate immune response via inhibition of purine biosynthesis, interference of cytotoxicity of natural killer cells and T cells, and reduction of suppressor T cell function and thus cell-mediated immunity. Upon administration, AZA is quickly metabolized nonenzymatically to 6-MP within red blood cells. 6-MP is then enzymatically converted to the active end products called 6-thioguanine nucleotides (6-TG). A competing enzyme, thiopurine methyltransferase (TPMT), also converts 6-MP to the inactive metabolites, 6-methylmercaptopurine (6-MMP) (Figure 13-6).

Clinical Efficacy

The benefit of AZA or 6-MP in the treatment of active CD has been demonstrated in controlled and uncontrolled studies. In a meta-analysis of seven randomized, placebo-controlled studies, AZA/6-MP was shown to be more efficacious than placebo in patients with active CD with an odds ratio of 3.09 (95% confidence interval [CI] 2.45 to 3.91). The overall response rate for the treatment of active CD is 55% with a dose response relationship. These immune modifiers also have important steroid-sparing effects in patients with CD, as well as benefits in the treatment of perineal disease.

A limiting factor in the use of these agents in the management of active disease is their delayed onset of action of 3 to 6 months. Recently, it was thought that the slow response to AZA might be avoided by the administration of an

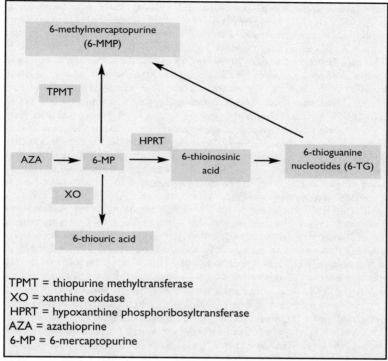

TPMT = thiopurine methyltransferase
XO = xanthine oxidase
HPRT = hypoxanthine phosphoribosyltransferase
AZA = azathioprine
6-MP = 6-mercaptopurine

Figure 13-6. Metabolism of azathioprine and 6-mercaptopurine.

intravenous loading dose; however, a recent controlled trial refuted this claim, illustrating that intravenous and oral AZA had similar time to onset of clinical efficacy.

There have been seven studies that have demonstrated efficacy of AZA/6-MP for maintenance of remission in patients with CD. A recent study of patients with CD in remission showed that the 5-year relapse rate of those who stopped AZA/6-MP was 75%, compared with 32% for those who continued these medications (p-value not available). Preliminary data suggest that 6-MP is also effective in preventing postoperative relapse of CD.

Indications, Dosing, and Toxicities

The use of AZA and 6-MP is indicated for the treatment of active CD, including perineal CD, and for the maintenance of remission in CD (see Table 13-1). Side effects of AZA and 6-MP include nausea, vomiting, allergic reactions, increased liver associated chemistry tests, and pancreatitis (see Table 13-3). An increased incidence of lymphoma and leukemia has been reported in patients with renal transplants taking AZA/6MP; however, the risk does not seem to be increased in patients with IBD who are treated with these agents. In patients with CD treated with AZA/6-MP, the development of lymphoma appears to be associated with Epstein-Barr virus infection. A common and important side effect associated with AZA or 6-MP is bone marrow toxicity. This dose-dependent toxicity occurs in 2% to 5% of patients. Patients should receive close monitoring of blood counts (and liver chemistries) for the entire duration of therapy with these agents. There have been several published suggested algorithms. It has been recommended that a complete blood count should be obtained weekly for 4 weeks, biweekly for 4 weeks, and then every 1 to 3 months for the duration of therapy. Concurrent use of allopurinol interferes with the metabolism of 6-MP and may increase the toxicity. Recent data also suggest that sulfasalazine may inhibit TPMT activity in vitro and may thus serve to augment efficacy of 6-MP or AZA at a given dose, when added to a standard regimen of 6-MP/AZA while limiting toxicity. This concept has yet to be proven in a prospective randomized fashion.

The optimal dose of 6-MP and AZA is currently unsettled. Induction of leukopenia (white blood cell count <5000 mm^3) has been shown to increase the likelihood of therapeutic response in some, but not all studies. Recent preliminary data (based on retrospective series) suggest that 6-TG levels >235 to 250 pmoles/8 x 10^8 RBCs correlate with a clinical response in patients with inflammatory bowel disease. At present, the recommended optimal doses for 6-MP and AZA are 1.5 mg/kg/day and 2.5 mg/kg/day, respectively; however, at these doses there may still be nonresponders and higher doses may be used. Some authorities suggest initiating the medications at 50 mg and increasing by 25 mg every 1 to 2 weeks, while others suggest initiating the medications at the anticipated optimal dose (1 to 1.5 mg/kg/day for 6-MP and 2.5 mg/kg/day for AZA) by weight. The incorporation of 6-TG metabolite measurement in the dose adjustment is controversial and is an area that is evolving. Measurement of 6-TG levels, however, may also be helpful in detecting noncompliance. If 6-TG levels are utilized, the test should be performed at least 2 to 4 weeks following any dose adjustment, given the time of 2 to 4 weeks for the metabolites to reach the steady state. Additional prospective trials will be necessary to determine whether an individual patient's AZA dose can be safely adjusted to achieve therapeutic metabolite levels and alter the future outcome of an individual patient's disease.

Since approximately 11% of the general population has mutant TPMT genotypes and consequent low or absent TPMT enzyme activity, AZA or 6-MP therapy in these individuals is associated with an increased bone marrow toxicity due to the shunting of 6-MP metabolism toward the excessive production of 6-TG nucleotides. The determination of TPMT genotype or enzyme activity prior to initiation of medications may allow appropriate dosing and minimize potential toxicities, although no controlled studies have evaluated such a practice. Continued investigation focusing on the importance and utility of monitoring TPMT genotype as well as 6-TG metabolite levels in IBD remains under intense investigation.

METHOTREXATE

Mechanism of Action and Pharmacology

Methotrexate (MTX) is a folic acid antagonist that has both antimetabolite and anti-inflammatory activities. It inhibits dihydrofolate reductase, thymidine synthetase, and other enzymes involving deoxyribonucleic acid (DNA) synthesis. It also interferes with the production of the proinflammatory cytokines IL-1 and IL-2.

The bioavailability of oral MTX is nearly 100% at low dose of MTX (<25 mg/week). It decreases at higher doses due to saturation of intestinal transport mechanism necessary for absorption of MTX into cells. Intramuscular MTX is given to increase compliance and bioavailability and decreases GI side effects, but it has not been proven to be superior to the oral form.

Clinical Efficacy

Intramuscular MTX (25 mg/week) has been shown to be beneficial in patients with active CD for the induction of remission and allowing withdrawal of corticosteroids in a large multicenter, double blind, placebo-controlled 16-week trial. In contrast, lower dose oral MTX has demonstrated less consistent results. Two studies failed to demonstrated statistically significant benefits of oral MTX (15 mg/week and 12.5 mg/week) over placebo for induction of remission in patients with active CD. It is unknown if the same dose given via different routes (either intramuscularly or subcutaneously) or higher doses of oral MTX would be effective.

In light of the findings in these trials, the typical scenario for treatment of patients with CD has been to treat with 25 mg intramuscularly or subcutaneously once a week with the intent of induction of remission. MTX should be considered in patients with CD who have refractory disease (have not responded or have had side effects to 6-MP or AZA), who are steroid dependent or have had adverse events related to the use of corticosteroids that have precluded their use, or in individuals who have used infliximab and have not benefited from therapy.

A randomized, placebo-controlled trial was recently published demonstrating maintenance benefit of MTX given intramuscularly at a dose of 15 once weekly to patients with quiescent CD. The duration of this particular study was 40 weeks.

Indications, Dosing, and Toxicities

MTX can be used for the treatment of active CD and maintenance of quiescent CD (see Table 13-1). The dose for treatment of active disease is 25 mg/week, and the dose for maintenance of remission is 15 mg/week (see Table 13-3). Potential toxicities of MTX include leukopenia, nausea, vomiting, and rarely, hypersensitivity pneumonitis (see Table 13-3). Hepatic fibrosis is one of the most serious potential sequela of long-term therapy with MTX. A pretreatment liver biopsy is indicated in patients who have abnormal liver associated laboratory chemistries and in those at potentially increased risk for hepatic toxicity (ie, obese individuals or individuals who consume ethanol). During the induction period (16 weeks), patients should receive liver associated laboratory chemistries frequently and a complete blood count perhaps every 2 to 4 weeks. The frequency can be reduced during the maintenance period. Patients should receive a complete blood count periodically every 4 weeks to every 12 weeks and liver-associated laboratory chemistries every 4 to 6 weeks to every 12 weeks while on MTX. Follow-up liver biopsy, although recommended by some clinicians for patients who have received a cumulative dose in excess of 1.5 g has not been assessed in controlled clinical trials in IBD nor is this widely accepted. Given the lack of consensus, it cannot be recommended at this point.

CYCLOSPORINE A

Mechanism of Action and Pharmacology

Cyclosporine A (CyA) is a lipophilic undecapeptide extracted from the soil fungus Tolypocladium infatum gams. It acts by binding to an endogenous peptide (cyclophilin), which blocks the entry of activated T lymphocytes into the S phase of the cell cycle, thus inhibiting the production of IL-2. It also alters B cell function by inhibiting T helper cells. Furthermore, it decreases recruitment of cytotoxic T cells and blocks other cytokines including IL-3, IL-4, gamma interferon, and TNF-alpha (a).

The absorption of CyA is dependent on a number of variables, including the small bowel transit time, the length of the small bowel, the integrity of intestinal mucosa, and the presence of bile. Thus, the absorption of oral CyA can be significantly impaired in patients with previous bowel resection and active CD.

Clinical Efficacy

Four randomized, controlled trials have evaluated the efficacy of oral CyA in active CD. One study demonstrated efficacy with a mean dose of 7.6 mg/kg, whereas the other three did not show any benefit over placebo with a mean dose of 5 mg/kg. Perhaps the higher dose is mandatory for CyA to be effective for the induction of remission in patients with active CD. As will be seen, however, the side effect profile may limit its use in patients with CD. A meta-analysis of these four randomized, controlled trials, however, illustrated that CyA had no therapeutic value in CD when compared to placebo.

There have been no randomized, controlled trials evaluating the efficacy of CyA for the treatment of fistulizing CD. Uncontrolled data, however, have shown efficacy of intravenous CyA (4 mg/kg/day) in the treatment of fistulous CD unresponsive to corticosteroids, antibiotics, or antimetabolites; 88% responded within a mean of 7.4 days. Half of those who responded had complete closure of the fistula.

Indications, Dosing, and Toxicities

There is currently no indication for the use of CyA in patients with CD, except for fistulous disease refractory to other medical therapies (antibiotics, AZA/6-MP, anti-TNF therapies as discussed below) (see Table 13-1). Side effects of CyA reported during the treatment of IBD include hypertension, seizures, paresthesias, tremor, gingival hyperplasia, hypertrichosis, electrolyte abnormalities, opportunistic infections, and nephrotoxicity. CyA blood levels should be regularly followed while on therapy, and careful monitoring for side effects is critical for those using CyA. Serum electrolytes, creatinine, cholesterol, and liver chemistry values should be measured prior to initiation of CyA therapy. Patients with an impaired creatinine clearance and a serum cholesterol <120 mg/dL at baseline should not receive CyA to minimize severe nephrotoxicity and risk of seizures, respectively. Patients receiving intravenous CyA should have high performance liquid chromatography (HPLC) CyA concentration and serum electrolytes determined daily, while patients receiving oral CyA should have these studies weekly. The CyA dose should be adjusted to achieve HPLC trough CyA concentrations between 200 and 300 ng/mL. Most centers use HPLC as the method to evaluate trough levels of CyA. When performing trough levels the levels need to be obtained 1 hour prior to the next dose and CyA needs to be administered every 12 hours in order to obtain valid trough levels. The dose should also be decreased when the serum creatinine increases by 30% from the baseline. Additionally, Pneumocystis carinii pneumonia prophylaxis with trimethoprim-sulfamethoxazole is recommended. The usual dose of trimethoprim-sulfamethoxazole is one double strength pill every Monday, Wednesday, and Friday.

ALTERNATIVE IMMUNOMODULATORS

Mycophenolate Mofetil

Mycophenolate mofetil (MMF), when administered orally, is converted to mycophenolic acid, the active ingredient that is a noncompetitive selective and reversible inhibitor of inosine monophosphate dehydrogenase (IMP). Inhibition of IMP depletes guanosine nucleotides in B and T lymphocytes, which reduces lymphocyte proliferation. MMF also inhibits the de novo pathway of purine synthesis and is predicted to have greater immunosuppression than AZA. It has a more rapid onset of action than AZA/6-MP.

A randomized study compared AZA 1.5 mg/kg/d to MMF 15 mg/kg/d with a tapering steroid course in 70 CD patients. Overall there was no difference observed in the number of patients who achieved remission in both groups; patients with severely active CD experienced a greater decrease in disease activity in the MMF group. In a recent open label prospective, uncontrolled multicenter study of MMF with steroids in 24 patients (both UC and CD), only 10 out of 24 patients achieved remission after 3 months and all but one CD patient had relapsed at 6 months. Further controlled trials are needed before considering use of MMF in CD patients in routine practice. In general, MMF should be reserved for patients who have failed or are intolerant to all medical therapies (eg, mesalamine, antibiotics, corticosteroids, 6-MP/AZA, infliximab, and MTX) and in whom surgery is not an option. However, it should also be noted that one study of 11 patients suggested that patients with resistance to AZA/6-MP might also be resistant to MMF.

Side effects that can be experienced with use of MMF include diarrhea, vomiting, leukopenia or thrombocytopenia, drug exanthema, and invasive CMV based upon experience from the transplant literature. Depression and migraine headaches necessitated drug withdrawal in two patients in the previously described study of 24 patients. The drug is considered teratogenic in animals, and patients are advised to avoid pregnancy while on MMF.

Tacrolimus

Tacrolimus is a macrolide antibiotic with actions similar to cyclosporine but with a 100-fold greater potency with rapid onset of action. It inhibits the transcription of interleukin-2 in T helper lymphocytes. It has improved bioavailability even in the presence of bowel inflammation or impaired bile flow. Hence, it can be used in those patients with complicated proximal small bowel and fistulizing CD as a bridge to long-term treatment with MTX or 6-MP. These patients would be expected to have poor absorption of standard oral cyclosporine.

Tacrolimus has been used in three CD patients with proximal small bowel disease, two of whom had fistulae, who showed rapid clinical improvement. Patients were then placed on maintenance treatment with MTX or 6-MP. In another small study of patients who had steroid-unresponsive acute attacks of IBD (six UC, two indeterminate colitis, two CD, one pouchitis), patients were first treated with intravenous tacrolimus followed by oral tacrolimus with concomitant AZA and mesalamine use. Seven of 11 patients achieved remission rapidly and modest improvement was noted in two. Two patients needed early colectomy. One patient who relapsed at follow-up needed a delayed colectomy. Tacrolimus has also been used in 13 steroid-resistant patients as long-term therapy, with reductions in CDAI scores at 6 months in 11 patients and at 1 year in nine patients.

Tacrolimus has also been used to treat fistulous CD in combination with AZA/6-MP; 11 patients were treated for a mean duration of 22 weeks, seven had a complete response, four a partial response, mean time to initial improvement was 2.4 weeks, and mean time to complete response was 12.2 weeks. Topical tacrolimus has also been used in oral and perianal CD with seven out of eight children showing improvement within 6 weeks and healing within 1 to 6 months.

Long-term use of tacrolimus in one CD patient with perianal fistula at a dose of 0.1 to 0.2 mg/kg/day for a total of 26 months without any adverse effects suggests that long-term treatment with tacrolimus may be an option in some CD patients.

Based on available data, tacrolimus cannot be recommended for routine use in patients with CD at the present time. It may be considered in patients who have failed or are intolerant to all medical therapies (eg, mesalamine, antibiotics, corticosteroids, 6-MP/AZA, infliximab, and MTX) and in whom surgery is not an option.

Side effects that can be seen with use of tacrolimus include nephrotoxicity, hyperkalemia, diarrhea, nausea, flushing, headache, tremor, paresthesias, insomnia, alopecia, hirsutism, and gingival hyperplasia.

BIOLOGICAL THERAPY

Cytokines are glycosylated proteins that are synthesized by a variety of cell types in response to tissue injury. Certain cytokines, such as TNF-a, IL-1, IL-6, IL-8, and IL-12, are categorized as "proinflammatory" owing to their ability to induce inflammation, while others such as IL-4, IL-10, IL-11, and IL-13 are categorized as "anti-inflammatory" due to their ability to reduce inflammation. There is increasing evidence that a disturbed balance between proinflammatory and anti-inflammatory cytokines is present in inflammatory bowel disease. For example, tissue levels of proinflammatory cytokines are elevated in active inflammatory bowel disease and correlate with the severity of the inflammation. This has led to the development of treatments directed at blocking the proinflammatory actions of these cytokines.

ANTI-TUMOR NECROSIS FACTOR THERAPY

Infliximab

MECHANISM OF ACTION AND PHARMACOLOGY

Infliximab (eg, Remicade [Centocor, Malvern, Pa]) is a chimeric (75% human, 25% murine) IgG1 monoclonal antibody directed against TNF-a. It binds to both the soluble and transmembrane forms of TNF-a and inhibits the binding of TNF-a with its receptor, thus neutralizing the biological activity of TNF-a. In addition, infliximab has also been shown to decrease the production of TNF-a and inhibit the induction of T cell and monocyte apoptosis. The pharmacokinetics of infliximab infusions in patients with CD are discussed below.

CLINICAL EFFICACY

In an initial open-label study, infusion of a single dose of infliximab (eight patients at a dose of 10 mg/kg and two patients at a dose of 20 mg/kg) resulted in remission of active CD in 8 of 10 patients (seven in the 10 mg/kg group and one in the 20 mg/kg group) previously unresponsive to steroid therapy. Maximal response was seen within 4 weeks and was maintained for at least 8 weeks in most patients. No side effects related to infliximab were observed. The efficacy and safety of infliximab was confirmed in a multicenter, randomized, placebo-controlled trial in 108 patients, showing that a single intravenous dose of infliximab (5, 10, or 20 mg/kg) resulted in clinical response in 65% of patients with steroid-resistant, moderate-to-severe CD, as compared with a response of 17% among patients given placebo within 4 weeks. The 5 mg/kg dose provided the best results, with 81% of treated patients demonstrating a clinical response. Clinical remission occurred in 33% of all patients (48% of the patients in the 5 mg/kg group) compared with 4% of patients receiving placebo. The mean duration of response was 8 to 12 weeks.

Infliximab has also proved to be efficacious in the treatment of CD-associated enterocutaneous fistulae. In one study, complete closure of more than half of all fistulae occurred in 62% of infliximab-treated patients, and complete closure of all fistulae was observed in 46% of infliximab-treated patients, compared with 13% of patients receiving placebo. The optimal dose of infliximab in this trial was 5 mg/kg given as three infusions at weeks 0, 2, and 6. Fifty-five percent of all patients who received infliximab at 5 mg/kg had complete closure of all fistulas for at least 1 month duration. The beneficial effect of infliximab was rapid (usually within 2 weeks) and persisted with reinfusion at 2-month intervals.

A recent study has demonstrated the long-term efficacy of infliximab. In this study, patients with moderately to severely active CD responding to an initial infusion of infliximab at 5 mg/kg were randomized to maintenance therapy with placebo, infliximab 5 mg/kg, or infliximab 10 mg/kg at 8-week intervals for 1 year. At the 54-week assessment, patients receiving infliximab maintenance therapy achieved significantly higher rates of both clinical remission and clinical response compared to those receiving placebo. Patients who received the 10 mg/kg maintenance dose appeared to have the best results, with remission and response rates of 38% and 53% at 54 weeks, respectively. In addition, a steroid-sparing effect was also observed with infliximab therapy.

INDICATIONS, DOSING, AND TOXICITIES

In August 1998, the Food and Drug Administration (FDA) approved infliximab for the treatment of patients with moderate-to-severe CD refractory to conventional medications and with draining enterocutaneous fistulae. Based on the currently available data, infliximab is indicated for induction of remission in patients with moderately to severely active CD, induction of remission in patients with active fistulous disease, and maintenance of remission in patients with quiescent CD induced by infliximab. Concurrent use of infliximab with 6-MP or AZA may be associated with prolonged remission in CD. The standard dose of infliximab is 5 mg/kg. The three-dose induction regimen, administered at weeks 0, 2, and 6, has been shown to be more effective than single-dose regimen for induction of remission.

Side effects of infliximab include upper respiratory tract infection, sinus congestion, headache, nausea, and myalgias. Some patients may develop antibodies against infliximab (formerly known as human antichimeric antibodies or HACA), although the clinical significance of these antibodies remains unclear. Delayed hypersensitivity-like reactions have been reported when prolonged periods (typically between 2 to 4 years) have elapsed between subsequent infusions. Antineutrophil antibodies and double stranded DNA antibodies may also occur as a result of therapy; however, the clinical significance of these findings remains under investigation. Only a small number of patients will develop a drug-induced, lupus-like syndrome in association with these serologies. Three lymphomas have been reported to date in patients with CD.

This is similar to the expected risk of lymphomas in the general population based upon the National Institute of Health SEER database, suggesting the risk for lymphoma is not substantially increased following infliximab infusions. Additional data are being collected to confirm the safety and determine if there is any long-term potential risk of lymphoproliferative disorders following infliximab infusion in CD. At present, it is believed that the risk for development of lymphoma is not higher in those receiving infliximab than the risk in the general population. It has recently been reported that in rheumatoid arthritis and CD patients, active tuberculosis may develop soon after initiation of treatment with infliximab. There have been 70 reported cases until May 2001; 64 of these were from countries with a low incidence of tuberculosis. Before considering the use of infliximab, physicians should screen patients for latent tuberculosis infection or disease.

Alternative Anti-TNF Therapies

Two other anti-TNF therapies, etanercept and thalidomide, have been investigated for their potential benefit in the treatment of CD. Etanercept is a genetically engineered fusion protein consisting of two identical chains of the recombinant human tumor necrosis factor receptor (TNFR or p75) fused with the human immunoglobulin IgG1 (Fc portion), which binds and inactivates TNF. In one study, 43 patients with moderate to severe CD were randomized to receive either an 8-week course of 25 mg of subcutaneous etanercept or placebo twice weekly. In this study, etanercept was safe but was not effective for treatment of moderate to severe CD compared to placebo. It is unknown whether a different dosing regimen of etanercept may result in efficacy for the treatment of CD. Thalidomide (Thalomid [Celgene Corp, Warren, NJ]), in contrast to infliximab and etanercept, is an oral agent known to inhibit TNF-a. Thalidomide has shown preliminary benefit in the treatment of intestinal and fistulizing CD patients unresponsive to standard therapies. In two open-label studies, about two thirds of patients who received thalidomide responded, 20% to 40% went into clinical remission, and 21% to 44% were able to discontinue steroids. Besides its known teratogenic properties, thalidomide often causes sedation, and may cause peripheral neuropathy. Controlled trials of thalidomide in inflammatory bowel disease are necessary to determine its utility in these patients. Based on currently available data, neither etanercept nor thalidomide can be recommended for routine clinical care of patients with CD. Their use should be reserved for clinical trials.

NUTRITIONAL THERAPY

Nutritional support is an important adjunct in the treatment of patients with CD. Nutritional therapy was initially derived from the theory that the antigenicity of the diet plays an important role in the pathogenesis of CD. Nutritional therapy, therefore, forms a mean to provide nutritional support while eliminating exposure of dietary antigens to the inflamed distal bowel. In addition, certain nutrients, such as glutamine, have been shown to be important in the maintenance of small intestinal metabolism, structure, and function.

An enteral route of nutritional support should be used whenever possible. Various forms of enteral nutrition have been evaluated. These can be classified into elemental and nonelemental forms. The elemental diets are amino acid based, while nonelemental diets consist of semielemental (oligopeptide) and polymeric (whole protein) contents. There is a large body of evidence in the pediatric and adult literature that suggests elemental enteral diets (composed primarily of L-amino acids) may be as effective as prednisone (particularly in small bowel disease) for the induction of remission. However, several meta-analyses upon formal analysis have failed to show superiority of enteral nutrition over corticosteroids in inducing remission. No significant difference between elemental and nonelemental diets has been demonstrated.

Elemental solutions have an unpleasant taste so they usually have to be given via some type of feeding tube, and this makes them an infeasible form of treatment in most patients. Elemental diets may be useful in treating small bowel disease that is refractory to corticosteroids and providing nutritional support in patients with borderline short-gut syndrome. Additionally, enteral nutritional support is important for insuring adequate caloric intake. Children or adolescents who have not completed their growth cycle are appropriate candidates for these supplements to their normal diet in order to ensure adequate nutrition. "Catch up" growth can be achieved with adequate nutrition.

Total parenteral nutrition should be reserved for patients in whom an enteral route is not feasible, as in high output fistula or obstructive disease. The use of growth hormone in conjunction with a high protein diet for the induction and maintenance of clinical remission of CD has been shown to be beneficial in preliminary trials and is under further investigation. Neither TPN nor elemental diets have proven efficacy for maintenance of remission in CD.

Despite the fact that food is a major source of intraluminal antigens, there is no consistent evidence that elimination diets or highly restrictive diets have a primary role in the treatment of patients with CD. Lactose restriction (or adequate supplementation with lactase supplements) may be helpful in eliminating symptoms that can be confused with symptoms of CD in some patients but is not mandatory in all patients. Patients with symptomatic fibrostenotic disease frequently benefit from a low-residue diet.

PROBIOTICS

Probiotics are living organisms in foods and dietary supplements that contribute to intestinal microbial balance. In patients with IBD, the actively inflamed areas are associated with high bacterial concentrations. Recent studies have also suggested a reduced tolerance toward individual intestinal flora in active disease in patients with IBD.

Lactobacillus has been used in four children with CD in an open-label pilot study for a 6-month period. A significant reduction in the pediatric CDAI (PCDAI) was seen at 1 week (indicative of less active disease). There was a 73% reduction in PCDAI at 4 weeks. In a larger study, 32 CD patients were treated with either mesalamine alone or mesalamine and nonpathogenic *Saccharomyces* for a 6-month period. A lower relapse rate of 6.25% versus 37.5% was noted in the group that received the probiotic compared to the group that did not receive the probiotic.

These preliminary results are encouraging, and it is likely that probiotics will emerge as adjunctive therapy to conventional medical treatments in CD. Recently, a new probiotic preparation (VSL#3) has shown potential benefit in patients with UC and pouchitis. VSL#3 contains eight bacterial species including *Streptococcus*, *Bifidobacterium*, and *Lactobacillus*. The benefit of VSL#3 in patients with CD is currently being evaluated.

GROWTH HORMONE

One recently investigated therapy that does not directly target a specific cytokine or mediator is growth hormone. This biological agent has been shown to have pleiotropic properties in the GI tract, including improvement of net protein anabolism and stimulation of wound healing. In a preliminary study of 37 patients, growth hormone (somatotropin) at a dose of 5 mg/day subcutaneously for 1 week followed by 1.5 mg/day for 4 months resulted in a significant reduction in disease severity compared to the placebo. A randomized-controlled trial is planned to confirm the clinical efficacy of this promising biological agent before it can be used in clinical practice. Table 13-5 lists various medications used in the induction and maintenance of clinical remission in CD and UC.

INDICATIONS FOR REFERRAL TO A SUBSPECIALIST

Given the complexity of CD, management of patients with IBD should be a joint venture between the nonsubspecialist primary physicians (eg, internists, family practitioners, gynecologists) and gastroenterologist. In general, all patients with IBD should be followed by a gastroenterologist, while their primary physicians can manage the systemic manifestations or complications of IBD, such as osteoporosis.

BIBLIOGRAPHY

Bickston SJ, Lichtenstein GR, Arseneau KO, et al. The relationship between infliximab treatment and lymphoma in Crohn's disease. *Gastroenterology.* 1999;117(6): 1433-1437.

Table 13-5

MEDICAL THERAPY FOR THE INDUCTION AND MAINTENANCE OF CLINICAL REMISSION

	Induction of Remission		Maintenance of Remission		
	UC	CD	UC	CD (med)*	CD (surg)*
5-ASA	+++	+	+++	+/-	+/-
Antibiotics	+/-	+	-	-	+/-[a]
Corticosteroids	+++	+++	-	-	-
AZA/6-MP	+++[b]	+++[b]	+++	+++	+
MTX	+/-[c]	++[b]	ND	++	ND
CSA	+++[d]	+/-	ND	+/-	ND
Infliximab	+[e]	+++[e]	+[e]	+++	ND

*Clinical remission induced by medical therapy or surgical resection, respectively

[a]Short-term efficacy (3 months) while antibiotics (metronidazole) continued; effect absent at 1 year

[b]Steroid-sparing effect also demonstrated

[c]Small, uncontrolled series suggest efficacy in steroid-refractory ulcerative colitis

[d]Clinical trials performed in patients refractory to corticosteroids and AZA/6-MP

[e]Data from preliminary studies (uncontrolled)

ND = no available data

Blam ME, Stein RB, Lichtenstein GR. Integrating anti-tumor necrosis factor-alpha therapy in inflammatory bowel disease: current and future perspectives. *Am J Gastroenterol.* 2001;96(7):1977-1997.

Egan LJ, Sandborn WJ, Tremaine WJ. Clinical outcome following treatment of refractory, inflammatory, and fistulizing Crohn's disease with intravenous cyclosporine. *Am J Gastroenterol.* 1998;93:442–448.

Ehrenpreis ED, Kane SV, Cohen LB, et al. Thalidomide therapy for patients with refractory Crohn's disease: an open-label trial. *Gastroenterology.* 1999;117(6): 1271-1277.

Feagan BG, Rochon J, Fedorak RN, et al. Methotrexate for the treatment of Crohn's disease. The North American Crohn's Study Group Investigators. *N Engl J Med.* 1995;332(5):292-297.

Greenberg GR, Feagan BG, Martin F, et al. Oral budesonide for active Crohn's disease. Canadian Inflammatory Bowel Disease Study Group. *N Engl J Med.* 1994;331(13):836-841.

Hanauer SB, Meyers S. Management of Crohn's disease in adults. *Am J Gastroenterol.* 1997;92(4):559-566.

Keane J, Gershon S, Wise RP, et al. Tuberculosis associated with infliximab, a tumor necrosis factor alpha-neutralizing agent. *N Engl J Med.* 2001;345(15):1098-1104.

Lewis JD, Schwartz JS, Lichtenstein GR. Azathioprine for maintenance of remission in Crohn's disease: benefits outweigh the risk of lymphoma. *Gastroenterology.* 2000;118(6):1018-1024.

Lichtenstein GR. Chemokines and cytokines in inflammatory bowel disease and their application to disease management. In: Bresalier R, ed. *Current Opinion in Gastroenterology.* London, England: Current Science; 2000: 83-88.

Lichtenstein GR. Treatment of fistulizing Crohn's disease. *Gastroenterology.* 2000; 119:1132-1147.

Lichtenstein GR. Approach to corticosteroid-dependent and corticosteroid-refractory Crohn's disease. *Inflamm Bowel Dis.* 2001;7(1):S23-S29.

Present DH, Rutgeerts P, Targan S, et al. Infliximab for the treatment of fistulas in patients with Crohn's disease. *N Engl J Med.* 1999;340(18):1398-1405.

Rutgeerts P, D'Haens G, Targan S, et al. Efficacy and safety of retreatment with anti-tumor necrosis factor antibody (infliximab) to maintain remission in Crohn's disease. *Gastroenterology.* 1999;117(4):761-769.

Sandborn WJ, Feagan BG, Hanauer SB, et al. An engineered human antibody to TNF (CDP571) for active Crohn's disease: a randomized, double-blind, placebo-controlled trial. *Gastroenterology.* 2001;120(6):1330-1338.

Sandborn WJ, Hanauer SB, Katz S, et al. Etanercept for active Crohn's disease: a randomized, double-blind, placebo-controlled trial. *Gastroenterology.* 2001;121(5):1088-1094.

Schwartz DA, Pemberton JH, Sandborn WJ. Diagnosis and treatment of perianal fistulas in Crohn's disease. *Ann Intern Med.* 2001;135(10):906-918.

Stein RB, Lichtenstein GR. Medical therapy for Crohn's disease: state of the art. *Surg Clin North Am.* 2001;81(1):71-101.

Su CG, Stein RB, Lewis JD, Lichtenstein GR. Azathioprine or 6-mercaptopurine for inflammatory bowel disease: do risks outweigh benefits? *Dig Liver Dis.* 2000;32(6):518-531.

Thomsen OO, Cortot A, Jewell D, et al. A comparison of budesonide and mesalamine for active Crohn's disease. International Budesonide-Mesalamine Study Group. *N Engl J Med.* 1998;339(6):370-374.

Vasiliauskas EA, Kam LY, Abreu-Martin MT, et al. An open-label pilot study of low-dose thalidomide in chronically active, steroid-dependent Crohn's disease. *Gastroenterology.* 1999;117(6):1278-1287.

Watts D, Campbell S, Ghosh S. Emerging therapies in Crohn's disease. *Infl Bowel Dis Monitor.* 2002;3:90-101.

Yang YX, Lichtenstein GR. Methotrexate for the maintenance of remission in Crohn's disease. *Gastroenterology.* 2001;120(6):1553-1555.

chapter **14**

Medical Therapy for Ulcerative Colitis

Radhika Srinivasan, MD; Chinyu G. Su, MD;
and Gary R. Lichtenstein, MD

INTRODUCTION

There are several goals of medical therapy of ulcerative colitis (UC) including inducing remission, maintaining remission, maintaining adequate nutrition, decrease disease- and treatment-related complications, and improving the patient's quality of life. In appropriate patients the optimal timing of a colectomy is also an important consideration.

At the time of initial presentation of patients with UC, 46% have proctosigmoiditis (ie, inflammation involving only the rectum and the sigmoid colon), 17% have left-sided colitis (ie, inflammation extending from the rectum up to the splenic flexure), and 37% have pancolitis (ie, inflammation involving the entire length of the colon). There are several factors that must be taken into account in order to effectively determine the appropriate medication and its route of administration. The extent of disease in any given patient is important. This data enable the physician to determine if topical, parenteral, or oral therapy is appropriate. Additionally, the severity of disease is important in assessing the medical therapy that is appropriate for a patient with UC. Another factor that must be taken into consideration is the previous experience a patient has had with a known medication or the presence of systemic complications that might favor or preclude the use of a specific agent(s).

There are a variety of scales (ie, disease activity indices) that can be used to assess disease severity in UC. An overall assessment of severity is derived from the patient's complaints, impact of the disease on daily function, pertinent physical examination findings (eg, fever, abdominal tenderness), and the presence of abnormal laboratory parameters (eg, anemia, hypoalbuminemia). Attention to these parameters and others frequently permits the clinician to categorize the patient as having mild, moderate, or severe disease activity. In addition, there are several endoscopic scales of disease activity used to grade the severity of colitis. One of the most widely used scales that combines patient symptoms and endoscopy is called the Mayo UC Gradation System. This consists of four subscales that assess stool frequency, rectal bleeding, findings at proctosigmoidoscopy, and the physician's overall assessment. The physician's global assessment acknowledged the first three criteria and in addition the patient's daily record of abdominal discomfort and general sense of well-being, physical findings, and performance status. A severely ill patient could have a total of 12 points (Table 14-1). A very similar scale used to assess disease activity in UC is the Sutherland Disease Activity Index. In general, it is taught that therapeutic decisions should be based primarily on the clinical status and not on endoscopic appearance. Currently, the Truelove and Witts classification of severity of disease continues to be one of the standard systems used for assessing systemic severity of UC (Table 14-2). Patients with toxic megacolon (a life-threatening form of UC) manifest signs of toxic colitis (fever >101°F, tachycardia, abdominal distention, and signs of localized or generalized peritonitis) with leukocytosis (ie, white blood cell count usually greater than 11,000 mL) and dilated colon on plain abdominal x-ray.

Tables 14-3 and 14-4 list the common side effects seen with medications used to treat UC and indications of these agents, respectively.

AMINOSALICYLATES

SULFASALAZINE

Mechanism of Action and Pharmacology

Sulfasalazine is comprised of a sulfapyridine moiety connected by an azobond to mesalamine (5-aminosalicylate [eg, 5-ASA]). The enzyme elaborated by colonic bacteria, azoreductase, is involved in the cleavage of this azobond. This activity releases the mesalamine derivative.

Clinical Efficacy

In mildly to moderately active UC, sulfasalazine will induce remission in 35% to 80% of patients when taken at a dose of 4 to 6 g/day. The rate of induction of remission is about twice that seen to occur with placebo. Approximately 15% of patients taking sulfasalazine have side effects significant enough to require discontinuation of the medication. Up to 90% of people

> *Table 14-1*
>
> ## MAYO CLINIC SCORING SYSTEM FOR ASSESSMENT OF ULCERATIVE COLITIS ACTIVITY
>
> ### Stool Frequency
> 0 = Normal number of stools for the patient
> 1 = 1 to 2 stools/day more than normal
> 2 = 3 to 4 stools/day more than normal
> 3 = 5 or more stools/day more than normal
>
> ### Rectal Bleeding
> 0 = None
> 1 = Streaks of blood with stool less than half the time
> 2 = Obvious blood with stools most of the time
> 3 = Mostly blood alone passed
>
> ### Mucosal Appearance
> 0 = Normal or inactive disease
> 1 = Mild disease (ie, erythema, decreased vascular pattern, mild friability)
> 2 = Moderate disease (ie, marked erythema, absent vascular pattern, friability, erosions)
> 3 = Severe disease (ie, ulceration, spontaneous bleeding)
>
> ### Physician's Rating of Disease Activity
> 0 = Normal
> 1 = Mild disease
> 2 = Moderate disease
> 3 = Severe disease
>
> **Maximum score = 12**

who are intolerant to sulfasalazine are tolerant of other mesalamine derivatives. Sulfasalazine is known to impair folate absorption by competitive inhibition with the jejunal enzyme folate conjugase. By inhibition of the enzyme folate conjugase this can contribute to anemia; thus, folate supplementation should be prescribed to patients receiving sulfasalazine. In the treatment of patients with active UC several studies have been performed assessing the efficacy of various medications for the induction of remission. These studies have looked at doses of sulfasalazine 1.5 to 3.0 g daily and compared them to 800 mg to 1.5 g of mesalamine. There is a trend in a recent meta-analysis (based upon

Table 14-2

TRUELOVE AND WITTS' ACTIVITY INDEX
FOR ULCERATIVE COLITIS

Severe
More than six bowel movements a day with blood
Temperature greater than 37°C
Heart rate greater than 90 beats per minute
Anemia with hemoglobin less than 75%
Erythrocyte sedimentation rate (ESR) greater than 30 mm/hr

Mild
Less than four bowel movements a day, nonbloody
No fever
Absence of tachycardia
Mild anemia
ESR less than 30 mm/hr

Moderate
Features in between those of mild and severe

Table 14-3

DOSING AND ADVERSE EFFECTS OF DRUGS USED
IN THE TREATMENT OF ULCERATIVE COLITIS

Agent	Route	Dose	Adverse Effects
Sulfasalazine	PO	4 to 6 g/day	Nausea, headache, rash, fever, hypersensitivity reactions, folate malabsorption, sperm abnormalities
5-ASA	PO, topical	2 to 4 g/day	Nausea, dyspepsia, headache, rare hypersensitivity reactions*

continued on next page

Table 14-3 (Continued)

DOSING AND ADVERSE EFFECTS OF DRUGS USED IN THE TREATMENT OF ULCERATIVE COLITIS

Agent	Route	Dose	Adverse Effects
Corticosteroids	IV, PO, topical	40 mg/day prednisone	Fat redistribution (47%), acne (30%), weight gain, striae (6%), mood changes, myopathy, hyperglycemia, cataracts (22%),[†] osteoporosis, osteonecrosis,[†] growth failure in children[†]
Ciprofloxacin	PO	1 g/d	Dyspepsia, diarrhea, headache, rash, abnormal liver chemistry, Achilles' tendon ruptures
AZA/6-MP	PO	AZA: 2.0 to 2.5 mg/kg/d 6-MP: 1.0 to 1.5 mg/kg/d	Nausea, fever, rash, pancreatitis (3% to 15%), infection (7%), bone marrow suppression[‡] (2% to 11%), increased LFTs (<1%)
Cyclosporine	IV, PO	4 mg/kg/d	Hypertension (11%), headache (5%), electrolyte abnormalities, tremor (7%), paresthesia (26%), increased LFTs, gingival hyperplasia (2%), nephrotoxicity (6%), seizure (rare), opportunistic infections (rare)

continued on next page

Table 14-3 (Continued)

DOSING AND ADVERSE EFFECTS OF DRUGS USED IN THE TREATMENT OF ULCERATIVE COLITIS

Agent	Route	Dose	Adverse Effects
Infliximab	IV	5 mg/kg	Nausea, abdominal pain, upper respiratory infection, myalgias, infusion reactions (0.5%), possible delayed hypersensitivity-like reactions, CHF exacerbation, tuberculosis

*5-ASA is usually well tolerated. Eighty percent of patients intolerant to sulfasalazine are able to tolerate 5-ASA.
†Subcapsular cataracts, osteonecrosis, and growth failure in children are usually associated with prolonged exposure to corticosteroids.
‡Bone marrow suppression with AZA or 6-MP may be delayed.

PO = by mouth, 5-ASA = 5-aminosalicylate, AZA = azathioprine, 6-MP = 6-mercaptopurine, IV = intravenous, IM = intramuscular, SC = subcutaneous, LFTs = liver function tests, CHF = congestive heart failure

---

Table 14-4

THERAPEUTIC INDICATIONS OF MEDICATIONS FOR ULCERATIVE COLITIS

Sulfasalazine
- Induction of remission for mildly to moderately active disease
- Maintenance of remission

Mesalamine
- Induction of remission for mildly to moderately active disease
- Induction of remission for active disease on concurrent corticosteroids (reducing steroid dependency)
- Maintenance of remission (most effective in surgically-induced remission)

continued on next page

Table 14-4 (Continued)

THERAPEUTIC INDICATIONS OF MEDICATIONS FOR ULCERATIVE COLITIS

Corticosteroids

- Induction of remission for moderately to severely active disease (intravenous for more severe disease)

Budesonide

- Induction of remission for mildly to moderately active disease

Ciprofloxacin

- For treatment of active disease

Azathioprine/6-Mercaptopurine

- Induction of remission for active UC
- Induction of remission for steroid dependent UC (allowing steroid withdrawal)
- Maintenance of medically-induced remission

Cyclosporine

- Severe UC refractory to other medical therapies (corticosteroids, 6-MP/AZA)

Infliximab

- Induction of remission for moderately to severely active UC

Short-Chain Fatty Acids and Oral Fish Oils

- Some benefit in treating active UC

data from two controlled trials suggesting that sulfasalazine is more effective for induction of remission than mesalamine; however, this did not reach statistical significance.

For maintenance of remission, a dose of 2 g daily is often seen as the dose that balances both efficacy and adverse events since the toxicity of sulfasalazine is dose-dependent.

ASACOL AND PENTASA

Mechanism of Action and Pharmacology

Given the toxicity and frequent intolerance to sulfasalazine that patients experience, oral mesalamine derivatives were developed. Asacol is mesalamine contained within a Eudragit-S coating, which is released in the region of the ileocecal region (above a pH of 7) and allows approximately 15% to 30% of the mesalamine to be taken up in the small bowel; Pentasa consists of ethyl-cellulose microgranules, which gives it a sustained release property. This allows the capsule to have approximately 50% release in the small bowel and approximately 50% delivery to the colon.

Clinical Efficacy

Oral mesalamine compounds have been shown to be superior to placebo for mildly to moderately active UC. A dose-response trend has also been observed, with the lack of significant effect for doses of mesalamine <2g/day compared to placebo, and increased response at doses of 4 to 4.8 g/day. At a Pentasa dose of 4 g/day the rate of remission is 59% versus 36% with placebo, whereas with Asacol at a dose of 4.8 g/day the response rate is 74% versus 18% with placebo. Asacol 4.8 g/day is actually comparable to sulfasalazine 12 g, the latter dose would not be used in clinical practice because of the extremely high probability of intolerance.

As with establishing remission, oral mesalamines exhibit a dose-response relationship without increasing toxicity when used to maintain remission. So with mesalamines, the same dose that was used to induce remission can be used to maintain remission. A 2002 meta-analysis of 11 trials examined the maintenance of remission with oral mesalamines (Asacol or Pentasa) or olsalazine (Dipentum) versus equimolar doses of sulfasalazine. Sulfasalazine was found to have a modest, but statistically significant benefit over 5-ASA in the trials of 6 months duration. Differences in response rates were not statistically significant when trials of 12-month duration were considered. There was also no apparent difference between the number of adverse events caused by sulfasalazine and 5-ASA.

OLSALAZINE

Mechanism of Action and Clinical Pharmacology

Olsalazine is a 5-ASA dimer linked by a diazobond, formulated as gelatin capsules, and released primarily in the colon. Approximately 98% of mesalamine is delivered to the colon with this agent.

Clinical Efficacy

Doses of 1 to 3 g daily are effective in inducing remission in approximately 70% of patients. The use of olsalazine for induction of remission in patients with IBD is associated with drug-induced diarrhea in up to 10% of patients and some would consider that it is not indicated for establishing remission in UC. The incidence is reduced to 3% if patients take olsalazine with meals. A systematic review of oral 5-ASA for maintenance of remission in UC concluded that olsalazine was significantly inferior to sulfasalazine. It appeared that the significantly higher proportions of withdrawals due to adverse events influenced the reduced efficacy.

BALSALAZIDE

Mechanism of Action and Clinical Pharmacology

Balsalazide is a relatively new mesalamine derivative that is a prodrug in which the 5-ASA is linked via a diazobond to 4-aminobenzoyl-b-alanine (4-ABA), an inert and biologically inactive carrier molecule. The azobond is cleaved by colonic bacterial azo reductases, and the mesalamine is released in the colon. Approximately 99% of the mesalamine is delivered to the colon. A significant difference between balsalazide and currently used prodrugs (eg, sulfasalazine) is that both the carrier molecule 4-ABA and the prodrug are pharmacologically inert and devoid of systemic effects.

Clinical Efficacy

Balsalazide has been shown to be more effective than placebo and most recently it has been compared to mesalamine in three prospective randomized trials. One of these recent studies demonstrated superiority of balsalazide over a pH-dependent formulation of mesalamine. In this randomized-controlled study, balsalazide 6.75 g daily (equivalent 5-ASA = 2.4 g daily) resulted in greater rates of both symptomatic and complete clinical remission at all points of evaluation (ie, 4, 8, and 12 weeks) compared to mesalamine 2.4 g daily. In addition, balsalazide was also better tolerated than mesalamine in the study, and the median time to complete relief of symptoms was shorter for patients in the balsalazide group than in the mesalamine group. Treatment with balsalazide in these trials has been shown to result in more rapid response when compared to mesalamine therapy. The greatest benefit of balsalazide appears to be in patients with newly diagnosed left-sided UC.

With regard to the use of balsalazide to maintain remission of UC, a double-blind, multicenter, randomized trial compared two doses of balsalazide (1.5 g twice daily and 3.0 g twice daily) with mesalamine 0.5 g three times daily. The higher dose of balsalazide resulted in a statistically significant higher clinical remission rate (77.5%) than the lower dose of balsalazide (43.8%) and mesalamine (56.8%). All three treatments were safe and well tolerated. Another randomized, double-blind study compared 3 g daily of balsalazide and 1.2 g daily of mesalamine for 12 months for maintenance of remission in UC. Remission at 12 months was 58% in both groups, but fewer balsalazide patients relapsed within the first 3 months. Adverse events were similar in both groups.

The most common adverse events reported with balsalazide were headache (8%), abdominal pain (6%), diarrhea (5%), respiratory infections (4%), arthralgia (4%), back pain (less than 3%), myalgia (less than 3%), and flu-like symptoms (less than 3%).

The use of any of the aminosalicylates for severely active UC has not been evaluated in controlled trials, but generally is not thought to provide benefit in these patients. Once remission is achieved, aminosalicylates have been shown to be quite effective as maintenance therapy. It has been demonstrated that doses of 1.5 to 4.8 g/day maintain remission in over half of patients with UC. Furthermore, these agents appear to be safe as long-term maintenance therapies.

TOPICAL AMINOSALICYLATES

Mechanism of Action and Pharmacology

Topical aminosalicylates can be administered in the form of 5-ASA enemas, 5-ASA suppositories, and, in Europe, 5-ASA foam. The use of enemas allows the medication to be administered up to the level of the splenic flexure in about 95% of individuals, and the suppositories are used to treat disease up to 15 to 20 cm from the anal verge. The foam has been shown to have a similar distribution as the enemas.

Clinical Efficacy

The standard dosing regimens used to induce remission are 1 to 4 g of topical mesalamine in the form of an enema nightly. Mesalamine suppositories 1.0 g/day (500 mg as needed twice a day [bid]) to 1.5 g/day (500 mg three times a day [tid]) either nightly or as divided doses are used to induce remission in those with distal disease. The treatment with mesalamine 500 mg per rectum bid is effective as 500 mg per rectum tid. Topical mesalamine is the most effective maintenance therapy to prevent relapse of distal colitis. The frequency of topical therapy is gradually decreased until the lowest frequency that maintains the patient's well-being is determined. Some patients prefer not to continue topical therapy, and for those patients a switch to oral mesalamine can be made at a dose of 2.4 g daily for maintenance of remission.

A recent meta-analysis reviewing 17 randomized, double-blind, controlled trials concluded that topical mesalamine was useful for both the induction and the maintenance of remission of mild to moderate distal UC. In such treatment, mesalamine enemas were as effective as oral sulfasalazine but were associated with fewer side effects. Similar efficacy has been demonstrated for 1 g, 2 g, and 4 g mesalamine enemas for the induction of remission of patients with mild-to-moderate left-sided UC not requiring concurrent corticosteroids. These were patients that were also not refractory to other medical therapies. A combined treatment of rectal and oral mesalamine may also be more effective than oral treatment alone for the induction and maintenance of remission of distal UC, suggesting a dose response effect. A significantly higher relapse rate of 69% was observed among patients who received oral therapy alone (p = 0.036). This finding is also consistent with a dose response phenomenon.

In the treatment of acute ulcerative proctitis, mesalamine administered as a 500 mg suppository twice daily has been shown to be beneficial. Mesalamine suppositories have also been shown to be effective in preventing relapse, and the dose may be titrated to patient response and tolerance. Mesalamine foam, not yet approved in the United States, has a more uniform distribution and longer persistence in the distal colon compared with mesalamine enemas and provided better patient acceptance than the enema preparation in one trial.

CORTICOSTEROIDS

MECHANISM OF ACTION AND PHARMACOLOGY

Corticosteroids have multiple effects on the immunoinflammatory pathway. They produce their effect by activating steroid receptors to regulate the expression of certain target genes. Thus, various steroid-responsive target genes are either induced or suppressed. They inhibit the release of proinflammatory cytokines like interleukin-1 (IL-1), IL-2, IL-8, IL-6, gamma interferon, and tumor necrosis factor alpha. The interaction between activated steroid receptors and other transcription factors like NF-kappa B may also be an important mechanism that mediates the anti-inflammatory action of steroids. NF-kappa B plays a vital role in signal transduction in the inflammatory process and thus inhibition of it by corticosteroids may be a crucial mechanism by which steroids exert their anti-inflammatory action. Corticosteroids can also suppress intestinal mucosal natural killer cell activity based on experimental data. It also reduces the exudation of plasma from postcapillary venules at sites of inflammation. Corticosteroids decrease the amount of diarrhea by stimulating water and sodium absorption. Prednisone is the most commonly administered glucocorticoid and has an 80% systemic bioavailability. Topical corticosteroids are available in liquid and foam formulations. Foam preparations are often better tolerated by patients and may be easier to retain. Cortifoam (Schwarz Pharma, Mequon, Wis) is available as 80 mg of 10% hydrocortisone acetate in the form of an aerosol with a rectal applicator. Hydrocortisone enemas are available in 100 mg dose in 60 mL of solution. Although absorption of corticosteroids after topical administration is less than absorption of corticosteroids after oral administration, prolonged treatment with topical steroids may still be associated with steroid-related side effects.

CLINICAL EFFICACY

Corticosteroids were the first agents demonstrated in controlled trials to have efficacy in UC. The data from that trial were published in 1955. They are efficacious for the treatment of active UC regardless of disease distribution. In moderate to severe flares of inflammatory bowel disease, corticosteroids in doses equivalent to 40 to 60 mg/day of prednisone are effective first-line therapy. The use of higher doses is associated with increased side effects without appreciable clinical benefit. In moderate to severely active UC, adding sulfasalazine to corticosteroids does not result in better overall efficacy as compared with corticosteroids alone.

Corticosteroids have no maintenance benefits in preventing relapse. Some patients may become steroid dependent, a term that applies to individual patients who are unable to taper off steroids without experiencing a disease flare. Steroid dependency has been reported to occur in approximately 22% of patients at 1 year based upon population-based data. Patients treated with steroids have a relatively poor prognosis for maintenance therapy with mesalamine. Based upon population-based data, approximately 29% of patients will undergo surgery within 1 year of initiation of steroids. Long-term remission rates in patients who required parenteral steroids for severe UC are approximately 50%. Most clinicians would consider the addition of immunomodulators in those patients who required two courses of steroids in a relatively short period of time to induce disease remission.

Faubion et al[1] determined the 1-year outcome after the first course of steroids in a cohort of patients with IBD in Olmstead County, Minn. A total of 185 UC patients were studied; 63 (34%) were treated with steroids. Complete remission was achieved in 54%, partial remission in 30%, and no response was noted in 16% of patients. Among the UC patients, 1-year outcomes were prolonged response in 49%, steroid dependence in 22%, and the need for operative intervention in 29% of patients.

SIDE EFFECTS OF CORTICOSTEROIDS

There is an increased incidence of toxicities involving the musculoskeletal system (ie, osteoporosis, aseptic necrosis), endocrine system (ie, hyperglycemia, obesity), gastrointestinal system (ie, nausea, vomiting, pancreatitis), eyes (ie, cataracts, hemorrhage), skin (ie, atrophy, striae), cardiovascular system (ie, hypertension, edema), hematological system (ie, leukocytosis, immunosuppression), and neuropsychiatric manifestations like mood disorders and impaired cognitive function (see Table 14-3).

BUDESONIDE

Mechanism of Action and Pharmacology

Budesonide, which was initially developed for treatment of asthma and allergic rhinitis, has recently been formulated into an oral preparation. Budesonide has enhanced topical anti-inflammatory activity, a very high affinity for the glucocorticoid receptor, stability in extra hepatic tissues, and a 90% first pass hepatic metabolism and is converted to metabolites that have little or no biologic activity. Because its systemic bioavailability is low it has a low potential for steroid-related side effects. No oral formulation of budesonide provides optimal release characteristics for the entire length of the colon.

Clinical Efficacy

Small, uncontrolled studies have suggested that Budenofalk (Dr Falk Pharma, Brussels, Belgium) (not the type that is available in the United States) 9 mg/d may be effective for prednisone-dependent universal UC. Studies have not shown the benefit of oral budesonide (eg, Entocort EC [Astra Zeneca, Wilmington, Del]) for the treatment of active UC.

TOPICAL CORTICOSTEROIDS

CLINICAL EFFICACY

Topical corticosteroids in liquid and foam formulations are effective therapy for induction of remission in patients with active UC distal to the splenic flexure. Foam preparations are often better tolerated by patients and may be easier to retain. In a meta-analysis, topical corticosteroids were found to be less effective than topical mesalamine for inducing remission of distal UC. However, the combination of topical corticosteroids with topical mesalamine is often more efficacious than either alone in the short-term treatment of distal UC. Although absorption of corticosteroids after topical administration is less than absorption of corticosteroids after oral administration, prolonged treatment with topical steroids may still be associated with steroid-related side effects.

ANTIBIOTICS

MECHANISM OF ACTION AND PHARMACOLOGY

The use of antibiotics is based on the demonstration of the importance of enteral microflora in murine models of enterocolitis. Increased intestinal wall permeability is thought to expose the colonic mucosa to the bacterial cell wall antigens like lipopolysaccharides. These antigens either initiate the colonic inflammation or sustain the inflammatory response of the host. Development of UC has been observed in some individuals after enteric infection with organisms such as *Salmonella* and *Shigella* species. It is thought that the infection initiates an inflammatory cascade in the genetically susceptible host. The exact mechanism by which antibiotics contribute to symptom improvement is not established.

Metronidazole is a synthetic antibacterial and antiprotozoal agent that belongs to the nitroimidazole class. It is bactericidal, and anaerobic organisms readily take it up. The reduced metronidazole then disrupts the DNA's helical structure and inhibits bacterial nucleic acid synthesis, which then results in bacterial cell death. Oral metronidazole is well absorbed with at least a 90% bioavailability. The primary site of metabolism is in the liver, and urinary excretion accounts for 60% to 80% of the administered dose. Peak concentrations are achieved 1 to 3 hours after oral administration of the drug. Decreased renal function does not alter the pharmacokinetic parameter of metronidazole. Accumulation of metronidazole and its metabolites can occur in patients with severe liver disease.

Ampicillin is an aminopenicillin and is primarily bactericidal. It inhibits the third and final stage of bacterial cell wall synthesis and autolytic enzymes mediated lysis. It has activity against both gram-positive and gram-negative organisms. Approximately 30% to 55% of an oral dose of ampicillin is absorbed. Peak serum levels occur within 1 to 2 hours of an oral dose and at 1 hour after an intramuscular dose. Parent drugs and metabolites are excreted into the urine. The dose has to be adjusted in patients with end-stage renal disease.

Gentamicin is an aminoglycoside antibiotic obtained from cultures of *Micromonospora purpurea*. It is most effective against gram-negative rods but is used in combination with other antibiotics to treat certain gram-positive organisms like *Staphylococcus aureus* and certain species of streptococcus. It is bactericidal and its mechanism of action is not fully understood though it does inhibit bacterial protein synthesis. Gentamicin is not absorbed orally, and serum levels are unpredictable after intramuscular administration. Peak serum concentrations after intravenous administration are proportional to the dose; a concentration of 6 to 8 mg/mL is usually achieved with an IV dose of 2 mg/kg infused over 30 minutes. It is not metabolized and is eliminated exclusively via glomerular filtration. In individuals with normal renal function the half-life is about 2 to 3 hours, while in those with impaired renal function it can be 24 hours or longer.

Third-generation cephalosporins like ceftazidime and ceftriaxone are more active and have a broader spectrum of activity against aerobic gram-negative bacteria when compared to first or second generation cephalosporins. They are beta-lactam antibiotics like penicillin and are mainly bactericidal. Ceftazidime is not absorbed from the GI tract, and peak serum levels occur within 1 hour following an intramuscular dose. About 5% to 24% of the drug is protein bound. The drug is excreted primarily via glomerular filtration with a 1.5- to 2-hour half-life. In patients with end-stage renal disease, the half-life can be as long as 35 hours; therefore, dosages should be adjusted accordingly. Ceftriaxone is also not absorbed from the GI tract, and peak serum concentrations occur within 1.5 to 4 hours following an intramuscular dose. It has a higher protein binding of 58% to 96%. The drug is excreted via urine and via bile in the feces. The elimination half-life is about 5.5 to 11 hours. Even though the elimination half-life increases as renal function declines, dose adjustments in patients with renal dysfunction are usually not necessary due to the extensive biliary excretion.

Another agent, ciprofloxacin, is a broad-spectrum anti-infective agent of the fluoroquinolone class. It is most effective against gram-negative organisms. It is also effective against gram-positive organisms but is not active against anaerobic organisms. It is bactericidal by inhibiting a DNA gyrase enzyme that is responsible for counteracting the excessive coiling of DNA during bacterial replication or transcription.

The drug can be administered orally or intravenously. When given orally it is rapidly absorbed from the GI tract and undergoes very little first pass metabolism. Peak serum concentrations are achieved within 2.5 hours. It is widely distributed in most tissues, as the protein binding is low. Plasma concentrations can be higher in individuals over the age of 65, which is thought to be partly related to decreased renal clearance. Elimination half-life varies between 3 and 5 hours, although it can be prolonged in those with renal failure. About one-half of the administered dose is excreted as unchanged drug via the urine; about 20% to 40% of the drug is eliminated via the feces. It appears that ciprofloxacin can be safely given to IBD patients who are receiving cyclosporine, although more data are needed.

CLINICAL EFFICACY

Metronidazole has not been shown to be beneficial as acute therapy for UC in controlled trials. One small trial has demonstrated the benefit of metronidazole for maintenance of remission in UC; however, the evidence is not compelling. A recent study suggested that 6 months of oral ciprofloxacin may be beneficial in the treatment of active UC when compared to placebo; however, additional confirmatory controlled trials are needed. Other similar quinolones and antibiotics (eg, clarithromycin) have been studied in uncontrolled trials and are currently being investigated in additional clinical trials. It is perceived that these medications are similar to placebo regarding their efficacy in patients with UC.

The general belief is that antibiotics should be used in patients who have severe disease and fever requiring hospitalization, especially if such patients have signs of transmural colitis, systemic toxicity, or fulminant colitis with or without megacolon. These individuals may have translocation of bacteria and bacterial products. A combination of intravenous ampicillin, gentamicin, and metronidazole or a third-generation cephalosporin and metronidazole are usually used even though there are no controlled trials that have confirmed the benefit of antibiotics in this setting.

SIDE EFFECTS OF COMMONLY USED ANTIBIOTICS

Acute psychoses and confusion can result when disulfiram and metronidazole are concurrently used. Metronidazole can inhibit alcohol dehydrogenase and other alcohol metabolizing enzymes. Metronidazole taken together with ethanol can result in the development of disulfiram-like side effects, including nausea, vomiting, headache, flushing, and abdominal cramps. Metronidazole can give rise to a metallic taste in the mouth (ie, dysgeusia), cause anorexia, cause nausea and vomiting in up to 12% of patients, cause constipation, cause headache, and result in peripheral neuropathy, which is usually reversible with discontinuation of the drug. Pancreatitis is a serious but rare side effect that occurs with use of metronidazole.

Ampicillin in large doses inhibits the renal tubular secretion of MTX and causes higher and more prolonged levels of MTX in the serum. Ampicillin can cause anaphylaxis, urticaria, skin rashes, GI upset, and blood dyscrasias. Diarrhea occurs more frequently with ampicillin than with other drugs in this class.

Gentamicin can cause nephrotoxicity, ototoxicity as manifested by high frequency hearing loss, tinnitus, vertigo, visual disturbances, elevated liver enzymes, and blood dyscrasias.

Ceftazidime can cause mild and transient neutropenia and eosinophilia. Seizures can occur but are rare. Elevated liver-associated laboratory chemistries, headache, malaise, abdominal pain, nausea, vomiting, and diarrhea can occur.

With use of ceftriaxone, the most common adverse effects are eosinophilia (6%), thrombocytosis (5%), and leukopenia (2%). Seizures are rare. Cholecystitis-like symptoms that develop are nausea, vomiting, epigastric distress, and right upper quadrant tenderness. Pseudocholelithiasis has been known to develop, especially in children, which is thought to be secondary to its high level of biliary excretion with subsequent formation of crystals of ceftriaxone that lodge in the biliary system.

Ciprofloxacin use can potentially be associated with the development of side effects. The gastrointestinal side effects of nausea, vomiting, diarrhea, and abdominal pain are noted in 1.7% to 5.2% of patients. Hepatotoxicity is rare. Central nervous system side effects of seizures, raised intracranial pressure, confusion, depression, and toxic psychosis have been reported. Tendon ruptures, which can occur unilaterally or bilaterally, have been reported. The Achilles' tendon and tendons of the hands and shoulder joint have been affected. Concomitant corticosteroid use in some patients who experienced this adverse effect may be a relevant risk factor. Hypersensitivity reactions, like rash, fever, eosinophilia, and interstitial nephritis, can be seen with use of ciprofloxacin. In less than 1% of patients, cardiovascular adverse effects, such as palpitations, atrial flutter, and premature ventricular contractions, can occur.

IMMUNOMODULATORS

Immunomodulator use is of value in the management of UC patients who are dependent on, refractory to, or intolerant of corticosteroids.

6-MERCAPTOPURINE AND AZATHIOPRINE

Mechanism of Action and Clinical Pharmacology

The most widely used immunomodulators are azathioprine (AZA) (eg, Imuran [Prometheus, San Diego, Calif]) and 6-mercaptopurine (6-MP) (eg, Purinethol [Glaxo Smith Kline, Research Triangle Park, NC]). These two agents are purine analogs that interfere with nucleic acid metabolism and cell growth. AZA is nonenzymatically converted to 6-MP, which is then metabolized through a series of pathways to 6-thioguanine nucleotides (6-TG). These end products are felt to be the active agents accounting for the efficacy of 6-MP/AZA. In addition to cell cycle inhibition, these agents also exert cytotoxic effects on lymphoid cells. Because of the delayed onset of action, a key factor when considering use of 6-MP and AZA in UC is whether the patient can tolerate an additional 3 to 6 months of symptoms and potential steroid toxicity. The usual doses used are 1 to 1.5 mg/kg for 6-MP and 2.0 to 2.5 mg/kg for AZA, while monitoring for potential side effects.

Side Effects and Drug Interactions

AZA and 6-MP can cause nausea, vomiting, pancreatitis, increase in liver chemistries, and leukopenia (see Table 14-3). Risk of leukemia and lymphoma does not seem to be increased in patients with IBD who are treated with these agents, although a higher incidence has been reported in renal transplant patients taking AZA/6-MP. Patients should be monitored for side effects by obtaining a complete blood count frequently. A typical periodicity would be weekly for 4 weeks, then biweekly for the next 4 weeks, and then every 1 to 3 months for the duration of therapy. Liver chemistries are also monitored at periodic intervals.

Both AZA and 6-MP interact with aminosalicylates. 5-ASA drugs inhibit thiopurine methyltransferase (TPMT), an important enzyme in the metabolism of AZA and 6-MP. Inhibition of this enzyme can increase the intracellular concentration of degradation product such as 6-TG metabolite levels to toxic levels, potentially leading to myelosuppression. This interaction can be advantageous in that lower doses of the immunomodulators can be used when patients are placed on concomitant 5-ASAs. Conversely, the dose of the immunomodulators may need to be increased when patients are taken off 5-ASA preparations.

The use of allopurinol concurrently with AZA and 6-MP can interfere with the metabolism of 6-MP by inhibition of the enzyme xanthine oxidase and thus increase the toxicity of the immunomodulators. Drug levels of AZA/6-MP can be monitored by measuring 6-TG levels; levels greater than 235 to 250 pmoles/8×10^8 RBCs have been demonstrated to correlate with a clinical response (based upon retrospective studies) in patients with IBD. Measurement of 6-TG levels can be helpful in detecting patient noncompliance with immunomodulator therapy. The test should be performed at least 2 to 4 weeks after any dosage adjustment, as it takes that long for the metabolites to reach a steady state.

Clinical Efficacy

There have been controlled studies that determined the efficacy of AZA in the treatment of active UC. Jewell and Truelove[2] treated 80 patients with acute UC with 40 mg of prednisolone and then patients were either placed on 2.5 mg/kg of AZA or placebo. There was no benefit to the addition of AZA when results[3] were evaluated at 1 month. Caprilli et al[3] undertook a double-blind comparison of the effectiveness of AZA and sulfasalazine in 20 patients with idiopathic proctocolitis. Both drugs produced similar improvement in clinical symptoms, laboratory findings, and endoscopic and biopsy findings, although radiological improvement was less evident (p = NS). In the trial by Kirk and Lennard-Jones,[4] 44 patients with chronic active disease were treated with 2.0 to 2.5 mg/kg of AZA for a 6-month period. Patients were on concurrent therapy at the discretion of the treating physician. The actual response rates were not reported but the activity of colitis, as judged by a numerical score, improved in the group that received AZA versus the group that received placebo (p <0.001). The mean dose reduction in prednisolone needed was greater in patients treated with AZA than in those treated with placebo (p = 0.001).

Furthermore, controlled trials have demonstrated efficacy of these agents for the maintenance of remission of UC. In one controlled trial of patients with UC who initially achieved remission on AZA, a 1-year relapse rate of 36% was seen in those who were continued on AZA, compared with a 59% relapse rate for those who were switched to placebo. Another study reported that more than 61% of patients with UC who were originally dependent on steroids were able to stop or reduce the steroid use when they were maintained on 6-MP. The relapse rate has been reported to be as high as 87% when patients discontinued use of 6-MP in one retrospective review of 105 patients treated with 6-MP for chronic refractory UC, in which a complete clinical remission was initially achieved in 65% of those patients. In contrast, in the trial by Jewell et al,[2] UC patients who were admitted with their first attack showed no benefit from a 1-year maintenance trial with 2.5 mg/kg AZA when compared to placebo (p = 0.18). In particular, there was no benefit for patients in their first attack of UC. It was, however, demonstrated that AZA reduces relapse in established disease. There was no benefit in patients on corticosteroids nor for maintenance of remission for the first year after administration of AZA. Similarly, in the study by Rosenberg et al,[5] there were no significant differences in clinical response in patients treated with AZA versus placebo, but AZA had a significant steroid sparing effect (p <0.05). The dose of AZA used in this trial was lower at 1.5 mg/kg.

CYCLOSPORINE

Mechanism of Action and Clinical Pharmacology

Cyclosporine A (CyA), an oral and parenteral agent, is a potent inhibitor of cell-mediated immunity. It is a cyclic polypeptide consisting of 11 amino acids and is produced by the fungus *Tolypocladium inflatum gams*. It inhibits the production of interleukin-2 and alters B cell function by inhibiting T helper cells. Cyclosporine binds to an immunophilin, which plays an important role in protein regulation. The cyclosporine-cyclophilin complex then binds to and inhibits the calcium-calmodulin activated phosphatase calcineurin. Calcineurin inhibition results in the blockade of signal transduction of the nuclear factor of activated T cells (NF-AT), thus causing a failure to activate NF-AT regulated genes. NF-AT activated genes include those required for B cell activation, including IL-4 and CD-40 ligand, and those required for T cell activation, including IL-2 and interferon gamma. Cyclosporine does not affect suppressor T cells or T cell independent, antibody mediated immunity. It is a substrate and inhibitor of P-glycoprotein, which is an energy-dependent drug-efflux pump located in intestinal epithelium and the blood brain barrier. There is an overlap between P-glycoprotein and the inhibitors and/or substrates of cytochrome P450 3A4. Granulocyte, monocyte, and macrophage function remain unaltered by CyA therapy.

Cyclosporine is administered orally, parenterally, and in enema form. It is extremely hydrophobic. Most clinicians use a 3:1 ratio when converting between oral and parenteral routes. Oral absorption is extremely unpredictable, especially with the nonmodified formulations of the oral preparation. In order to improve the bioavailability of cyclosporine, a microemulsion formulation (ie, Neoral [Novartis Pharmaceuticals Corp, East Hanover, NJ]) was FDA approved in 1995. Following oral administration, the Tmax for cyclosporine ranges from 1.5 to 2 hours. It is widely distributed throughout the body, but a preferential uptake occurs in the liver, pancreas, and adipose tissue. The elimination half-life can vary over 16 to 40 hours. The drug undergoes enterohepatic recycling and about 6% is excreted renally. In subjects with hepatobiliary diseases, the half-life can be prolonged. Patients receiving intravenous CyA should have a high performance liquid chromatography (HPLC) CyA concentration and serum electrolytes determined daily, while patients receiving oral CyA should have these studies performed at least weekly. The usual IV dose is 4 mg/kg/day by continuous infusion and the usual oral dose is 5 to 7 mg/kg/day. Recent data suggest that an initial dose of 2 mg/kg is more appropriate to use with patients with active UC. The CyA dose should be adjusted to achieve HPLC trough CyA concentrations between 200 and 300 ng/mL. Most centers use HPLC as the method to evaluate trough levels of CyA. When performing trough levels the levels need to be obtained 1 hour prior to the next dose and CyA needs to be administered every 12 hours in order to obtain valid trough levels. The dose should also be decreased when the serum creatinine increases by 30% from the baseline. Additionally, Pneumocystis carinii pneumonia prophylaxis with trimethoprim-sulfamethoxazole is recommended at a dose of one double strength pill three times a week.

Drug interaction with other nephrotoxic agents can potentiate the nephrotoxicity of cyclosporine. It can cause hyperkalemia; hence, its use with potassium sparing diuretics can be problematic. Several drugs that inhibit hepatic cytochrome P450 can decrease the clearance of cyclosporine. The metabolism of cyclosporine can be inhibited. Its use with IBD is primarily in severe steroid-refractory UC and with those patients who do not respond to 6-MP/AZA or are intolerant to these agents.

Clinical Efficacy

There have been three randomized, double-blind, placebo-controlled studies evaluating the efficacy of intravenous CyA in UC. The first report in 1994 studied patients with severe UC who failed IV corticosteroids. In 11 patients who failed at least 7 days of IV hydrocortisone, nine (82%) responded favorably to continuous IV infusion of CyA (4 mg/kg/day) within a mean of 7.1 days, compared to none of the patients receiving placebo. During a 6-month follow-up period, 44% of those who were successfully treated with intravenous CyA ultimately required colectomy despite being maintained on oral CyA.

The addition of AZA or 6-MP appears to be beneficial in patients who have responded to intravenous CyA and may lead to a reduced rate of relapse or colectomy. This finding is substantiated from data in several retrospective studies. These findings suggest that CyA may be used as a "bridge" for control of disease until AZA or 6-MP becomes efficacious or until elective surgery is performed at a later date.

In addition to the above landmark study evaluating the efficacy of CyA in patients with severe steroid-refractory UC, the combination therapy with IV CyA and corticosteroids for 14 days appears to be more effective in inducing remission in patients with severely active UC refractory to 1 week of IV steroids. In this study of 30 patients by Svaoni et al,[6] approximately 70% of the patients on IV cyclosporine monotherapy responded compared to 92% of those who received the combination therapy of cyclosporine and steroids.

A recent study by D'Haens et al[7] suggested that IV CyA monotherapy is equally effective as IV corticosteroids in patients with severely active UC. In this randomized controlled trial, 53% of patients with severely active UC receiving IV CyA at 4 mg/kg/d for 8 days had a clinical response compared to 64% of patients receiving IV methylprednisolone. With the addition of AZA, 78% of patients who initially responded to CyA remained in remission at 12 months compared to 37% of patients who initially responded to corticosteroids (the p-value is not available).

There have been uncontrolled studies evaluating the use of cyclosporine enemas for refractory proctosigmoiditis. Twenty-one of 36 patients (58%) responded to initial therapy, and 36% of these remained in remission after therapy. The one controlled study of 40 patients on 350 mg of cyclosporine enema appears to be ineffective (no more effective than placebo) in treatment with the endpoint of induction of remission of active left-sided UC.

Side Effects

Nephrotoxicity is the most common side effect (20% to 38% of renal transplant recipients) thought to be secondary to intense renal vasoconstriction. Mild to moderate hypertension, seizures (especially in those with serum cholesterol levels less than 120 mg/dL), paresthesias, tremor (55%), hepatotoxicity (4% to 7%), anorexia, nausea, vomiting, gingival hyperplasia (4% to 16%), and hypertrichosis are also noted. Mild encephalopathy has been reported in 30% of patients. Infections reported in 1% to 3% of patients receiving cyclosporine include abscesses, cellulitis, folliculitis, moniliasis, and tonsillitis. Hypersensitivity reactions, including anaphylaxis, have been reported during administration of cyclosporine; castor oil vehicle is thought to be responsible.

METHOTREXATE

Mechanism of Action and Clinical Pharmacology

Methotrexate (MTX) is a folic acid antagonist and has both immunomodulatory and anti-inflammatory properties. It inhibits DNA synthesis by inhibiting dihydrofolate reductase, thymidine synthase, and other enzymes. It is cycle-specific, inhibiting cells primarily in the S-phase. It also inhibits the production of proinflammatory cytokines like IL-1, interferon gamma, and tumor necrosis factor; impairs the release of histamine from basophils; and decreases chemotaxis of neutrophils. Methotrexate can be give orally, intravenously, intramuscularly, subcutaneously, and intrathecally. It is absorbed from the GI tract by active transport mechanism. When given orally, the mean bioavailability of MTX is 60% and there is an extensive first pass metabolism in the liver. It is well absorbed intramuscularly with a Tmax in 30 to 60 minutes. When administered subcutaneously at doses of 15 mg/wk and 25 mg/wk, the drug reaches steady state concentrations at approximately week 6. The elimination of MTX is triphasic; the first half-life is 45 minutes, which reflects the distribution phase. The second half-life is due to renal clearance and is about 3.5 hours, while the terminal half-life is about 10 to 12 hours and possibly reflects enterohepatic circulation of the drug. The primary route of elimination is via the kidneys.

Coadministration of nonsteroidal anti-inflammatory drugs (NSAIDs) and penicillins can decrease the clearance of MTX. Prednisone has been shown to block the MTX-induced inhibition of DNA synthesis, while dexamethasone and prednisolone do not interfere with the cytotoxicity of MTX.

Clinical Efficacy

In a prospective nonblinded pilot trial 21 patients (seven with UC and 14 with CD) were given 12 once-a-week injections of intramuscular MTX 25 mg/wk. Treatment of these patients led to a reduction in mean UC activity index from 13.3 to 6.3, and the mean prednisone dose was reduced from 38.6 mg to 12.9 mg at the end of the study period. Five of seven patients with UC responded as did 11 of 14 patients with CD. Based upon the aforementioned trial, there was a subsequent prospective, randomized, double-blind, placebo-controlled trial demonstrating no benefit to the administration of oral MTX at 12.5 mg/week over placebo for the treatment of active UC. Subcutaneous administration or intramuscular administration of MTX has not been examined in any controlled study of patients with active or quiescent UC to date. Additionally, oral doses above 12.5 mg/week have not been critically examined in a prospective, randomized fashion. No maintenance benefit has been tested or proven in UC by means of controlled clinical trials.

Side Effects

Stomatitis, esophagitis, oral ulcerations, nausea, vomiting, and abdominal distress are most commonly reported acute side effects. It can suppress bone marrow and cause anemia, leukopenia, and thrombocytopenia. The above toxicities can be minimized by the use of leucovorin. Elevation in liver enzymes (15%), with acute use and portal fibrosis and cirrhosis with chronic use (cumulative dose over 1.5 g) can be seen. Pretreatment liver biopsy may be indicated in patients who are obese and use alcohol. There are no firm, published guidelines regarding the need for liver biopsy when IBD patients are treated with MTX and a cumulative dose of 1.5 g is reached.

NEWER IMMUNOMODULATORS

These are used in patients who are intolerant of AZA or 6-MP or do not respond to traditional immunomodulators.

MYCOPHENOLATE MOFETIL

Mechanism of Action and Pharmacology

Mycophenolate mofetil (MMF) is the ester prodrug of mycophenolic acid (MPA). It was isolated from a *Penicillium* culture in 1898 but was not studied as an immunosuppressive agent until the 1970s. MMF, when converted to its active metabolite, inhibits lymphocyte purine synthesis by reversibly inhibiting the enzyme inosine monophosphate dehydrogenase. It thus inhibits the de novo pathway of purine synthesis and also the synthesis of lymphocyte DNA, ribonucleic acid (RNA), proteins, and glycoproteins. Subsequently, lymphocyte proliferation is inhibited. It has a greater immunosuppression than AZA and a quicker onset of action. It can be administered orally or intravenously. Peak plasma levels of MPA occur within 36 to 42 minutes, and the absolute bioavailability is about 94%. MPA is excreted in bile and undergoes extensive enterohepatic circulation, which results in a second plasma peak concentration about 6 to 12 hours after the initial dose. The mean elimination half-life after oral and intravenous administration is about 18 hours and 16 hours, respectively.

Coadministration of MMF with antacids or cholestyramine decreases its bioavailability. When given concurrently with salicylates, the protein binding of MPA is decreased and thus increased clinical effects of MMF can be seen as well as additive GI side effects.

Clinical Efficacy

A 12-month pilot study of MMF in UC patients (n = 12 patients) versus AZA (n = 12 patients) with concomitant prednisolone use showed that the rate of remission was higher with AZA/prednisolone combination at all time points, 100% versus 88% after 1 year. There were two serious adverse events noted in the MMF group: recurrent upper respiratory tract infection that resulted in drug discontinuation in one patient and a second patient developed bacterial meningitis. Two other patients had a worsening of their UC and had to discontinue the use of MMF.

In a recent open-label prospective and uncontrolled multicenter study of MMF with steroids in 24 patients (both UC and CD), 10 patients achieved remission after 3 months and all but one CD patient had relapsed at 6 months. Depression and migraine necessitated drug withdrawal in two patients. Further controlled investigations of the use of MMF in UC patients are needed.

Side Effects

GI side effects are the most common (>10%) and can consist of nausea, vomiting, diarrhea, flatulence, abdominal pain, constipation, dyspepsia, oral candidiasis, and anorexia. Generalized body pain, back pain, chest pain, asthenia, fever, and headache are also seen. An absolute neutrophil count of less than 500/mm^3 can develop in 2% to 3.6% of patients on MMF. Interstitial pneumonitis, including fatal pulmonary fibrosis, has been rarely reported.

TACROLIMUS

Mechanism of Action and Pharmacology

Tacrolimus is a macrolide antibiotic derived from the fungus *Streptomyces tsukubaensis* and has actions similar to cyclosporine. It is 10 to 100 times more potent than cyclosporine. It inhibits the first phase of T cell activation, thus inhibiting the transcriptional activation of IL-2, IL-3, IL-4, granulocyte-macrophage colony stimulating factor, and interferon gamma. It binds to a binding protein called FK binding protein. This complex inhibits the phosphatase activity of calcineurin, which then results in the blockade of signal transduction of the nuclear factor of activated T cells (NF-AT). NF-AT activated genes include those that are required for B and T cell activation. Like cyclosporine, tacrolimus is a substrate and inhibitor of P-glycoprotein. A topical formulation is also available for treatment of atopic dermatitis, and it exerts its mechanism of action by inhibiting T cells, releasing mast cell mediators, and down regulating IL-8 receptors. There is a down regulation of the entire inflammatory cascade.

The absorption of oral tacrolimus is poor and very variable. The bioavailability of oral tacrolimus is approximately 17% to 22%. The drug is highly protein bound, and metabolism is by hepatic cytochrome P450 3A4 enzyme with an elimination half-life of about 12 hours. This increases to 28 to 140 hours in those patients with mild hepatic dysfunction. Any drug that inhibits cytochrome P450 3A4 enzyme can increase the drug level of tacrolimus, while those that induce the enzyme can cause a decrease in the whole blood levels of tacrolimus. Use of other nephrotoxic agents along with tacrolimus should be avoided.

Clinical Efficacy

Steroid-unresponsive acute attacks of IBD (six UC, two indeterminate colitis, two CD, one pouchitis) were treated with IV tacrolimus followed by oral tacrolimus with concomitant AZA and mesalamine. Seven of 11 patients achieved rapid remission and modest improvement was noted in two patients. Two patients needed early colectomy. One patient who relapsed at follow-up needed a delayed colectomy.

Side Effects

Nephrotoxicity occurs in approximately 36% to 52% of transplant patients as does hyperkalemia in 13% to 45% of patients. Neurotoxicity consisting of headache (64%), tremor (56%), paresthesias (40%), and dizziness (19%) are other common side effects noted with the use of tacrolimus. Hypertension occurs in almost half the patients treated with this drug. Insulin-dependent diabetes mellitus is also seen in about 20% of transplant patients. GI side effects of abdominal pain, constipation, dyspepsia, elevated liver enzymes, nausea, and vomiting are seen in 24% to 72% of patients. Hematologic adverse reactions (15% to 59%) include anemia, leukocytosis, leukopenia, and thrombocytopenia.

ANTI-TUMOR NECROSIS FACTOR THERAPY

INFLIXIMAB

Mechanism of Action and Pharmacology

Infliximab is a chimeric IgG-1 monoclonal antibody directed against tumor necrosis factor alpha (TNF-α). It consists of approximately 75% human protein and 25% murine protein. The murine portion is the antigen recognition region. It neutralizes both the soluble and transmembrane TNF-α. Infliximab inhibits several biological activities of TNF-α, such as induction of proinflammatory cytokines IL-1 and IL-6, enhancement of leukocyte migration, expression of adhesion molecules by endothelial cells and leukocytes, activation of neutrophil and eosinophil functional activity, proliferation of fibroblasts, and synthesis of prostaglandins. In patients with IBD, infliximab reduces infiltration of inflammatory cells and TNF-α production in inflamed areas of the intestine. In addition, the proportion of mononuclear cells in the lamina propria that can express TNF-α and gamma interferon is reduced.

Infliximab is administered intravenously, and a single infusion of 5 mg/kg results in a median Cmax of 118 mg/mL. It is predominantly distributed in the vascular compartment and has an elimination half-life of about 8 to 9.5 days. No specific drug interaction studies have been conducted with infliximab.

Clinical Efficacy

No large randomized-controlled study to date has evaluated the efficacy of infliximab for UC. There are currently two large ongoing studies to help answer the question as to how well infliximab works for patients with UC. In a pilot study, Sands et al[8] evaluated patients with severe steroid-refractory UC. Patients received a single infusion of either 5, 10, or 20 mg/kg dose of infliximab. Fifty percent (four of eight patients) had clinical improvement at week 2 compared to none (zero of three) of those who received the placebo. This was a study that evaluated the effect of a single dose only. There was no long-term follow-up of patients.

Chey et al[9] conducted another open label study in which eight patients with severe refractory UC were given a single 5 mg/kg infusion of infliximab and then endoscopically and histologically assessed. All eight patients responded without significant complications or side effects; the mean duration of remission has not been assessed because none of the patients had relapsed at the time of publication.

Su et al[10] reported on 27 UC patients who received either single or multiple infusions of infliximab either as an inpatient or as an outpatient. Twelve patients (44%) achieved remission and six patients (22%) had a partial response. Five out of nine patients who had no response subsequently underwent colectomy. The median duration of response was 8 weeks; steroid refractory patients were less likely to respond when compared to those patients who were steroid-responsive (33% vs. 83%; p = 0.026).

A large, ongoing, randomized-controlled trial is now being conducted to confirm these preliminary findings.

Side Effects

The most common adverse effect is headache, which is experienced by 23% of patients. GI side effects, seen in 3% to 17% of patients, include nausea, vomiting, diarrhea and abdominal pain. An acute infusion reaction occurs within 1 to 2 hours of administration of the drug in about 19% of patients; fever and chills are the most common manifestations and cardiopulmonary symptoms such as chest pain, dyspnea, hypotension, and hypertension also occur. A syndrome of delayed hypersensitivity consisting of headache; sore throat; urticaria; pruritus; dysphagia; and edema of the lips, hands, and face has been reported in 25% patients who were retreated with infliximab after a long drug holiday (2 to 4 years). Antibodies against infliximab (ATI), formally called human antichimeric antibodies (HACA), occur in 13% of patients, although some studies have reported higher percentages. Some treated patients developed ANA, and some of these patients developed a drug-induced lupus-like picture but it was rare. Serious infections, such as tuberculosis, histoplasmosis, listeriosis, and aspergillosis, can occur in infliximab-treated patients. Tuberculin skin testing and chest x-ray in those with a positive skin test are recommended prior to treatment with infliximab, although many of these patients may be anergic. There are some preliminary data on the outcome of pregnancies in women receiving infliximab, but firm conclusions cannot be drawn at this time.

NUTRITIONAL THERAPY AND PROBIOTICS

Bowel rest and TPN are often effective as primary therapy for the treatment of active Crohn's disease but have not proven effective in UC. Use of short-chain fatty acids, which serve as important nutrients of the colonic epithelium, may be beneficial in some patients with active UC, and oral fish oil preparations have shown modest benefit in active and quiescent UC.

PROBIOTICS

Description and Mechanism of Action

Probiotic effect refers to the ingestion of a living organism to favorably affect the health of a host. Probiotics help to re-establish normal intestinal flora. These create an environment that is unfavorable to potentially pathogenic bacteria. Probiotics prevent overgrowth of potentially pathogenic bacteria and maintain the integrity of the gut mucosal barrier. The mechanism of these actions is not well understood, but it has been shown that probiotics produce an antibiotic-like substance and also reduce the luminal colonic pH. In vitro studies have suggested that they stimulate the intestinal immune system by enhancing macrophage and natural killer activities and proliferation of lymphocytes. *Lactobacilli* species adhere to the gut mucosal surface and inhibit the attachment of gram-negative aerobic bacteria. VSL#3 consists of four strains of lyophilized *Lactobacilli,* three strains of *Bifidobacterium,* and one strain of *Streptococcus salivarius.*

Two maintenance trials in UC have demonstrated potential benefits of the Nissle strain of *E. coli* in preventing relapse of UC compared to low dose of mesalamine. Placebo-controlled trials or trials using higher doses of mesalamine are needed before the more widespread use of probiotics in preventing UC relapse becomes a part of the treatment armamentarium.

Side Effects

Some patients report increased flatulence at the start of therapy with the use of lactobacillus tablets, which tends to subside with continued treatment. Constipation, hiccups, rash, and vomiting have been reported but causality has not been determined.

OTHER INVESTIGATIONAL THERAPIES

NICOTINE

Mechanism of Action and Pharmacology

Nicotine is a naturally occurring alkaloid and by itself is not considered a health threat. There are multiple potential mechanisms of action for the beneficial effect of smoking and/or the use of nicotine in UC. Smoking suppresses both humoral and cellular immunity in healthy controls. Experimental studies have shown that nicotine, tobacco extract, and smoking decrease the production of several inflammatory cytokines like IL-1, IL-2, IL-8, IL-10, and TNF-a. This reduction is evident in both peripheral mononuclear cells and colonic mucosa of both UC patients and normal controls. In vivo studies have shown a similar effect in both men and mice. Nicotine also has eicosanoid effects as evidenced by decreased production of prostaglandin E and leukotrienes B4, C4, D4, and E4. Though in vitro studies have shown increased mucus production by colonic mucosa in smokers with UC, this has not been noted in *in vivo* studies; therefore, this mechanism is not thought to contribute to the protective effect of nicotine in UC patients. Both smoking and nicotine increase levels of endogenous corticosteroids, which may have a beneficial effect in controlling symptoms of UC. Another possible mechanism is decreasing neutrophil-mediated inflammation by inhibiting the neutrophil production of oxygen-free radicals.

Nicotine can be delivered via chewing gum or a transdermal patch. During 20 to 30 minutes of rhythmic chewing, about 50% to 90% of the content of the gum can be absorbed. Nicotine has an extensive first pass metabolism through the liver. Chewing gum produces peak plasma concentrations within 15 to 20 minutes while time to peak plasma concentrations from transdermal patches can vary from 4 to 9 hours after application. A 30-mg nicotine patch delivers about 22 mg of nicotine and results in peak and trough plasma concentrations that are approximately two-thirds of that achieved with smoking. Nicotine and its metabolites cotinine and nicotine-1'-oxide are excreted by the kidneys; about 10% to 20% of unchanged nicotine is eliminated through the urine.

Clinical Efficacy

The observation that smoking appears to have a protective effect in patients with UC prompted the use of nicotine in these patients. Six uncontrolled trials using either nicotine gum or transdermal patches suggested that nicotine was beneficial in patients with active and steroid-dependent UC, although patients who had never smoked did not tolerate it. These observations led to six controlled trials. Lashner et al[11] reported on seven patients with active UC who were treated with 2 mg of nicotine gum administered five to seven times a day versus placebo. Three of four ex-smokers benefited from the treatment while three nonsmokers did not benefit. Two randomized, placebo-controlled trials of transdermal nicotine reported that a dose of 22 to 25 mg/24 hours was efficacious when compared to placebo. In contrast, a fourth study that used 25 mg/24 hours of transdermal nicotine showed equivalence to use of prednisolone 15 mg/day, with a trend for the latter being more beneficial. In keeping with this above study, another controlled trial showed equivalent results when patients were randomized to treatment with 15 mg/24 hours of nicotine for 5 weeks or prednisone 30 mg/day that was tapered over 5 weeks, once again with a trend toward better treatment response with use of prednisone. At the 6-month follow-up, among the patients who initially achieved remission with either drug and who were then placed on mesalamine, significantly fewer patients relapsed in the group who achieved remission on nicotine. The sixth study demonstrated that a dose of 15 mg/16 hours of nicotine when compared to placebo was not efficacious for maintenance of remission in UC patients.

Side Effects

The physiological actions of nicotine include tachycardia, an increase in blood pressure, and a greater sense of alertness due to central nervous system stimulation. The nicotine patch may cause localized erythema, pruritus, rash, or urticaria. Nicotine gum is stickier and heavier than regular chewing gum and can affect artificial teeth or other dental work. Minor side effects include mild headache, nausea, vomiting, appetite stimulation, constipation, diarrhea, dysmenorrhea, flushing, insomnia, and irritability.

HEPARIN

Mechanism of Action and Pharmacology

Heparin is a glycosaminoglycan composed of chains of D-glucosamine and an uronic acid. It is derived from porcine or bovine tissue and is available as a calcium or sodium salt. Therapeutic doses of heparin prolong the clotting time but the bleeding time is unaffected. Heparin exerts its anticoagulant action by accelerating the activity of antithrombin III to inactivating thrombin (factor IIa). It also inactivates factor Xa and factor IXa. In addition to its anticoagulant effect, heparin may also interfere with the inflammatory cascade by blocking adhesion molecules involved in leukocyte recruitment. By restoring binding of antiulcerogenic factors it may also promote healing of intestinal lesions. After IV administration of heparin, the response is almost immediate, whereas after subcutaneous administration its anticoagulant activity is delayed for 1 to 2 hours. It is cleared and metabolized by the reticuloendothelial system. Most available data indicate that heparin elimination is not adversely affected by the presence of renal or hepatic dysfunction.

Efficacy

There is evidence that abnormalities within the microcirculation of the GI tract play a crucial role in the development of IBD. Prothrombotic abnormalities within the circulatory system and the presence of inflammatory vasculitis and microthrombi within the bowel mucosa suggest that a hypercoagulable state is an important contributor to the pathogenesis of IBD. Uncontrolled studies suggested that unfractionated heparin reduces symptoms and improves healing in patients with steroid resistant UC. Other uncontrolled studies have shown that heparin reduces the concentration of TNF-a and C-reactive protein. Dwarakanath et al[12] showed that heparin is beneficial against pyoderma gangrenosum, and Brazier et al[13] have shown that it is useful in treatment of erythema nodosum. Panes et al[14] reported on a multicenter randomized trial in 25 hospitalized moderate or severe UC patients comparing continuous heparin infusion versus methylprednisolone at 0.75 to 1 mg/kg/day. The proportion of patients with persistent rectal bleeding at day 10 was 31% in the steroid-treated group versus 90% in the heparin-treated group (p <0.05). Three patients in the heparin group were withdrawn from the study because of rectal bleeding; one needed transfusion and one underwent surgery. In the other randomized study (N = 20), Ang et al[15] compared IV heparin (25,000 to 45,000 IU daily) for 5 days followed by subcutaneous heparin for 5 weeks (10,000 IU bid for 2 weeks and then 5000 IU bid for 3 weeks) with high-dose IV hydrocortisone (200 mg) for 5 days followed by 40 mg of oral prednisone daily and the dose was reduced by 5 mg per day each week. The response rate was similar in both treatment groups when authors monitored clinical activity index, stool frequency, and endoscopic and histopathological grading. Both treatments were well tolerated with no serious adverse effects.

Side Effects

Bleeding is the most serious adverse effect associated with the use of heparin, which can either be minor or major hemorrhage. The incidence of thrombocytopenia is between 0% and 30%. It can occur as an early, benign, reversible nonimmune form or as a late, more serious, IgG mediated immune thrombocytopenia. One should monitor for osteoporosis in patients who receive heparin for more than a month. Skin lesions, such as ulceration, hematoma, erythema, plaques, and necrosis, can occur. Abnormalities of liver associated laboratory chemistries have also been noted.

SPECIFIC CLINICAL SCENARIOS

Algorithms for treatment of mild to moderate and severe ulcerative colitis are presented in Figures 14-1 and 14-2.

POUCHITIS

A total abdominal colectomy with ileal pouch-anal anastomosis (IPAA) is the surgical treatment of choice for most patients with medically uncontrolled UC. The most common long-term complication of this operation is chronic inflammation of the pouch, which is referred to as pouchitis. Up to 50% of patients will develop at least one episode of pouchitis and 15% of these patients will need maintenance therapy and are thought to have chronic pouchitis.

The mainstay of therapy for acute and chronic pouchitis is antibiotics that have anaerobic coverage. The usual treatment dose is oral metronidazole at 10 to 20 mg/kg/day for a 14-day period.

Two placebo-controlled trials of metronidazole treatment of pouchitis have been performed. The first study was a single patient who either received the antibiotic or the placebo, and this patient's clinical course was worse when receiving the placebo. Madden et al[16] conducted a randomized, double-blind, placebo-controlled crossover trial of oral metronidazole or placebo. Eleven of 13 patients completed the trial. The mean stool frequency decreased significantly in these patients while they received the active drug.

Topical metronidazole is an option to reduce the side effects of oral metronidazole. In an open-label study of 11 patients, liquid suspension of 40 mg of metronidazole was instilled into the pouch. All 11 improved and none experienced any side effects. Another option is to use vaginal preparations of metronidazole and to administer them through the anus. All six patients thus treated had improvement of symptoms. One patient experienced side effects similar to that occurring with use of oral metronidazole.

Alternatives to the use of metronidazole are ciprofloxacin or amoxicillin/clavulanic acid. For those patients who are on maintenance therapy, cycling of multiple antibiotics at weekly intervals can help overcome bacterial resistance. There have been no controlled trials using these agents.

Second-line treatment options for pouchitis include use of topical mesalamine, oral mesalamine, and sulfasalazine. The bacterial concentrations in the pouch are sufficient to break down the azobond of sulfasalazine. The use of these agents is based on uncontrolled studies and anecdotal experiences.

Corticosteroids are options to consider, although use of corticosteroids in a topical fashion (as opposed to oral) will help reduce systemic side effects. Ten patients showed improvement with the use of budesonide suppositories (not currently available in the United States). Caution must be borne in the long-term use of topical steroids for chronic pouchitis, since a significant amount of systemic absorption may potentially occur.

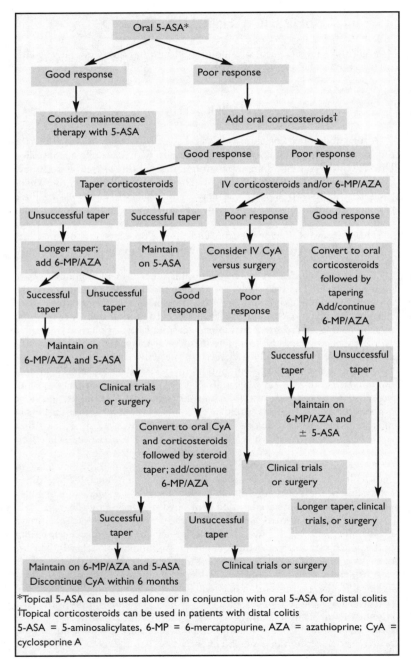

Figure 14-1. Management algorithm for mildly to moderately active ulcerative colitis.

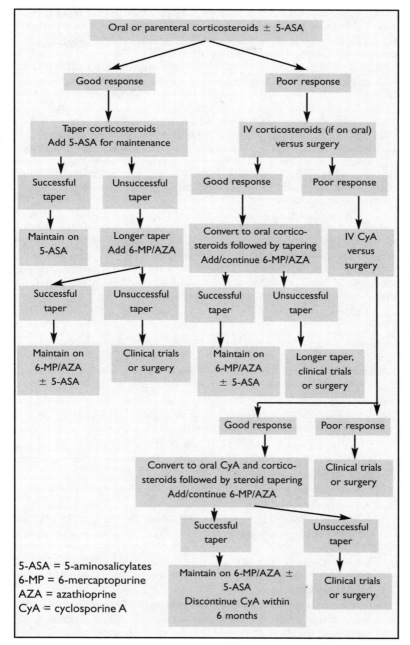

Figure 14-2. Management algorithm for severely active ulcerative colitis.

Some have reported benefit with the use of AZA. However, in 11 patients who had both an IPAA and had undergone liver transplantation for primary sclerosing cholangitis, 45% still experienced symptoms of chronic pouchitis even though they were heavily immunosuppressed.

Use of probiotics is another option. A recent study randomized 40 patients with quiescent chronic pouchitis to either placebo or an oral probiotic bacterial formula (VSL#3 is currently available at www.VSL3.com in the United States) for a 9-month period. Fifteen percent of the treatment group versus 100% of the placebo group experienced a flare of pouchitis.

No benefit has been shown with the use of short-chain fatty acid enemas in chronic pouchitis. This is possibly related to the fact that it is not as important in maintenance of ileal mucosal homeostasis in contrast to colonic mucosal homeostasis. Butyrate, propionate, and acetate account for 90% of the short-chain fatty acids present in the colon. Butyrate accounts for 70% of the oxygen utilization of the colonocytes.

Even though an open label study showed benefit with the use of bismuth carbomer enemas, a randomized, double-blind, placebo-controlled study failed to show benefit. In contrast use of chewable bismuth subsalicylate showed symptom improvement in 11 of 13 patients during a 4-week treatment trial.

Allopurinol, which prevents the formation of oxygen-free radicals, has been shown to be beneficial in seven of 14 patients treated. This was an uncontrolled, non-randomized, nonplacebo controlled trial.

REFERENCES

1. Faubion WA, Loftus EV, Harmsen WS, Zinsmeister AR, Sandborn WJ. The natural history of corticosteroid therapy for inflammatory bowel disease: a population based study. *Gastroenterology.* 2001;121:255-260.

2. Jewell DP, Truelove SC. Azathioprine in ulcerative colitis: final report on controlled therapeutic trial. *Br Med J.* 1974;4:627-630.

3. Caprilli R, Carratu R, Babbini M. Double blind comparison of the effectiveness of azathioprine and sulfasalazine in idiopathic proctocolitis. Preliminary report. *Am J Dig Dis.* 1975;20:115-120.

4. Kirk AP, Lennard-Jones JE. A controlled trial of azathioprine in chronic ulcerative colitis. *Br Med J.* 1982;284:1291-1292.

5. Rosenberg JL, Wall AJ, Levin B, Binder HJ, Kirsner JB. A controlled trial of azathioprine in the management of chronic ulcerative colitis. *Gastroenterology.* 1975;69:96-99.

6. Svaoni F, Bonassi U, Bagnolo F, et al. Effectiveness of cyclosporine A (CsA) in the treatment of active refractory ulcerative colitis (UC). *Gastroenterology.* 1998;114:A1096.

7. D'Haens G, Lemmens L, Geboes K, et al. Intravenous cyclosporine versus intravenous corticosteroids as single therapy for severe attacks of ulcerative colitis. *Gastroenterology.* 2001;120:1323-1329.

8. Sands BE, Tremaine WJ, Sandborn WJ, et al. Infliximab in the treatment of severe, steroid-refractory ulcerative colitis: a pilot study. *Inflamm Bowel Dis.* 2001;7:83-88.

9. Chey WY, Hussain A, Ryan C, Potter GD, Shah A. Infliximab for refractory ulcerative colitis. *Am J Gastroenterol.* 2001;96:2373-2381.

10. Su C, Salzberg BA, Lewis JD, et al. Efficacy of anti-tumor necrosis factor therapy in patients with ulcerative colitis. *Am J Gastroenterol.* 2002;97:2577-2584.

11. Lashner BA, Hanauer SB, Silverstein MD. Testing nicotine gum for ulcerative colitis patients. Experience with single-patient trials. *Dig Dis Sci.* 1990;35:827-832.

12. Dwarakanath AD, Yu LG, Brookes C, et al. "Sticky" neutrophils, pathergic arthritis, and response to heparin in pyoderma gangrenosum complicating ulcerative colitis. *Gut.* 1995;37:585-588.

13. Brazier F, Yzet T, Duchman J, et al. Effect of heparin treatment on extraintestinal manifestations associated with inflammatory bowel disease. *Gastroenterology.* 1996;110:A872.

14. Panes J, Esteve M, Cabre E, et al. Comparison of heparin and steroids in the treatment of moderate and severe ulcerative colitis. *Gastroenterology.* 2000;119:903-908.

15. Ang YS, Mahmud N, White B, et al. Randomized comparison of unfractionated heparin with corticosteroids in severe active inflammatory bowel disease. *Aliment Pharmacol Ther.* 2000;14:1015-1022.

16. Madden MV, McIntyre AS, Nicholls RJ. Double-blind crossover trial of metronidazole versus placebo in chronic unremitting pouchitis. *Dig Dis Sci.* 1994;39:1193-1196.

BIBLIOGRAPHY

Alder DJ, Korelitz BI. The therapeutic efficacy of 6-mercaptopurine in refractory ulcerative colitis. *Am J Gastroenterol.* 1990;85:717-722.

Baron JH, Connell AM, Lennard-Jones JE, Jones FA. Sulfasalazine and salicylazosulfadimidine in ulcerative colitis. *Lancet.* 1962;1:1094-1096.

Cohen RD, Stein R, Hanauer SB. Intravenous cyclosporin in ulcerative colitis: a five-year experience. *Am J Gastroenterol.* 1999;94:1587-1592.

D'Albasio G, Pacini F, Camarri E, et al. Combined therapy with 5-aminosalicylic acid tablets and enemas for maintaining remission in ulcerative colitis: a randomized double-blind study. *Am J Gastroenterol.* 1997;92:1143-1147.

Fellermann K, Ludwig D, Stahl M, David-Walek T, Stange EF. Steroid-unresponsive acute attacks of inflammatory bowel disease: immunomodulation by Tacrolimus (FK506). *Am J Gastroenterol.* 1998;93:1860-1866.

George J, Present DH, Pou R, Bodian C, Rubin PH. The long-term outcome of ulcerative colitis treated with 6-mercaptopurine. *Am J Gastroenterol.* 1996;91:1711-1714.

Gionchetti P, Rizzello F, Venturi A, et al. Oral bacteriotherapy as maintenance treatment in patients with chronic pouchitis: a double-blind, placebo-controlled trial. *Gastroenterology.* 2000;119:305-309.

Green JRB, Lobo AJ, Holdsworth CD, Abacus Investigator Group, et al. Balsalazide is more effective and better tolerated than mesalamine in the treatment of acute ulcerative colitis. *Gastroenterology.* 1998;114:15-22.

Hanauer SB. Dose-ranging study of mesalamine (Pentasa) enemas of acute ulcerative proctosigmoiditis: results of a multicentered placebo-controlled trial. *Inflamm Bowel Dis.* 1998;4:79-83.

Hawthorne AB, Logan RFA, Hawkey CJ, et al. Randomized controlled trial of azathioprine withdrawal in ulcerative colitis. *Br Med J.* 1992;305:20-22.

Kam L, Cohen H, Dooley C, Rubin P, Orchard J. A comparison of mesalamine suspension enema and oral sulfasalazine for treatment of active distal ulcerative colitis in adults. *Am J Gastroenterol.* 1996;91:1338-1342.

Katz J, Lichtenstein G, Kennan G, Healy D, Jacobs S. Outcome of pregnancy in women receiving Remicade (infliximab) for the treatment of Crohn's disease or rheumatoid arthritis. *Gastroenterology.* 2001;120:A69.

Kornbluth A, Present DH, Lichtiger S, et al. Cyclosporin for severe ulcerative colitis: a user's guide. *Am J Gastroenterol.* 1997; 92:1424-1428.

Kornbluth A, Sachar DB. Ulcerative colitis practice guidelines in adults. *Am J Gastroenterol.* 1997;92:204-211.

Lichtiger S, Present DH, Kornbluth A, et al. Cyclosporin in severe ulcerative colitis refractory to steroid therapy. *N Engl J Med.* 1994;330:841-845.

Lofberg R, Dannielsson A, Suhr O, et al. Oral budesonide versus prednisolone in patients with active extensive and left-sided colitis. *Gastroenterology.* 1996;110:1713-1718.

Marshall JK, Irvine EJ. Rectal aminosalicylate therapy for distal ulcerative colitis: a meta-analysis. *Aliment Pharmacol Ther.* 1995;9:293-300.

Marshall JK, Irvine EJ. Rectal corticosteroids versus alternative treatment in ulcerative colitis: a meta-analysis. *Gut.* 1997;40:775-781.

Neurath MF, Wanitschke R, Peters M, et al. Mycophenolate mofetil for treatment of active inflammatory bowel disease. Clinical and immunological studies. *Ann N Y Acad Sci.* 1998;859:315-318.

Nygaard K, Bergan T, Bjorkneklett A, et al. Topical metronidazole treatment in pouchitis. *Scand J Gastroenterol.* 1994;29:462-467.

Oren R, Arber N, Odes S, et al. Methotrexate in chronic active ulcerative colitis: a double-blind, randomized, Israeli multi-center trial. *Gastroenterology.* 1996;110:1416-1421.

Present DH, Meltzer SJ, Krumholz MP, Wolke A, Korelitz BI. 6-mercaptopurine in the management of inflammatory bowel disease: short- and long-term toxicity. *Ann Intern Med.* 1989;111:641-649.

Rembacken BJ, Snelling AM, Hawkey PM, et al. Nonpathogenic E. coli versus mesalazine for the treatment of ulcerative colitis: a randomized trial. *Lancet.* 1999;354:635-639.

Safdi M, DeMicco M, Sninsky C, et al. A double-blind comparison of oral versus rectal mesalamine versus combination therapy in the treatment of distal ulcerative colitis. *Am J Gastroenterol.* 1997;92:1867-1871.

Sandborn WJ. Nicotine therapy for ulcerative colitis: a review of rationale, mechanisms, pharmacology, and clinical results. *Am J Gastroenterol.* 1999;94:1161-1171.

Sandborn WJ, McLeod R, Jewell DP. Medical therapy for the induction and maintenance of remission in pouchitis: a systematic review. *Inflamm Bowel Dis.* 1999;5:33-39.

Sandborn WJ, Tremaine WJ, Schroeder KW, et al. A placebo-controlled trial of cyclosporine enemas for mildly to moderately active left-sided ulcerative colitis. *Gastroenterology.* 1994;106:1429-1435.

Schreiber S, Fedorak RN, Wild G, et al. Safety and tolerance of rHuIL-10 treatment in patients with mild/moderate active ulcerative colitis. *Gastroenterology.* 1998;114:A1080.

Schroeder KW, Tremaine WJ, Ilstrup DM. Coated oral 5-aminosalicylic acid therapy for mildly to moderately active ulcerative colitis. *N Engl J Med.* 1987;317:1625-1629.

Srinivasan R. Infliximab treatment and pregnancy outcome in active Crohn's disease. *Am J Gastroenterol.* 2001;96:2274-2275.

Sutherland LR, Martin F, Greer S, et al. 5-aminosalicylic acid enema in the treatment of distal ulcerative colitis, proctosigmoiditis, and proctitis. *Gastroenterology.* 1987;92:1894-1898.

Sutherland LR, May GR, Shaffer EA. Sulfasalazine revisited: a meta-analysis of 5-aminosalicylic acid in the treatment of ulcerative colitis. *Ann Intern Med.* 1993;118:540-549.

Sutherland L, Roth D, Beck P, May G, Makiyama K. Oral 5-aminosalicylic acid for inducing remission in ulcerative colitis. *Cochrane Database Syst Rev.* 2000;(2):CD000543.

Torkvist L, Thorlacius H, Sjoqvist U, et al. Low molecular weight heparin as adjuvant therapy in active ulcerative colitis. *Aliment Pharmacol Ther.* 1999;13:1323-1328.

Truelove SC, Witts LJ. Cortisone in ulcerative colitis: final report on a therapeutic trial. *Br Med J.* 1955;2:1041-1048.

Turunen UM, Farkkila MA, Hakala K, et al. Long-term treatment of ulcerative colitis with ciprofloxacin: a prospective, double-blind, placebo-controlled study. *Gastroenterology.* 1998;115:1072-1078.

Vrij AA, Jansen JM, Schoon EJ, de Bruine A, Hemker HC, Stockbrugger RW. Low molecular weight heparin treatment in steroid refractory ulcerative colitis: clinical outcome and influence on mucosal capillary thrombi. *Scand J Gastroenterol Suppl.* 2001;234:41-47.

chapter 15

Disease Modifiers in Inflammatory Bowel Disease

Jaime Oviedo, MD and Francis A. Farraye, MD, MSc

INTRODUCTION

In addition to the diagnosis and medical management of patients with inflammatory bowel disease (IBD), careful attention should be paid to the environmental, health maintenance, and lifestyle factors that can modify the course, complications, and severity of the disease. Several of these factors have been identified and have become increasingly relevant for physicians, as well as for patients who often seek to assume a more active role in the management of their disease. An approach that includes discussion and education on lifestyle and environmental issues affecting IBD patients should be part of our routine practice. This chapter reviews the available evidence surrounding the influence of such factors on the natural history and course of IBD.

INFECTIONS AND IBD

Clinical observations and animal experiments have suggested that intestinal bacteria may trigger and perpetuate chronic bowel inflammation. It is now

---

Table 15-1

INFECTIOUS AGENTS POSSIBLY LINKED TO THE OCCURRENCE OF IBD

Bacterial

- *Mycobacterium paratuberculosis*[3]
- *Listeria*[4]
- Pharyngitis and otitis media[15]

Viral

- Unspecified childhood gastroenteritis
- Measles[5]
- Mumps[7]
- Influenza[6]
- Varicella[6]

Parasites

- Helminthic parasites[1]

---

increasingly clear that IBD represents the outcome of three essential interactive cofactors: host susceptibility, enteric microflora, and mucosal immunity. In addition to the capacity to respond to episodic challenge from pathogens, the mucosal immune system has the ability to recognize, tolerate, and avoid reacting against nonpathogenic intestinal bacteria. In susceptible individuals, a breakdown in the regulatory constraints of the mucosal immune responses to enteric bacteria may result in the development of IBD.[1]

Since the 1950s infectious agents have been proposed to be causally related to the occurrence of IBD.[2] A wide range of different microorganisms, including *Mycobacterium paratuberculosis*[3]; *Listeria*[4]; unspecified childhood gastroenteritis; and viral infections such as measles,[5] influenza, and varicella,[6] have been linked with either ulcerative colitis (UC), Crohn's disease (CD), or both (Table 15-1).

The association between exposure to measles and other viruses and the onset of IBD was described as early as 1950; however, the data supporting these associations have become increasingly controversial. In a British cohort study,[7] mumps infection before 2 years of age was found to be a risk for UC (odds ratio [OR], 25.12; 95% confidence interval [CI], 6.35 to 99.36). Similarly, measles and mumps infections in the same year of life were significantly associated with UC and CD (OR 7.47, CI 2.42 to 23.06 and 4.27, and CI 1.24 to 14.46, respectively). These relationships were reported to be independent of each other as well as of sex, social class at birth, household crowding in childhood, and family history of IBD. No significant relationship between measles infection or vaccination at a young age and later IBD was found in this cohort. However, mumps infection and exposure to monovalent measles vaccination within the same year was associated with a significantly increased risk of CD. An increased incidence of IBD following concurrent epidemics of mumps and measles has also been reported in other parts of the world.[8] However, the findings from other populations,[9] as well as microbiologic studies, do not support the relationship between viral infections or vaccinations and IBD. A recent study showed no significant differences in the titers of serum antimumps IgG in IBD patients when compared to healthy controls.[10,11] Similarly, studies using amplification techniques found no evidence of mumps viral genome in intestinal mucosa or peripheral lymphocytes of patients with IBD.[12-14]

Other childhood infections have also been postulated as a potential factor associated with the development of IBD. In a population study from North Carolina, patients with CD were more likely to report an increased frequency of childhood infections in general (OR 4.67, 95% CI 2.65 to 8.23), and pharyngitis specifically (OR 2.14, 95% CI 1.30 to 3.51), as well as treatment with antibiotics for both otitis media (OR 2.07, 95% CI 1.03 to 4.14) and pharyngitis (OR 2.14, 95% CI 1.20 to 3.84). Persons with UC also reported an excess of infections in general (odds ratio 2.37, 95% CI 1.19-4.71), but not an excess of specific infections or treatments with antibiotics. Persons who reported an increased frequency of infections tended to have an earlier onset of CD (p <0.0001) and UC (p = 0.04).[15]

Reduced immunologic exposure to helminthic parasites has also been proposed as a potential factor to explain the increased incidence of CD in industrialized societies when compared to developing countries.[1] Colonization with pathogenically attenuated helminths has been used to switch the mucosal cytokine profile in patients with CD and was associated with improvement in Crohn's disease activity index (CDAI) scores in a small open-label trial.[16]

The role of the normal intestinal flora in the development and progression of IBD has generated considerable interest. It is possible that products of the commensal flora promote inflammation in the presence of an impaired mucosal barrier or injury to the mucosa. Growing evidence suggests that a change in the quantity or quality of bacterial luminal content may lead to the induction or persistence of mucosal inflammation.[17] The manipulation of the normal intestinal flora with antibiotics or with other nonpathogenic organisms (ie, probiotics) appears to be the obvious method to modify mucosal cytokine balance and inflammatory response. Antibiotics have been shown to be beneficial in the treatment of perianal and colonic CD and pouchitis[1]; however, their efficacy in the treatment of uncomplicated CD is less clear. The role of antibiotics in the therapy of IBD is discussed in Chapter 18.

In general, the available evidence does not suggest that IBD is an infectious disease or a self-antigen-specific autoimmune disease. Recent findings increasingly suggest that tissue damage might be caused by nonspecific inflammation, which is driven by common, ubiquitous microbial agents derived from the bacterial flora in the intestinal lumen.[18]

INFECTIONS THAT MAY MIMIC IBD

Infectious causes should always be considered in the differential diagnosis of patients presenting with diarrhea. The initial distinction between infectious diarrhea and IBD may be difficult because the symptoms may be very similar. Diarrhea can be bloody or nonbloody and associated with abdominal pain or cramps, fever, and occasionally arthralgias. An acute onset of diarrhea, large number of bowel movements, and early fever are typically in favor of an infectious etiology. Conversely, IBD has a more insidious onset with less frequent bowel movements, and early fever is uncommon. Although the endoscopic appearance is rarely diagnostic, mucosal biopsies may be useful in distinguishing acute self-limited, infectious-type colitis from IBD. Biopsies of patients with infectious colitis typically show a preserved mucosal architecture. IBD, on the other hand, leads to chronic architectural changes and infiltration of the lamina propria by inflammatory cells.[19] A careful examination of the biopsy specimens by an experienced pathologist is instrumental to assure the correct diagnosis and avoid the use of unnecessary treatments with potential serious side effects in cases of self-limited colitis. In certain situations, only time and a close follow-up—both clinical, and occasionally endoscopic—will provide the correct diagnosis.

In general, any pathogen that causes invasive enterocolitis can present with bloody diarrhea that may mimic IBD (Table 15-2). The infectious agents commonly seen in practice are discussed next.

Campylobacter jejuni

Campylobacter jejuni is the most commonly identified bacterial pathogen in cases of diarrhea in the United States, accounting for over 2.4 million cases annually.[20] *Campylobacter* is usually acquired from contaminated food or water, and most often from undercooked poultry, particularly grilled, barbecued, or fried broiler chicken. Ileal disease can simulate appendicitis, and up to 50% of patients may present with rectal bleeding and tenesmus similar to ulcerative proctitis. The demonstration of *C. jejuni* or other *Campylobacter* species by stool culture is the single most important diagnostic test. Therapy for acute *Campylobacter* infections should be based on the severity of the disease. Mild symptoms in healthy adults can be treated at home, while severe infections in infants, elderly, or immunosuppressed patients may require aggressive inpatient therapy.[21,22]

SALMONELLA

Salmonella sp invade and replicate in the ileal mucosa. Bacteremia can develop following replication, resulting in infection at distal sites. Several distinctive syndromes, including typhoid fever, gastroenteritis, septicemia, arteritis, as well as various focal infections and chronic carrier states, may occur. The source of the organism is usually contaminated water, poultry, eggs, milk, and foods containing raw or powdered eggs or milk, such as mayonnaise. The most

Table 15-2

INFECTIONS THAT MAY MIMIC IBD

Bacteria

- *Campylobacter jejuni*
- *Salmonella sp*
- *Shigella sp*
- *E. coli 0157:H7*
- *Yersinia sp*
- *Aeromonas* and *Plesiomonas*
- *Clostridium difficile*
- Chlamydia
- *Listeria monocytogenes*

Parasites

- Entamoeba histolytica
- Anisakis simplex

Viruses

- Cytomegalovirus

Fungi

- Histoplasm capsulatum

common manifestation of salmonella infection is diarrhea, which is usually watery. Less commonly, a colitis picture with frequent, small volume, bloody diarrhea and tenesmus may occur. Antibiotic therapy is indicated in severe illness, septicemia, extremes of age, and immunosuppression.[22,23]

SHIGELLA

Shigella sp are transmitted by the fecal-oral route, which make them highly contagious for humans. Outbreaks related to contaminated food and water occasionally occur. The most common vehicle for foodborne transmission is salad, usually related to a breech in hygienic practices by an infected food handler. A dramatic decline in the incidence of shigellosis in the United States has followed the improvements in hygiene and socioeconomic conditions. Most cases of shigellosis in the United States are due to *S. sonnei*. *Shigella* locally invades the colon, especially the left colon, causing watery diarrhea that progresses within a few hours or days to frank dysentery with abdominal cramps and tenesmus. In severe cases, patients may pass 20 or more bowel movements per day. Antibiotic therapy may have a role in interrupting person-to-person transmission and has been shown to reduce disease severity and duration.[22,24]

ESCHERICHIA COLI

E. coli 0157:H7 has been implicated in multiple foodborne epidemics of bloody diarrhea and hemorrhagic colitis associated with ingestion of under-cooked ground beef, hamburgers, unpasteurized apple juice, lettuce, milk, and salami. Colitis is due to both bacterial invasion and toxin production causing watery diarrhea, which later becomes bloody and may be associated with severe abdominal pain. In addition to IBD, the differential diagnosis includes ischemic colitis, especially in elderly individuals. Hemolytic-uremic syndrome (HUS) is a potential complication and occurs in 5% of the cases, mostly children.[22,25] The use of antidiarrheals and antibiotics appears to be a risk factor for the development of HUS.[26] Although it is recommended to avoid antibiotic therapy, antibiotics are frequently given empirically to seriously ill individuals before the results of stool cultures reveal the presence of the organism.

YERSINIA

Y. enterocolitica and *Y. pseudotuberculosis* are uncommon in the United States but frequent in northern Europe. The organisms cause ileocolitis and can simulate appendicitis. The clinical presentation is indistinguishable in up to 20% of patients subsequently shown to have *Yersinia* infection. The diarrhea due to *Y. enterocolitica* is usually watery. Bloody diarrhea may occur in up to 25% of cases. Due to the invasive nature of the organism and the potential to cause serious systemic illness, antibiotic therapy is indicated for prolonged cases. Diarrhea may sometimes be accompanied by a large joint arthropathy simulating the arthritis of IBD.[22]

AEROMONAS and PLESIOMONAS

A. hydrophila, a waterborne pathogen, and *P. shigelloides,* from shellfish, most frequently raw oysters, can cause acute colitis. Cases of chronic colitis following infection with either of these pathogens have also been reported.[22]

CLOSTRIDIUM DIFFICILE

C. difficile colitis occurs either as a hospital-acquired infection or as a complication of antibiotics that have altered the normal flora allowing the overgrowth and toxin production by the bacteria. The diarrhea is usually watery, but blood can be seen in severe cases. Typical pseudomembranes are not always present. The diagnosis is usually confirmed by the detection of the toxin in the stool.[22]

CHLAMYDIA

Lymphogranuloma venereum (LGV) serotypes of of *Chlamydia trachomatis* are transmitted by anoreceptive sexual activity and may produce rectal infections presenting with fever, pain, tenesmus, and a mucoid or bloody discharge. Persistent disease, especially in homosexual men, may lead to rectal strictures. Less virulent non-LGV strains cause a milder form of proctitis. Endoscopic findings are varied and may be confused with those seen in IBD, especially CD. The rectal mucosa may appear nodular or cobblestoned with erythema, friability, and ulceration. The histopathological features include crypt abscesses, granulomata, and giant cells; these findings are similar to those seen in CD.[27]

LISTERIA

Listeria monocytogenes has been increasingly implicated as a cause of febrile gastroenteritis with about 2500 cases per year in the United States. Neonates, the elderly, pregnant women, and patients with cell-mediated immune deficiency, such as those with HIV infection or on steroid therapy, appear to be at increased risk. However, there have also been reports of outbreaks in the immunocompetent host. Diarrhea usually lasts 1 to 2 days and is typically watery. *Listeria* outbreaks have been associated with a wide range of food products, including pasteurized milk, soft cheeses, shellfish, raw vegetables, and hotdogs. Early reports suggested that *Listeria monocytogenes* may have the potential to cause IBD.[4,28] Recently, this theory has lost strength when studies utilizing tissue culture and polymerase-chain reaction (PCR) have not found the bacteria in biopsy specimens from IBD patients.[29]

AMEBIC COLITIS

Entamoeba histolytica can cause an acute colitis that may simulate IBD. Amebic colitis should be considered in the diagnosis of bloody diarrhea, especially in travelers, homosexual males, or immigrants from endemic areas. Occasionally, fulminant amebic colitis and bowel perforation may follow the administration of steroids in individuals previously infested with the parasite. Diagnosis is usually made by the combination of stool examination, serology, and colonoscopy with biopsies.[22]

CYTOMEGALOVIRUS

Gastrointestinal cytomegalovirus (CMV) infection is uncommon in immunocompetent individuals. Immunocompromised patients, especially those with HIV/AIDS or bone marrow or organ transplantation, cancer patients receiving chemotherapy, elderly patients, and patients on chronic steroid therapy are at risk for CMV infection. Infections of the anorectal area can cause ulcerative lesions or diffuse proctocolitis. The diagnosis of CMV may require several tests. Serology is helpful in assessing acute or chronic infection. An elevated or rising IgM titer suggests current infection. The presence of intranuclear inclusion bodies within endothelial cells, histiocytes, and macrophages in colonic biopsy specimens is pathognomonic. When CMV infection is documented, antiviral therapy with ganciclovir should be instituted and concurrent immunosuppressive therapy discontinued.[22,27]

ANISAKIDAE

Consumption of raw fish, which has become increasingly popular, may result in infection with larval nematodes of the family *Anisakidae*. Commonly infected fish include mackerel, rockfish, salmon, and true herring. Ingestion of raw fish contaminated with *Anisakis simplex* results in acute severe abdominal pain, which is often violent and may require laparotomy. Clinically, anisakiasis may mimic appendicitis or even CD. There is no effective medical treatment; however, endoscopic removal of the larvae with biopsy forceps is therapeutic.[25]

HISTOPLASMOSIS

Histoplasma capsulatum may invade the terminal ileum in patients with disseminated histoplasmosis. Initial symptoms usually include diarrhea, fever, and abdominal pain. Ileocecal involvement leads to obstructive symptoms and weight loss. The diagnosis should be considered in immunocompromised hosts or in travelers from endemic areas such as the Ohio River Valley. Endoscopy reveals discrete ileal and colonic ulcers and biopsy specimens may show granulomata. The diagnosis is confirmed by identification of the organism by biopsy, culture, or serology.[30]

INFECTIONS THAT MAY AGGRAVATE IBD

Although there is no evidence suggesting that patients with IBD are more susceptible to gastrointestinal (GI) infections than healthy subjects, infections with any of the common enteric pathogens previously mentioned may worsen or exacerbate pre-existing IBD.

Similarly, due to the frequent use of antibiotics, steroids, and immunosuppressive therapy for the treatment of patients with IBD, infections such as *C. difficile* and CMV are commonly seen in these patients and should be considered when dealing with exacerbations of the disease.

C. difficile

Patients with IBD are not more likely to carry *C. difficile*, unless they have recently received antibiotics. Early reports implicated *C. difficile* in the development of IBD exacerbations.[31,32] However, other studies[33,34] have not confirmed this association. Patients with IBD, especially those with complications of CD including abscesses, fistulas, and perianal disease, are frequently treated with antibiotic therapy; therefore, they may be more likely to develop antibiotic-associated diarrhea and *C. difficile* infection. The course of *C. difficile* related disease may also be more severe in IBD patients receiving concurrent steroid or immunosuppressive therapy.

CYTOMEGALOVIRUS

CMV infection may aggravate the course of refractory IBD and should be suspected in patients who fail to respond or experience worsening of symptoms despite immunosuppressive therapy.[35] CMV disease in immunocompromised IBD patients can present as a typical exacerbation of IBD, or less commonly, as a mononucleosis-like syndrome or atypical pneumonitis. Unrecognized CMV infection in patients with IBD may lead to fulminant disease, requiring colectomy. CMV infection should be considered in IBD patients with systemic symptoms and signs such as high fevers, dyspnea, lymphadenopathy, or splenomegaly, as well as in those whose bowel disease is unresponsive to steroids and those who develop worsening of clinical symptoms following an initial improvement on immunosuppressive therapy.[35]

A high index of suspicion, early diagnosis, and prompt intervention are thus necessary to prevent major complications and possibly mortality. Treatment with ganciclovir leads to significant clinical improvement in about 70% of the cases.[36] Foscarnet is indicated in the treatment of ganciclovir-resistant patients.

In general, it is possible that GI infection may either precipitate, unmask, or worsen IBD in otherwise predisposed individuals. There is also a small proportion of cases in which a previously healthy patient developed a documented infectious colitis in which symptoms do not resolve despite the eradication of the inciting organism and may evolve into UC or CD.[37]

Infectious factors may significantly modify the course and severity of IBD. Accordingly, patients with newly diagnosed UC or acute flares of CD should be evaluated for the possibility of a complicating enteric infection.[38] Active infections should be treated, and the medical regimen should be adjusted to control acute flares. The recommendations for treatment of selected enteric pathogens are summarized in Table 15-3. Individuals with IBD, like any other person, should be instructed to adopt simple measures to assure food safety (Table 15-4).

PROBIOTICS

Based on their ability to prevent the overgrowth of potentially pathogenic organisms and stimulate the intestinal immune defense system,[39] probiotics are being increasingly used as an adjuvant or alternative therapy for intestinal disorders particularly IBD, *C. difficile* infection, and antibiotic-associated diarrhea. Probiotics are live, nonpathogenic microbial food ingredients, usually of the genera *Bifidobacterium* or *Lactobacillus*, that alter the enteric flora and have been associated with beneficial effects on human health. Some noninvasive coliforms and nonbacterial organisms such as *Saccharomyces boulardii* may also be categorized as probiotics.[1] In two controlled studies,[40,41] a nonpathogenic strain of *E. coli* was as effective as a 5-aminosalicylic acid (5-ASA) preparation maintaining remission in patients with UC. Probiotic combinations have also shown impressive results in the treatment of chronic pouchitis, reducing the

Table 15-3

SUGGESTED TREATMENT OF SELECTED ENTERIC PATHOGENS

Campylobacter s.	Rehydration, fluoroquinolones[a], macrolides, or doxycycline
Salmonella sp.	Rehydrate, avoid antibiotics in uncomplicated cases; treat bacteremia, focal infections, or high risk hosts[b] with fluoroquinolones[a] or third-generation cephalosporin
Shigella spp.	Rehydration, TMP-SMX, or erythromycin
E. coli 0157:H7	Rehydration, supportive care
Yersinia enterocolitica	Rehydration, fluoroquinolones[a], TMP-SMX, or doxycycline, if not severe
Aeromonas and Plesiomonas	Fluoroquinolones[a], TMP-SMX, or third-generation cephalosporin
C. difficile	Metronidazole 250 mg orally four times a day (qid) or 500 mg IV every 8 hours for 10 days. Oral vancomycin 125 mg orally qid for 10 days in severe or fulminant colitis, or metronidazole intolerance/treatment failure
Chlamydia	Azithromycin 1 g oral single dose or doxycycline 100 mg orally twice a day (bid) for 7 days
Listeria monocytogenes	Ampicillin
Entamoeba histolytica	Metronidazole 750 mg orally three times a day (tid) for 10 days, followed by diiodohydroxyquin 650 mg orally tid for 20 days
Cytomegalovirus	Ganciclovir or foscarnet

[a]Fluoroquinolones are contraindicated for pregnant women and children under 17 years of age
[b]High-risk patients include those with HIV infection and lymphoproliferative disease

Adapted from LaMont JT. *Gastrointestinal Infections. Diagnosis and Management.* New York, NY: Marcel Dekker Inc; 1997.

Table 15-4

MEASURES TO PREVENT FOODBORNE INFECTIONS

- Wash hands and cooking surfaces often
- Separate raw meat, poultry, and seafood to avoid cross-contamination
- Cook at proper temperatures
- Do not consume raw or undercooked food
- Refrigerate perishables, prepared food, and leftovers

Adapted from Partnership for Food Safety Education. *Four steps.* Available at: http://www.fightbac.org. Accessed August 29, 2002.

relapse rate by up to 85% when compared to placebo.[42] In CD, an open-label study of approximately 20 patients with mildly to moderately active disease showed that probiotics reduced the need for corticosteroid therapy in over 75% of the cases and were safe and well tolerated.[43]

Although patients find the concept of using dietary probiotic supplements appealing, more well-designed, controlled clinical trials are required to clarify the role of these agents in the management of IBD. Based on the available evidence, probiotics should not be routinely recommended for the treatment of IBD but may be considered in patients with pouchitis. Patients should also be cautioned to avoid excessive expense and potential risks from dubious sources of probiotic preparations.[1]

ENVIRONMENTAL FACTORS

SMOKING

Smoking is the best characterization of an environmental factor that can affect the severity and natural history of IBD. Smoking cigarettes is associated with an increased prevalence of CD, while nonsmoking is associated with UC. There is also strong evidence suggesting that smoking cigarettes has a negative effect on the course of CD, and may improve the disease severity or have a "protective" effect in some patients with UC.[44]

Smoking and UC

UC is predominantly a disease of nonsmokers. Several meta-analysis as well as observational and case-control studies have confirmed that the relative risk of colitis is reduced in smokers when compared to people who have never smoked and to individuals who have quit smoking.[45] The incidence of UC in the Mormon community in which smoking is discouraged is five-fold higher than the general population.[46,47] Lifetime nonsmokers are almost three times more likely to have UC than current smokers.[48] Furthermore, approximately two-thirds of former smokers with UC develop the disease after quitting smoking with a particularly high incidence in the first few years.[49-51]

Smoking appears to have an effect in the clinical course of UC. A significant proportion of patients report that their colitis improves while smoking 20 cigarettes daily. Similarly, smokers with UC report fewer bowel complaints than their nonsmoking counterparts.[52] Most of the available evidence also supports the concept that smoking is a significant disease modifier in UC. Several studies have found lower hospitalization rates in patients smoking at the onset of colitis, higher colectomy rates in ex-smokers who gave up smoking before the onset of their colitis,[53] reduced rates of clinical relapse in patients who began smoking after diagnosis,[54] and reduced incidence of pouchitis in smokers following proctocolectomy.[55] Conversely, smoking cessation is usually followed by a statistically significant increase in disease severity, hospitalization rate, and need for major medical therapy, when compared to smoking continuation.[56]

Smoking and CD

Smoking is a well-recognized risk factor for CD.[48] Compared with nonsmokers, patients with CD who smoke suffer more clinical relapses,[52,57,58] develop more complications,[59] are operated on more often,[44,60] and require more immunosuppressive therapy.[61,62] Conversely, patients with CD have higher rates of tobacco use than than the general population.[48,63]

There is also some evidence suggesting that the harmful effects of smoking in CD abate after smoking cessation. Patients who quit smoking have a decreased risk of relapse,[64,65] and postoperative recurrence when compared to current smokers.[60] On the basis of these associations, smoking cessation is a potential therapy for CD. However, many patients are unaware of the risk of worsening their CD by smoking and do not recall their physician ever telling them about these risks.[66] Although it has been suggested that CD patients are poorly receptive to smoking cessation advice,[67] which may explain why more efforts are not made to get these patients to quit, the percentages of people considering and attempting to quit are similar to those reported in other groups of smokers in the general population. Therefore, there is no evidence to conclude that patients with CD are any more refractory to smoking cessation than smokers in the general population.

Although remaining abstinent is also as difficult for people with CD as it is for the smokers in the general population, the benefits of smoking cessation in individuals with CD justify every effort involved in achieving smoking cessation. Patients who successfully quit smoking for more than 1 year seem to significantly reduce their risk of experiencing a flare, as well as the need for the use of steroids or immunomodulators when compared to continuing smokers.[68]

Table 15-5

EFFECTS OF SMOKING AND SMOKING CESSATION ON IBD

	Crohn's Disease	*Ulcerative Colitis*
Smoking	Increased prevalence Negative effect • More relapses • Increased complications • More surgeries • Increased need for use of immuno-modulators	Decreased prevalence "Protective effect" • Less flare-ups • Reduced hospitalizations • Reduced colectomy rates • Reduced incidence of pouchitis
Smoking cessation	• Decreased risk of relapse and post-operative recurrence • Decreased risk for steroids and immuno-modulators	• Increased disease activity • Increased need for hospitalization, steroids, and immunomodulators • Increased need for colectomy

Despite these well-described associations, the mechanism by which cigarette smoking affects UC and CD in opposite ways is not known. Table 15-5 summarizes the effects of smoking and smoking cessation on IBD.

Based on the known effects of cigarette smoking in the incidence and course of UC, nicotine has been studied as a potential therapeutic alternative. The role of nicotine therapy in the management of UC is discussed in Chapter 18.

Smoking and IBD in Clinical Practice

Patients with CD should be strongly encouraged to quit smoking. Like any other smokers, Crohn's patients will have low abstinence rates without help. Counseling, smoking cessation groups, and pharmacotherapy should be offered by physicians treating these patients.

Although most evidence supports a beneficial effect of cigarette smoking on the course of UC, these patients should not be encouraged to smoke and should, as any other smoker, receive education about the health risks of nicotine use. Patients with UC should be educated about the relationship between smoking and their disease and be allowed to make their own decision based on the facts. Smokers with UC who plan to stop smoking should be informed of the potential risk of increase in disease activity, and accordingly, therapy should be adjusted to prevent a flare of their colitis.

NONSTEROIDAL ANTI-INFLAMMATORY DRUGS

At least 13 million people with various arthritides use prescription non-steroidal anti-inflammatory drugs (NSAIDs) regularly in the United States. In addition, more than 30 billion NSAID tablets are sold over the counter.[69]

A large body of evidence supports the relationship between NSAIDs and multiple types of mucosal injury to the distal small intestine and colon, including acute lesions and exacerbation of pre-existing disease.[70] More than 80% of patients with IBD interviewed for one study reported use of NSAIDs within the previous month. Approximately one-third of these patients thought that there was an association between their IBD symptoms and NSAID use. Only 2% of the IBS population used as control reported worsening symptoms following NSAID use.[71,72]

Although most of the available clinical evidence points toward an adverse influence of NSAIDs on the course of IBD, the exact mechanism by which NSAIDs can lead to exacerbations of the disease is not fully understood. Inhibition of colonic prostaglandin (PG) synthesis is likely a contributing factor.[73] The key enzyme in this pathway is cyclooxygenase (COX), which exists in two isoforms: COX-1, the constitutive enzyme involved in maintaining mucosal integrity in the GI tract and COX-2, an inducible enzyme that is expressed at sites of inflammation. COX-2 appears to have a beneficial effect in healing experimental colitis,[73] and COX-2 expression is significantly increased in the colonic mucosa of patients with active IBD when compared to inactive disease or healthy controls.[74] Theoretically, inhibition of COX-2 might negatively affect healing of colitis.[75]

There is some evidence suggesting that COX-2 specific inhibitors are less toxic to the GI tract. Consequently, patients and physicians assumed that these agents would not increase the risk of exacerbation of IBD. However, cases of flare-ups of IBD associated with use of COX-2 inhibitors have been reported in the literature.[76] Although controlled trials have not been performed, the general expert consensus is that the use of COX-2 specific inhibitors in patients with IBD should be viewed with the same caution as the use of traditional NSAIDs.[77]

There is no simple solution for the small number of patients who require NSAIDs and have significant IBD activity. When patients are using NSAIDs to control the pain from IBD-related arthritis, the intestinal disease should be treated aggressively. It is hoped that the severity of the arthritis will decrease as the intestinal inflammatory activity resolves. Non-NSAID analgesics can be prescribed in the interim to control joint pain. In rheumatoid arthritis or other arthritides, this strategy may not be as successful because the course of the arthritis is independent of the activity of the intestinal disease.[78] Non-NSAID analgesics and local measures can be used for the treatment of trauma-related pain and inflammation in patients with IBD. If these fail, a short course of NSAIDs may be prescribed, with close monitoring of symptoms and side effects.

Table 15-6

POSSIBLE EFFECTS OF EXERCISE ON IBD

- Decreased incidence of CD and UC
- Possible reduction in incidence of colon cancer
- Increased bone density
- Improvement in quality of life with CD
- Reduction in flare-ups and activity index with CD

EXERCISE

There is growing evidence that suggests that frequent exercise is beneficial in the prevention and management of chronic diseases such as cardiovascular disease, diabetes mellitus, and rheumatoid arthritis.[79] Accordingly, most physicians are now including recommendations to increase physical activity as an important element in the management of these entities.

There is also some data supporting an association of exercise with beneficial effects involving the GI tract. Despite the common occurrence of GI symptoms such as nausea, heartburn, diarrhea, and occasionally GI bleeding during vigorous exercise,[80-83] physical activity has also been consistently associated with a reduction of colon cancer risk.[84,85] More intense activity appears to confer greater protection than less intense activity.[84] It seems likely that these risk reduction benefits would extend to patients with IBD who exercise regularly.

Sedentary and physically less demanding occupations have been associated with a higher incidence of IBD.[86,87] Similarly, regular exercise was associated with significant improvements in quality of life and activity index scores, as well as a reduction in the frequency of flares in a small group of patients with CD (Table 15-6).[88]

While the preventive effect of physical activity remains inconclusive, it seems clear that physical activity is not harmful for patients with IBD. Another important reason to recommend regular physical activity is that IBD patients, especially those on chronic steroids, are at risk for osteoporosis and osteopenia.[85,89] A low-impact exercise program can potentially increase bone density in these patients.[90] Exercise may also alleviate stress and allow people to deal with stressful events more effectively, increasing their sense of general well-being and quality of life.[88] Physical activity should be promoted, keeping in mind that there is limited data regarding exactly how much exercise is appropriate.[77]

Stress

The disability caused by the symptoms of IBD and the uncertainty regarding disease outcomes can be worrisome and stress-producing for patients.[91] It has been suggested that psychological stress plays a significant role increasing disease activity and frequency of relapses, as well as the use of medical services in patients with IBD.[91-95]

The issue of stress initiating or exacerbating CD remains controversial. Although many patients and family members are convinced that stress is an important factor in the onset and course of the illness, it has not been possible to correlate the development of disease with any psychological predisposition or exacerbations to stressful life events.[96] While short-term stress does not appear to trigger disease flares in patients with UC in remission, long-term perceived stress has been associated with an increased risk of exacerbation.[97]

The possibility of overlapping irritable bowel syndrome (IBS)-related symptoms and their relation to stressful events should also be recognized to minimize the use of potent anti-inflammatory or disease-modifying therapies in the absence of a documented inflammatory component.

Strategies that improve social support, including local groups in which individuals can share their experiences, can have a favorable impact on psychological distress and can ultimately improve health outcomes in patients with IBD.[95] Patients should be encouraged to ask about disease-related worries and concerns, including fear of cancer and diagnostic procedures. The overall quality of life and adaptation to the illness as well as the individual emotional responses to the disease should be assessed and addressed. Empathy, understanding, positive regard, and psychological support improve the patient-physician relationship and lead to better quality of life for the patient. The importance of psychotherapy and psychopharmacology in patients with psychiatric comorbidity cannot be overlooked.[98] A close working relationship between the gastroenterologist and a mental health provider is essential in meeting the needs of these patients.

Complementary or Alternative Medicine

The use of alternative therapies for both bowel disease and general health by patients with IBD is common.[99,100] Consequently, gastroenterologists will frequently encounter patients who are using or want to use nontraditional treatments to manage their IBD. Managing these situations can be difficult, as we may not be familiar with these therapies and would be hesitant to support them without strong scientific evidence of their efficacy and safety.

In many alternative medical regimens, the emphasis is placed on health and well-being, rather than on disease. This allows patients to play a more active role in their treatment, which increases their sense of self-control. This approach may be particularly appealing to patients.[101]

In general, there are no major safety concerns with the common forms of therapy (herbs and nutritional supplements) used by patients with IBD. Potential risks include allergic reactions, contamination or mislabeling of herbal products, and nutritional deficiencies resulting from restrictive diets. Serious side effects, such as hepatic veno-occlusive disease and toxicity with heavy metals after the use of herbs prepared in Asia, have been reported.[77]

Most alternative therapies are based on traditional healing practices; however, there is little, if any, direct scientific evidence supporting their benefit. Much of the evidence to which patients and physicians have access is anecdotal. The Chinese literature has reported studies in which a combination of 11 Chinese herbs was beneficial for patients with UC. Response rates were as high as 60% and relapse rates as low as 10%.[102] Randomized controlled studies with strict methodology should be performed before these therapies can be recommended in the United States.

In general, patients do not substitute conventional medicine for alternative therapies. Instead, they tend to use both, often hoping for a synergistic effect. In an attempt to reduce or prevent the side effects from the conventional medicine, many herbs and supplements can affect the absorption or metabolism of conventional medicines. Patients on immunomodulators or other medications with a narrow therapeutic window should be especially careful.[101]

Counseling patients about alternative therapies is important and can help the patient make a more informed choice. Patients are more likely to follow recommendations and avoid self-prescription if a sensitive, nonjudgmental approach with an open discussion of the potential value and risks associated with a therapy is used.[103] Determining specific areas of concern or dissatisfaction with conventional treatments could allow modifications to be made. Realistic expectations for improvement, basis for these expectations, and the cost of the treatments should also be discussed before embarking on complementary therapies. Unrealistic goals and expectations for a quick cure should be discouraged, and many times this is easier to obtain with an open, nonauthoritative approach.

REFERENCES

1. Shanahan F. Inflammatory bowel disease: immunodiagnostics, immunotherapeutics, and ecotherapeutics. *Gastroenterology.* 2001;120:622-635.

2. Whorwell PJ, Holdstock G, Whorwell GM, Wright R. Bottle feeding, early gastroenteritis, and inflammatory bowel disease. *Br Med J.* 1979;1:382.

3. Morgan KL. Johne's and Crohn's. Chronic inflammatory bowel diseases of infectious aetiology? *Lancet.* 1987;1:1017-1019.

4. Van Kruiningen HJ, Colombel JF, Cartun RW, et al. An in-depth study of Crohn's disease in two French families. *Gastroenterology.* 1993;104:351-360.

5. Pardi DS, Tremaine WJ, Sandborn WJ, et al. Early measles virus infection is associated with the development of inflammatory bowel disease. *Am J Gastroenterol.* 2000;95:1480-1485.

6. Ekbom A, Adami HO, Helmick CG, Jonzon A, Zack MM. Perinatal risk factors for inflammatory bowel disease: a case-control study. *Am J Epidemiol.* 1990;132:1111-1119.

7. Montgomery SM, Morris DL, Pounder RE, Wakefield AJ. Paramyxovirus infections in childhood and subsequent inflammatory bowel disease. *Gastroenterology.* 1999;116:796-803.

8. Montgomery SM, Bjornsson S, Johannsson JH, Thjodleifsson B, Pounder RE, Wakefield AJ. Concurrent measles and mumps epidemics in Iceland are a risk factor for later inflammatory bowel disease. *Gut.* 1998;42:A41.

9. Anonymous. Case control study finds no link between measles vaccine and inflammatory bowel disease. *Commun Dis Rep CDR Wkly.* 1997;7:339.

10. Iizuka M, Saito H, Yukawa M, et al. No evidence of persistent mumps virus infection in inflammatory bowel disease. *Gut.* 2001;48:637-641.

11. Peltola H, Patja A, Leinikki P, Valle M, Davidkin I, Paunio M. No evidence for measles, mumps, and rubella vaccine-associated inflammatory bowel disease or autism in a 14-year prospective study. *Lancet.* 1998;351:1327-1328.

12. Haga Y, Funakoshi O, Kuroe K, et al. Absence of measles viral genomic sequence in intestinal tissues from Crohn's disease by nested polymerase chain reaction. *Gut.* 1996;38:211-215.

13. Afzal MA, Armitage E, Begley J, et al. Absence of detectable measles virus genome sequence in inflammatory bowel disease tissues and peripheral blood lymphocytes. *J Med Virol.* 1998;55:243-249.

14. Folwaczny C, Jager G, Schnettler D, Wiebecke B, Loeschke K. Search for mumps virus genome in intestinal biopsy specimens of patients with IBD. *Gastroenterology.* 1999;117:1253-1255.

15. Wurzelmann JI, Lyles CM, Sandler RS. Childhood infections and the risk of inflammatory bowel disease. *Dig Dis Sci.* 1994;39:555-560.

16. Summers RW, Urban J, Elliott D, Qadir H, Thompson J, Weinstock J. TH2 conditioning by trichuris suis appears safe and effective in modifying the mucosal immune response in inflammatory bowel disease. *Gastroenterology.* 1999;116:A828.

17. Fiocchi C. Inflammatory bowel disease: etiology and pathogenesis. *Gastroenterology.* 1998;115:182-205.

18. Merger M, Croitoru K. Infections in the immunopathogenesis of chronic inflammatory bowel disease. *Semin Immunol.* 1998;10:69-78.

19. Surawicz CM, Haggitt RC, Husseman M, McFarland LV. Mucosal biopsy diagnosis of colitis: acute self-limited colitis and idiopathic inflammatory bowel disease. *Gastroenterology.* 1994;107:755-763.

20. Preliminary FoodNet data on the incidence of foodborne illnesses—selected sites, United States, 2000. *Morb Mortal Wkly Rep.* 2001;50:241-246.

21. LaMont JT. Campylobacter infections. In: LaMont JT, ed. *Gastrointestinal Infections. Diagnosis and Management.* New York, NY: Marcel Dekker Inc; 1997: 247-263.

22. Lee SD, Surawicz CM. Infectious agents as aggravating factors in inflammatory bowel disease. In: Bayless TM, Hanauer SB, eds. *Advanced Therapy of Inflammatory Bowel Disease*. London, England: BC Decker Inc; 2001: 95-98.

23. Acheson DW, Keusch GT. Intestinal infections with salmonella and yersinia species. In: LaMont JT, ed. *Gastrointestinal Infections. Diagnosis and Management*. New York, NY: Marcel Dekker Inc; 1997: 149-189.

24. Kotloff KL, Levine MM. Shigella infections. In: LaMont JT, ed. *Gastrointestinal infections. Diagnosis and Management*. New York, NY: Marcel Dekker Inc; 1997:265-291.

25. Oldfield III EC. Emerging foodborne pathogens: keeping your patients and your family safe. *Reviews in Gastroenterological Disorders*. 2001;1:177-186.

26. Wong CS, Jelacic S, Habeeb RL, Watkins SL, Tarr PI. The risk of the hemolytic-uremic syndrome after antibiotic treatment of *Escherichia coli* O157:H7 infections. *N Engl J Med*. 2000;342:1930-1936.

27. Bailen L, Peppercorn MA. Sexually transmitted anorectal infections. In: LaMont JT, ed. *Gastrointestinal Infections. Diagnosis and Management*. New York, NY: Marcel Dekker Inc; 1997:411-451.

28. Liu Y, van Kruiningen HJ, West AB, Cartun RW, Cortot A, Colombel JF. Immunocytochemical evidence of *Listeria, Escherichia coli*, and *Streptococcus* antigens in Crohn's disease. *Gastroenterology*. 1995;108:1396-1404.

29. Swidsinski A, Ladhoff A, Pernthaler A, et al. Mucosal flora in inflammatory bowel disease. *Gastroenterology*. 2002;122:44-54.

30. Legnani PE, Kornbluth A. Difficult differential diagnosis in IBD. *Seminars in Gastrointestinal Disease*. 2001;12:211-222.

31. Bolton RP, Sherriff RJ, Read AE. *Clostridium difficile* associated diarrhea: a role in inflammatory bowel disease? *Lancet*. 1980;1:383-384.

32. Lee DK, Cooper BT, Barbezat GO. *Clostridium difficile* toxin in chronic idiopathic colitis. *N Z Med J*. 1986;99:620-622.

33. Rolny P, Jarnerot G, Mollby R. Occurrence of *Clostridium difficile* toxin in inflammatory bowel disease. *Scand J Gastroenterol*. 1983;18:61-64.

34. Hyams JS, McLaughlin JC. Lack of relationship between *Clostridium difficile* toxin and inflammatory bowel disease in children. *J Clin Gastroenterol*. 1985;7:387-390.

35. Papadakis KA, Tung JK, Binder SW, et al. Outcome of cytomegalovirus infections in patients with inflammatory bowel disease. *Am J Gastroenterol*. 2001;96:2137-2142.

36. Karasik MS, Afdhal NH. Small and large bowel infections in AIDS. In: LaMont JT, ed. *Gastrointestinal Infections. Diagnosis and Management*. New York, NY: Marcel Dekker Inc; 1997:212-215.

37. Wright CL, Riddell RH. Acute infectious colitis. Diagnostic dilemmas. In: Allan RN, Rhodes JM, Hanauer SB, eds. *Inflammatory Bowel Disease*. New York, NY: Churchill-Livingstone; 1997: 359-368.

38. Hanauer SB. Therapy for inflammatory bowel disease. In: Wolfe MM, ed. *Therapy of Digestive Disorders*. Philadelphia, Pa: WB Saunders; 2000: 565-589.

39. Bengmark S. Colonic food: pre- and probiotics. *Am J Gastroenterol.* 2000;95:S5-S7.

40. Kruis W, Schulz T, Fric P, et al. Double blind comparison of an oral Escherichia coli preparation and mesalazine in maintaining remission of ulcerative colitis. *Aliment Pharmacol Ther.* 1997;11:853-858.

41. Rembacken BJ, Snelling AM, Hawkey PM, et al. Non-pathogenic Escherichia coli versus mesalazine for the treatment of ulcerative colitis: a randomized trial. *Lancet.* 1999;354:635-639.

42. Gionchetti P, Rizzello F, Venturi A, Campieri M. Probiotics in infective diarrhea and inflammatory bowel diseases. *J Gastroenterol Hepatol.* 2000;15:489-493.

43. Shanahan F. Probiotics: science or snake oil. *Clin Persp Gastroenterol.* 2001;4:47-50.

44. Sutherland LR, Ramcharan S, Bryant H, Fick G. Effect of cigarette smoking on recurrence of Crohn's disease. *Gastroenterology.* 1990;98:1123-1128.

45. Gareth AO, Thomas BS, Rhodes J, Green JT. Inflammatory bowel disease and smoking—a review. *Am J Gastroenterol.* 1998;93:144-149.

46. Penny WJ, Penny E, Mayberry JF, et al. Mormons, smoking and ulcerative colitis. *Lancet.* 1983:2(8362):1315.

47. Penny WJ, Penny E, Mayberry JF, al. e. Prevalence of inflammatory bowel disease amongst Mormons in Britain and Ireland. *Soc Sci Med.* 1985;21:287-290.

48. Calkins BM. A meta-analysis of the role of smoking in inflammatory bowel disease. *Dig Dis Sci.* 1989;34:1841-1854.

49. Motley RJ, Rhodes J, Ford GA, et al. Time relationship between cessation of smoking and onset of ulcerative colitis. *Digestion.* 1987;37:125-127.

50. Boyko EJ, Koepsell TD, Perera DR, al. e. Risk of ulcerative colitis among former and current cigarette smokers. *N Eng J Med* 1987; 316:707-710.

51. Lindberg E, Tysk C, Anderson K, et al. Smoking and inflammatory bowel disease. A case-control study. *Gut.* 1988;29:352-357.

52. Russel MG, Nieman FH, Bergers JM, Stockbrugger RW. Cigarette smoking and quality of life in patients with inflammatory bowel disease. South Limburg IBD Study Group. *Eur J Gastroenterol Hepatol.* 1996;8:1075-1081.

53. Boyko EJ, Perera DR, Koepsell TD, et al. Effects of cigarette smoking on the clinical course of ulcerative colitis. *Scand J Gastroenterol.* 1988;23:1147-1152.

54. Fraga XF, Vergara M, Medina C, Casellas F, Bermejo B, Malagelada JR. Effects of smoking on the presentation and clinical course of inflammatory bowel disease. *Eur J Gastroenterol Hepatol.* 1997;9:683-687.

55. Merrett MN, Mortensen N, Kettlewell M, Jewell DO. Smoking may prevent pouchitis in patients with restorative proctocolectomy for ulcerative colitis. *Gut.* 1996;38:362-364.

56. Beaugerie L, Massot N, Carbonnel F, et al. Impact of cessation of smoking on the course of ulcerative colitis. *Am J Gastroenterol.* 2001;96:2113-2116.

57. Breuer-Katschinski BD, Hollander N, Goebell H. Effect of cigarette smoking on the course of Crohn's disease. *Eur J Gastroenterol Hepatol.* 1996;8:225-228.

58. Cosnes J, Carbonnel F, Carrat F, Beaugerie L, Gendre JP. Oral contraceptive use and the clinical course of Crohn's disease: a prospective cohort study. *Gut.* 1999;45:218-222.

59. Lindberg E, Jarnerot G, Huitfeldt B. Smoking in Crohn's disease: effect on localization and clinical course. *Gut.* 1992;33:779-782.

60. Cottone M, Rosselli M, Orlando A, et al. Smoking habits and recurrence in Crohn's disease. *Gastroenterology.* 1994;106:643-648.

61. Cosnes J, Carbonnel F, Beaugerie L, Le Quintrec Y, Gendre JP. Effects of cigarette smoking on the long-term course of Crohn's disease. *Gastroenterology.* 1996;110:424-431.

62. Russel MG, Volovics A, Schoon EJ, et al. Inflammatory bowel disease: is there any relation between smoking status and disease presentation? European Collaborative IBD Study Group. *Inflamm Bowel Dis.* 1998;4:182-186.

63. Hilsden RJ, Hodgins D, Czechowsky D, Verhoef MJ, Sutherland LR. Attitudes toward smoking and smoking behaviors of patients with Crohn's disease. *Am J Gastroenterol.* 2001;96:1849-1853.

64. Cosnes J, Carbonnel F, Carrat F, Beaugerie L, Cattan S, Gendre J. Effects of current and former cigarette smoking on the clinical course of Crohn's disease. *Aliment Pharmacol Ther.* 1999;13:1403-1411.

65. Timmer A, Sutherland LR, Martin F. Oral contraceptive use and smoking are risk factors for relapse in Crohn's disease. The Canadian Mesalamine for Remission of Crohn's Disease Study Group. *Gastroenterology.* 1998;114:1143-1150.

66. Shields PL, Low-Beer TS. Patients' awareness of adverse relation between Crohn's disease and their smoking: questionnaire survey. *Br Med J.* 1996;313:265-266.

67. Cosnes J, Beaugerie L, Carbonnel F, Gendre JP. Decreased severity of Crohn's disease after smoking cessation: preliminary results of a prospective intervention study. *Gastroenterology.* 2000;118:A870.

68. Cosnes J, Beaugerie L, Carbonnel F, Gendre JP. Smoking cessation and the course of Crohn's disease: an intervention study. *Gastroenterology.* 2001;120:1093-1099.

69. Wolfe MM, Lichtenstein DR, Singh G. Gastrointestinal toxicity of nonsteroidal anti-inflammatory drugs. *N Eng J Med.* 1999;340:1888-1899.

70. O'Brien J. Nonsteroidal anti-inflammatory drugs in patients with inflammatory bowel disease. *Am J Gastroenterol.* 2000;95:1859-1861.

71. Felder JB, Korelitz BI, Rajapakse R, Schwarz S, Horatagis AP, Gleim G. Effects of nonsteroidal anti-inflammatory drugs on inflammatory bowel disease: a case-control study. *Am J Gastroenterol.* 2000;95:1949-1954.

72. Bonner GF, Walczak M, Kitchen L, Bayona M. Tolerance of nonsteroidal anti-inflammatory drugs in patients with inflammatory bowel disease. *Am J Gastroenterol.* 2000;95:1946-1948.

73. Wallace JL. Nonsteroidal anti-inflammatory drugs and gastroenteropathy: the second hundred years. *Gastroenterology.* 1997;112:1000-1016.

74. Hendel J, Nielsen OH. Expression of cyclooxygenase-2 mRNA in active inflammatory bowel disease. *Am J Gastroenterol.* 1997;92:1170-1173.

75. Oviedo JA, Wolfe MM. Clinical potential of cyclo-oxygenase-2 inhibitors. *BioDrugs*. 2001;15:563-572.

76. Bonner GF. Exacerbation of inflammatory bowel disease associated with use of celecoxib. *Am J Gastroenterol*. 2001;96:1306-1308.

77. Oviedo J, Farraye FA. Self-care for the inflammatory bowel disease patient: what can the professional recommend? *Semin Gastrointest Dis*. 2001;12:223-236.

78. Smale S, Bjarnason I. Nonsteroidal anti-inflammatory drugs, enterocolonic ulceration and inflammatory bowel disease. In: Bayless-Hanauer, ed. *Advance Therapy of Inflammatory Bowel Disease*. London, England: BC Decker; 2001: 625-627.

79. Harkcom TM, Lampman RM, Figley-Banwell B, et al. Therapeutic value of graded aerobic exercise training in rheumatoid arthritis. *Arthritis Rheum*. 1985;1985:32-38.

80. Oktedalen O, Lunde OC, Opstad PK, et al. Changes in the gastrointestinal mucosa after long-distance running. *Scand J Gastroenterol*. 1992;27:270-274.

81. Peters HP, Bos M, Seebregts L, et al. Gastrointestinal symptoms in long-distance runners, cyclists, and triathletes: prevalence, medication, and etiology. *Am J Gastroenterol*. 1999;94:1570-1581.

82. Peters HP, Zweers M, Backx FJ, et al. Gastrointestinal symptoms during long-distance walking. *Med Sci Sports Exerc*. 1999;31:767-773.

83. Lucas W, Schroy PC. Reversible ischemic colitis in a high endurance athlete. *Am J Gastroenterol*. 1998;93:2231-2234.

84. Oliveria SA, Christos PJ. The epidemiology of physical activity and cancer. *Ann N Y Acad Sci*. 1997;833:79-90.

85. Peters HP, De Vries WR, Vanberge-Henegouwen GP, Akkermans LM. Potential benefits and hazards of physical activity and exercise on the gastrointestinal tract. *Gut*. 2001;48:435-439.

86. Sonnenberg A. Occupational distribution of inflammatory bowel disease among German employees. *Gut*. 1990;31:1037-1040.

87. Persson PG, Leijonmarck CE, Bernell O, Hellers G, Ahlbom A. Risk indicators for inflammatory bowel disease. *Int J Epidemiol*. 1993;22:268-272.

88. Loudon CP, Corroll V, Butcher J, Rawsthorne P, Bernstein CN. The effects of physical exercise on patients with Crohn's disease. *Am J Gastroenterol*. 1999;94:697-703.

89. Robinson RJ, al-Azzawi F, Iqbal SJ, et al. Osteoporosis and determinants of bone density in patients with Crohn's disease. *Dig Dis Sci*. 1998;43:2500-2506.

90. Robinson RJ, Krzywicki T, Almond L, et al. Effect of a low-impact exercise program on bone mineral density in Crohn's disease: a randomized controlled trial. *Gastroenterology*. 1998;115:36-41.

91. Drossman DA, Leserman J, Mitchell M, et al. Health status and healthcare use in persons with inflammatory bowel disease: a national sample. *Dig Dis Sci*. 1991;36:1746-1755.

92. Porcelli P, Zaka S, Centonze S, Sisto G. Psychological distress and levels of disease activity in inflammatory bowel disease. *Ital J Gastroenterol*. 1994;26:111-115.

93. Porcelli P, Leoci C, Guerra V. A prospective study of the relationship between disease activity and psychologic distress in patients with inflammatory bowel disease. *Scand J Gastroenterol.* 1996;31:792-796.

94. North CS, Alpers DH, Helzer JE, et al. Do life events or depression exacerbate inflammatory bowel disease? a prospective study. *Ann Intern Med.* 1991;114:381-386.

95. Sewitch MJ, Abrahamowicz M, Bitton A, et al. Psychological distress, social support, and disease activity in patients with inflammatory bowel disease. *Am J Gastroenterol.* 2001;96:1470-1479.

96. Hanauer SB, Sandborn WJ. Management of Crohn's disease in adults. *Am J Gastroenterol.* 2001;96:635-643.

97. Levenstein S, Prantera C, Varvo V, et al. Stress and exacerbation in ulcerative colitis: a prospective study of patients enrolled in remission. *Am J Gastroenterol.* 2000;95:1213-1220.

98. Moser G, Drossman DA. Managing patients' concerns. In: Bayless-Hanauer, ed. *Advanced Therapy of Inflammatory Bowel Disease.* London, England: BC Decker Inc; 2001: 527-529.

99. Hilsden RJ, Scott CM, Verhoef MJ. Complementary medicine use by patients with inflammatory bowel disease. *Am J Gastroenterol.* 1998;93:697-701.

100. Rawsthorne P, Shanahan F, Cronin NC, et al. An international survey of the use and attitudes regarding alternative medicine by patients with inflammatory bowel disease. *Am J Gastroenterol.* 1999;94:1298-1303.

101. Hilsden RJ. Alternative patient care methods. In: Bayless-Hanauer, ed. Advanced *Therapy of Inflammatory Bowel Disease.* London, England: BC Decker Inc; 2001.

102. Diehl DL, Lerner DS. Chinese herbal medicine. *Clin Persp Gastroenterol.* 2000:100-104.

103. Eisenberg DM. Advising patients who seek alternative medical therapies. *Ann Intern Med.* 1997;127:61-69.

chapter 16

Evaluation of the Patient Suspected of Having Inflammatory Bowel Disease

L. Arturo Batres, MD and Robert N. Baldassano, MD

Table 16-1 summarizes the initial evaluation of a patient with inflammatory bowel disease (IBD).

APPROPRIATE TESTING

LABORATORY EVALUATION

The evaluation of a patient suspected of having IBD should include a complete blood count (CBC), electrolytes, liver function tests, erythrocyte sedimentation rate (ESR), and C-reactive protein (CRP). Other nonspecific tests for inflammation (acute phase reactants), such as ferritin and platelet count, can also be elevated in IBD. It is important to rule out stool infection, especially *Clostridium difficile*.

Serologic markers are another tool that can help diagnose and characterize patients with IBD. The perinuclear antineutrophil cytoplasmic antibody (pANCA) is expressed in the majority of patients with ulcerative colitis (UC) and can be found in 10% to 30% of patients with Crohn's disease (CD). The

Table 16-1

Appropriate Testing for the Initial Evaluation of IBD

Laboratory Evaluation

Laboratory Evaluation	Findings
Complete blood cell count (CBC)	Leukocytosis, anemia, thrombocytosis
Erythrocyte sedimentation rate (ESR), C-reactive protein (CRP), ferritin	Elevated acute phase reactants
Stool studies	Infection (eg, *C. difficile*) needs to be ruled out
pANCA	Expressed in the majority of UC 10% to 30% of CD (left-sided colitis)
ASCA	50% to 70% of CD 6% to 14% of UC

Radiology

Radiology	Findings
Plain abdominal x-ray	Rule out toxic megacolon or obstruction
Contrast studies UGI/SBFT and enteroclysis	Help delineate places not reached by endoscopy
Barium enema	Superior to colonoscopy for distribution of disease, fissures, fistulas, and subtle strictures
Computed tomography (CT)	Demonstrates the bowel wall, adjacent abdominal organs, mesentery, and retroperitoneum

Endoscopy

Endoscopy	Findings
CD	Rectum is spared, skipped areas with the formation of pseudopolyps, aphthous ulcerations, and fistulas
UC	Loss of vascular markings, diffuse erythema, mucosal friability and granularity, ulceration with an inflamed mucosa, and continuous involvement

continued on next page

Table 16-1 (Continued)

APPROPRIATE TESTING FOR THE
INITIAL EVALUATION OF IBD

Histology	Findings
CD	Noncaseating granulomas, skipped lesions, polymorphonuclear infiltration of the crypts, crypt abscesses, and distortion of the crypt architecture
UC	Infiltrate of neutrophils in the mucosa, crypt abscesses, goblet cell mucus depletion, and neutrophils in the crypt lumen

subset of pANCA-positive patients with CD can have features similar to UC, such as left-sided colitis. The other antibody used in IBD is the anti-*Saccharomyces cerevisiae* antibodies (ASCA); 50% to 70% of patients with CD and 6% to 14% of patients with UC are ASCA positive. ASCA reactivity is characterized by immunoglobulin subtype in IgA and IgG. Patients with CD who express both the IgA and IgG-type ASCA are much more likely to have fibrostenosing disease. Serologic markers to bacterial antigens, such as *Escherichia coli* and a bacterial sequence called I2, are currently under investigation for the initial evaluation of IBD.

RADIOGRAPHY

Radiologic examination of the colon can differentiate UC from CD. UC is characterized by disease extending retrogradely from the anorectal junction in a continuous symmetric fashion. In contrast, CD is characterized by a discontinuous, asymmetric, and patchy involvement of the colon.

Contrast radiography and computed tomography (CT) scanning are the most common radiologic tests in IBD. Plain films of the abdomen serve two principal functions in the evaluation of a patient with IBD. The first is the assessment of colonic distention when toxic megacolon is suspected. The second is in the evaluation of intestinal obstruction.

Magnetic resonance imaging and sonography are inferior to contrast radiography and CT scanning in the initial evaluation of IBD.

Barium Studies

Barium studies include an upper gastrointestinal series with small bowel follow-through (UGI/SBFT), enteroclysis (small bowel enema), barium enema, and retrograde ileostomy examinations. Early radiographic findings of CD in the small bowel include a coarse villous pattern of the mucosa, thickened folds, aphthous ulcerations, and cobblestoning. The upper gastrointestinal series with small bowel follow-through and the enteroclysis help delineate the small bowel in places that cannot be reached by endoscopy. The UGI/SBFT is limited by the rate of gastric emptying. If barium passage through the pylorus is too slow, the small bowel may not distend completely and short or skipped lesions may not be visualized. The enteroclysis procedure consists of the passage of a nasal or oral catheter to the small bowel. In bypassing the pylorus with the catheter, the radiologist can control the rate of barium entering the small bowel.

A double-contrast barium enema examination gives detailed contrast images of the colon. Reflux of barium and air into the distal small bowel occurs in 85% of patients. The barium enema is superior to colonoscopy in demonstrating the distribution of the disease, fissures, fistulas and subtle strictures. A retrograde ileostomy examination is shorter and achieves better distention of the distal small bowel than the UGI/SBFT but lacks value for the proximal intestine.

Computed Tomography

CT should be performed in patients with acute symptoms suspected of having CD. The ability to directly demonstrate the bowel wall, adjacent abdominal organs, mesentery, and retroperitoneum makes CT superior to barium studies in the diagnosis of CD. Extraintestinal complications of CD, such as gallstones, urinary tract calculi, and osteomyelitis, may also be detected on CT scan. CT scan findings of UC include target appearance of the rectum, adenopathy, increased perirectal and presacral fat, heterogeneous wall density, and absence of thickening of the small bowel. CD findings on CT scan include mural thickening (>2 cm); homogeneous wall density; mesenteric fat stranding; perianal disease; adenopathy; and the presence of abscesses, fistulas, or sinus tracts.

ENDOSCOPY

Endoscopy provides direct mucosal visualization and tissue sampling. Colonoscopy with ileum biopsy has been shown to be helpful in the diagnosis of inflammatory disorders when radiology of the terminal ileum was abnormal or inconclusive.

Endoscopic features of UC include loss of vascular markings, diffuse erythema, mucosal friability and granularity, ulceration with an inflamed mucosa, and continuous involvement (including the rectum). In CD the rectum is spared, there are skipped areas with the formation of pseudopolyps and apthous ulcerations, and there is the presence of fistulas. Terminal ileal intubation is imperative in making the diagnosis of CD. Obvious contraindications would be the presence of acute severe colitis, in which case a limited colonoscopy is indicated to avoid the risk of precipitating toxic megacolon or perforation.

Performing an esophagogastroduodenoscopy (EGD) is useful in CD because the disease may involve the proximal gastrointestinal tract. Common lesions include aphthous ulcers, mucosal nodularities, and strictures.

HISTOLOGY

Mucosa that appeared normal on endoscopy often reveal histologic abnormalities such as edema and increased mononuclear cell density in the lamina propria. CD can affect all the layers of the bowel wall, while UC is confined to the mucosa (except in fulminant colitis). Because endoscopic biopsies do not go beyond the submucosa, sometimes mucosal changes of CD may resemble UC or infectious colitis.

The pathogenesis of ulcer formation in CD is not mucosally based. Submucosal lymph follicles expand and penetrate through the mucosa, giving the typical picture of aphthous ulcers. The mucosa that surrounds the ulcers most of the time has normal histology. The presence of fibrosis and histiocytic proliferation in the submucosa suggests CD. The skipped lesions are also seen in histology. Other mucosal features include polymorphonuclear infiltration of the crypts, crypt abscesses, and distortion of the crypt architecture. Noncaseating granulomas are diagnostic of CD and are noted in 10% to 30% of biopsy specimens.

The pathologic findings of UC include an intense infiltrate of neutrophils in the mucosa, crypt abscesses, goblet cell mucus depletion, and neutrophils in the crypt lumen. In quiescent UC the inflammatory infiltrate is less intense, but the mucosa usually remains abnormal. Crypts are reduced in number, shortened, and branched.

DIFFERENTIAL DIAGNOSIS OF IBD

The differential diagnosis of IBD is summarized in Table 16-2. A good clinical history and physical examination are important to elucidate the diagnosis. The following categories constitute the differential diagnosis:

INFECTIOUS

Intestinal infections may mimic Crohn's ileitis or UC. A good clinical history, proper culture techniques, and a high index of suspicion are essential in making the correct diagnosis.

Mycobacterium tuberculosis

Over 40% of patients with intestinal tuberculosis will have ileocecal involvement that can mimic CD. Patients can present with ileitis, fistulae and abscess formation, bleeding, and perforation. The diagnosis is confirmed by

---

Table 16-2

DIFFERENTIAL DIAGNOSIS OF IBD

Infectious

Mycobacterium tuberculosis
Histoplasma capsulatum
Yersinia enterocolitica
Campylobacter jejuni
Entamoeba histolytica
Cytomegalovirus (CMV)
Clostridium difficile

Inflammatory

Acute appendicitis
Cecal diverticulitis

Functional

Irritable bowel syndrome

Vascular

Ileal ischemia
Systemic lupus erythematosus
Henoch-Schönlein purpura
Churg-Strauss syndrome
Behçet's disease

Gynecologic

Tubo-ovarian abscesses
Pelvic inflammatory disease
Ovarian cysts
Ectopic pregnancy
Endometriosis

Neoplastic

Carcinoid
Cecal carcinoma
Lymphosarcoma of the ileum
Non-Hodgkin's lymphoma
Metastatic disease

Infiltrative

Amyloidosis
Eosinophilic gastroenteritis

Medications

Nonsteroidal anti-inflammatory drugs
(NSAIDs)

Adapted from Legnani PE, Kornbluth A. Difficult differential diagnoses in IBD: ileitis and indeterminate colitis. *Semin Gastrointest Dis.* 2001;12(4):211-222.

---

caseating granulomas on mucosal biopsy, although granulomas are rarely noted and may not reveal caseation. The yield of the biopsy in making the diagnosis is 30% to 50%. The mucosal biopsy sensitivity by PCR is 70% to 90%.

Histoplasma capsulatum

Histoplasma involves the terminal ileum in approximately one third of patients with gastrointestinal disease. The diagnosis should be considered in immunocompromised hosts or in travelers from endemic areas. Biopsy may show granulomas and the organism can be identified by serology, culture, or by deoxyribonucleic acid (DNA) probe.

Yersinia enterocolitica

Y. enterocolitica is a foodborne infection that may lead to symptoms of abdominal pain, fever, and diarrhea. Extraintestinal symptoms such as arthritis, erythema nodosum, and aphthous stomatitis can also be present. The bacteria can invade the intestine, particularly the distal ileum, and cause a granulomatous reaction in the bowel wall and regional nodes. Colonoscopy may reveal colonic and ileal ulcerations. The diagnosis is made by stool cultures or serology.

Campylobacter jejuni

This gram-negative organism requires special medium and temperature for isolation. Patients can present with recurrent episodes of abdominal pain and bloody diarrhea. Twenty percent of patients with *Campylobacter* infection may relapse or have a prolonged illness that may mimic IBD.

Entamoeba histolytica

Isolated ileal involvement with amebiasis is rare; however, when the infection is in the right lower quadrant, symptoms can be indistinguishable from CD. The diagnosis of amebiasis can be made by biopsy, stool culture, or serology.

Cytomegalovirus

Cytomegalovirus (CMV) occurs mostly in immunocompromised patients. Colonic involvement is more common than ileal involvement. Symptoms include right lower quadrant pain, diarrhea, and fever. Colonoscopy may reveal erythema, granularity, and ulcerations. CMV inclusion bodies or positive viral cultures on biopsy confirm the diagnosis.

Clostridium difficile

This infection can mimic the symptoms of both UC and CD. It is important to culture the stool several times and to test for both toxins A and B. There are high recurrence and relapse rates.

INFLAMMATORY

The most common condition that mimics ileitis is acute appendicitis. An appendiceal abscess can have features similar to CD on CT scan and small bowel series.

Cecal diverticulitis can present with cecal thickening, pericecal fluid, and inflammation that can mimic IBD.

FUNCTIONAL

Irritable bowel syndrome (IBS) can present with symptoms similar to IBD, such as abdominal distention, abdominal pain, and diarrhea. Weight loss is usually absent in IBS. The physical examination and the radiographic and endoscopic studies in IBS are normal.

VASCULAR

Ileal ischemia may mimic CD. This condition occurs in hypercoagulable states (protein C and protein S deficiency), antiphospholipid syndrome, vasculopathy, medications (oral contraceptives), malrotation, and after embolism. Systemic vasculitides such as systemic lupus erythematosus (SLE), Henoch-Schönlein purpura, and Churg-Strauss syndrome have been reported to have ileal involvement. Behçet's disease may involve the gastrointestinal tract in 15% to 65% of cases, with ileocecal involvement being the most common. The diagnosis of Behçet's disease is suspected by prominent oral, ocular, and genital ulcerations. Patients with Behçet's disease usually respond to glucocorticosteroids and immunomodulators.

GYNECOLOGIC

Tubo-ovarian abscesses, pelvic inflammatory disease, ovarian cysts, ectopic pregnancy, and endometriosis may all present with chronic, intermittent lower abdominal pain with inflammatory symptoms.

NEOPLASTIC

Carcinoid is the most common tumor of the ileum. The desmoplastic reaction associated with carcinoid can simulate transmural involvement, mimicking CD. Cecal carcinoma and lymphosarcoma of the ileum can produce obstructive symptoms and diarrhea similar to IBD. The gastrointestinal tract is the most common site of primary extranodal involvement of non-Hodgkin's lymphoma. Twenty-five percent of the involvement is ileal. Metastatic disease from breast, stomach, pancreas, and skin cancers may mimic ileitis.

INFILTRATIVE

Primary and secondary amyloidosis may present with ileal disease. Early symptoms are nonspecific, but progressive amyloid deposition in the ileum may lead to obstruction, perforation, ulceration, or bleeding. Eosinophilic infiltration of the ileum, seen in eosinophilic gastroenteritis, can be confused with CD.

MEDICATIONS

NSAIDs may produce small bowel ulceration, stricture formation, and intermittent obstruction that can mimic IBD.

BIBLIOGRAPHY

Abreu M, Vasiliauskas EA, Kam LY, Dubinsky MC. Use of serologic tests in Crohn's disease. *Clinical Perspectives in Gastroenterology.* 2001;4(3):155-164.

Feller ER, Ribaudo S, Jackson ND. Gynecologic aspects of Crohn's disease. *Am Fam Physician.* 2001;64(10):1725-1728.

Horvath KD, Whelan RL. Intestinal tuberculosis: return of an old disease. *Am J Gastroenterol.* 1998;93(5):692-696.

Horwitz BJ, Fisher RS. The irritable bowel syndrome. *N Engl J Med.* 2001;344(24):1846-1850.

Hsu EY, Feldman JM, Lichtenstein GR. Ileal carcinoid tumors stimulating Crohn's disease: incidence among 176 consecutive cases of ileal carcinoid. *Am J Gastroenterol.* 1997;92(11):2062-2065.

Keidar S, Pappo I, Shperber Y, Orda R. Cecal diverticulitis: a diagnostic challenge. *Dig Surg.* 2000;17(5):508-512.

Legnani PE, Kornbluth A. Difficult differential diagnoses in IBD: ileitis and indeterminate colitis. *Semin Gastrointest Dis.* 2001;12(4):211-222.

Markowitz JE, Brown KA, Mamula P, Drott HR, Piccoli DA, Baldassano RN. Failure of single-toxin assays to detect clostridium difficile infection in pediatric inflammatory bowel disease. *Am J Gastroenterol.* 2001;96(9):2688-2690.

Rubesin SE, Scotiniotis I, Birnbaum BA, Gingseng GG. Radiologic and endoscopic diagnosis of Crohn's disease. *Surg Clin North Am.* 2001;81(1):39-70, viii.

Scotiniotis I, Rubesin SE, Ginsberg GG. Imaging modalities in inflammatory bowel disease. *Gastroenterol Clin North Am.* 1999;28(2):391-421, ix.

chapter 17

Special Considerations for Pediatric and Adolescent Patients With Inflammatory Bowel Disease

L. Arturo Batres, MD and Robert N. Baldassano, MD

INTRODUCTION

The first patient Dr. Crohn described with regional enteritis was a 16-year-old boy. Twenty-five percent to 30% of all patients with Crohn's disease (CD) and 20% of those with ulcerative colitis (UC) present before the age of 20 years. Four percent of pediatric inflammatory bowel disease (IBD) occurs before the age of 5, with a peak age of onset in the late adolescent years. With the increasing recognition of IBD among pediatric patients, it has become one of the most significant chronic diseases affecting children and adolescents.

In IBD, growth failure may be the only clinical presentation; it is imperative to perform a detailed history and physical examination to search for other systemic and gastrointestinal manifestations of the disease. IBD can have a significant impact on linear growth, weight gain, and bone mineralization and can cause delays in the onset of puberty. Delays in growth and sexual development can be early indicators of disease activity, so assessment of growth and development should be done frequently.

Nutritional therapy is important; it corrects undernutrition and serves as therapy for IBD. Delayed puberty can have a significant impact on the self-esteem of the adolescent patient and diminish final adult height. Loss of bone mineral density is especially significant during a period in which the majority of bone accretion is expected to occur. Weight loss can be documented in approximately 85% of children with CD and 65% with UC at time of diagnosis. These unique problems that are encountered in the pediatric population necessitate a different medical approach than that used for adult onset IBD.

CROHN'S DISEASE

EPIDEMIOLOGY

The age-specific incidence rates in North America for 10 to 19 year olds are approximately 3.5/100,000 for CD. Most studies have reported an equal incidence of CD in males and females. Multiple familial occurrences are well documented in 15% to 20% of patients. This is particularly common with early-onset IBD. Recently, the first gene for CD, Nod2, has been mapped on chromosome 16. This gene is most likely to be present in patients diagnosed with CD before the age of 20. A high rate of concordance for CD between monozygotic twins (44.4%) compared with dizygotic twins (3.8%) has been reported. Since monozygotic twins share identical genomic material and yet may be discordant for CD, no combination of genes is sufficient for the development of CD. Rather, some environmental trigger is likely to be also involved.

CLINICAL MANIFESTATIONS

The clinical manifestations of CD in children are summarized in Table 17-1. The intestinal involvement in CD may occur in any segment of the gastrointestinal tract. The presentation is primarily determined by the location and extent of the disease involvement. The majority of children (50% to 70%) have disease involving the terminal ileum. More than half of these patients also have inflammation in variable segments of the colon, usually the ascending colon. Ten percent to 20% of children have isolated colonic disease, and 10% to 15% have diffuse small bowel disease involving the more proximal ileum or jejunum. Isolated gastroduodenal disease is uncommon (fewer than 5% of patients), but there may be endoscopic and histologic evidence of gastroduodenal inflammation in up to 30% to 40% of children with CD.

There is a higher incidence of large bowel involvement in children with CD younger than 5 years of age. Presenting symptoms in this age group include failure to thrive, vomiting, and fever.

CD involving the small intestine usually presents with evidence of malabsorption including diarrhea, abdominal pain, growth deceleration, weight loss, and anorexia. Initially, these symptoms may be quite subtle, and any one may dominate the clinical picture. Small bowel mucosal disease may result in malabsorption of iron, zinc, folate, or vitamin B_{12} deficiency. CD involving the colon may be clinically indistinguishable from UC with symptoms of bloody mucopurulent diarrhea, crampy abdominal pain, and urgency to defecate.

Table 17-1

CLINICAL MANIFESTATIONS OF PEDIATRIC IBD

	Ulcerative Colitis	*Crohn's Disease*
Abdominal pain	+ +	+ +
Hematochezia	+ +	+ +
Diarrhea	+ +	+ +
Growth deceleration	+	+ +
Weight loss and anorexia	+	+ +
Malabsorption	–	+ +
Perianal disease	–	+ +
Bone disease	+	+ +
Delayed puberty	+	+ +

Extraintestinal Manifestations

- Skin: erythema nodosum and pyoderma gangrenosum
- Oral: aphthous ulcerations
- Ophthalmic: episcleritis and anterior uveitis
- Rheumatologic: arthralgias, arthritis, and ankylosing spondylitis
- Hepatobiliary: chronic active hepatitis, granulomatous hepatitis, amyloidosis, fatty liver, pericholangitis, cholelithiasis and sclerosing cholangitis nephrolithiasis, hydronephrosis, and enterovesical fistulae
- Vascular: deep vein thrombosis, pulmonary emboli, neurovascular disease, and vasculitis
- Other: pancreatitis, fibrosing alveolitis, interstitial pneumonitis, pericarditis, and peripheral neuropathy

---

Symptoms of painful defecation, bright red rectal bleeding, and perirectal pain may signal perianal disease, which may occur without symptomatic involvement in any other area of the intestinal tract. Perianal involvement includes simple skin tags, fissures, abscesses, and fistulae. The perineum should be inspected in all patients presenting with signs and symptoms of CD because abnormalities detectable in this region will substantially increase the clinical suspicion of IBD.

GROWTH FAILURE

Growth failure is usually insidious, and any child or adolescent with persistent alterations in growth should have an appropriate diagnostic evaluation for IBD. Growth failure may precede the onset of intestinal symptoms by years. There are multiple causes of growth failure in patients with CD, but inadequate nutrient intake is usually present. Anorexia, reduced intake, malabsorption, increased losses, and increased metabolic demands all contribute to poor growth. Recent studies have evaluated the growth of children with CD, and it is clear that impairment of linear growth is common prior to diagnosis, as well as during subsequent years, and that height at maturity is often compromised.

Height velocity is the most sensitive parameter by which to diagnose impaired growth and follow the effects on growth following therapy. A decrease in height velocity prior to onset of intestinal symptoms has been reported. Height velocity continues to decrease after the development of symptoms. The greater the height deficit at diagnosis, the greater the demands for catch-up growth. Multiple factors contribute to growth impairment in children with CD. Greater emphasis has been placed on the importance of chronic undernutrition as the primary cause of growth retardation. Serum IGF-1 levels are low in most patients with growth abnormalities and likely reflect a poor nutritional state. The nutritional insufficiency, although multifactorial, results primarily from inadequate intake rather than increased losses or requirements. Disease-related anorexia and exacerbation of abdominal cramps while eating can limit intake. Most studies have found resting energy expenditure to be normal in patients with CD. Caloric intake during relapse is less than in healthy siblings, whereas caloric intake during remission is normal; however, consumption of vegetables is less and of sweets is greater than that of siblings.

The impact of inadequate nutrition is more apparent in the growing child or adolescent than in adults. The pubertal growth spurt accounts for about 16% of adult height and is associated with nearly a doubling of body weight. This acceleration in growth velocity results in increased nutritional requirements, which are unlikely to be met. Undernutrition leads to delays in skeletal maturation, onset of menarche, and epiphyseal fusion in long bones.

Endocrine testing is generally normal, with normal cortisol levels and thyroid function. Serum growth hormone levels may be depressed but respond to stimulation testing. Somatomedin-C values are depressed in some patients with growth failure but respond to nutritional intervention.

DELAYED PUBERTY

Children with CD often have delays in the onset of pubertal development, and careful evaluation of pubertal staging should be part of their routine evaluation. Active disease uncontrolled by medical therapy could potentially delay the onset of puberty indefinitely with a deleterious effect on pubertal growth. The duration of puberty could also be affected in children with CD. Active or relapsing disease during the years following the onset of puberty may slow down or even arrest the progression of puberty. Arrest of pubertal development in children with CD may be an early indication of disease relapse, and in the same manner delay in pubertal onset may indicate persistent occult disease.

Inducing disease remission before the onset of puberty and maintaining it during the pubertal years is crucial in order to avoid loosing valuable height as a consequence of a missed pubertal growth spurt. Patients that are in remission by the time they go into puberty can experience good catch-up growth with peak height velocities greater than 12 cm/year. The potential for catch-up growth may be severely compromised in those children who suffered relapse or whose disease activity is not controlled in the peripubertal years. Differing from healthy children, delayed puberty in CD may not allow future prolonged and/or greater linear growth.

Factors affecting pubertal development in children with Crohn's disease include nutritional deprivation, the inflammatory process, hormonal disturbances, and the effects of therapy. Severe protein-calorie malnutrition and weight loss can be associated with prepubertal levels of sex steroids despite previous evidence of pubertal progression. Secondary amenorrhea is also observed following severe weight loss in these patients, similar to patients with anorexia nervosa in which there is suppression of gonadotrophin secretion.

Delayed puberty in patients with CD may affect the normal bone mineral accumulation peak that follows the pubertal growth spurt, being another factor contributing to osteoporosis. Estrogen and testosterone are important for normal bone mineralization, as shown by the osteopenia found in estrogen and androgen-resistant syndromes.

BONE DISEASE

Bone disease in IBD has been widely described. Bone turnover in IBD is characterized by suppressed bone formation and normal bone resorption. A high prevalence of low BMD in children with CD has been reported.

The pathogenesis and risk factors of bone loss in IBD have not been well characterized. It has been reported to be secondary to the use of medication (mainly corticosteroids), malnutrition, and after an intestinal resection. Newly diagnosed patients, especially children and young adults, can present with bone disease that is independent from nutritional and therapeutic side effects; several genetic factors have been proposed.

Genetic variations in the IL-6 and IL-1ra gene can identify patients at risk for increase bone loss. Increased urinary N-telopeptide cross-linked type I collagen (NTx) levels can predict spinal bone loss in IBD. Vitamin K status is also associated with low bone mineral density (BMD) in CD.

Most of the bone mass accumulation occurs during childhood and adolescence. Growth failure is common feature in CD patients, especially in males; therefore, bone mineralization can be compromised. Osteoporosis presenting as vertebral compression fractures can be the only manifestation of CD in childhood.

Bone mass can be estimated by dual-energy x-ray absorptiometry (DXA) (in the pediatric population it is important to use the low-density array software for the interpretation of the results). The bone mineral density should be reported as z-score, which differs from the standards typically employed in adults. Treatment modalities for osteoporosis include calcium and vitamin D supplementation and the use of biphosphonates. The safety of biphosphonates in the pediatric population has yet to be determined. It is important to emphasize that weight-bearing exercises represent one of the most important therapies for osteoporosis.

ULCERATIVE COLITIS

EPIDEMIOLOGY

The age-specific incidence rates in North America for 10 to 19 year olds are approximately 2/100,000 for UC.

CLINICAL MANIFESTATIONS

The clinical manifestations of UC in children are summarized in Table 17-1. UC is a diffuse mucosal inflammation limited to the colon. It invariably affects the rectum and may extend proximally in a symmetric uninterrupted pattern to involve parts or all of the large intestine. Since UC is a mucosal disease limited to the colon, the most common presenting symptoms are rectal bleeding, diarrhea, and abdominal pain. The cumulative colectomy probability of 6% after 1 year and 29% after 20 years is not different from that of adults. They also reported that when a child presents with proctitis at diagnosis there is a 65% chance of further spread of the disease to other parts of the large intestine during the course of the disease.

There are multiple patterns of presentation of UC in the pediatric age group. Mild disease is seen in 50% to 60%. The onset of diarrhea is insidious and later associated with hematochezia. There are no systemic signs of fever, weight loss, or hypoalbuminemia in these patients. The disease is usually confined to the distal colon and responds well to therapy. Thirty percent of pediatric patients present with moderate disease characterized by bloody diarrhea, cramps, the urge to defecate, and abdominal tenderness. These patients have associated systemic signs, such as anorexia, weight loss, low-grade fever, and mild anemia. Severe colitis occurs in approximately 10% of patients. This presentation is characterized by more than six bloody stools per day, abdominal tenderness, fever, anemia, leukocytosis, and hypoalbuminemia. Severe hemorrhage, toxic megacolon, and perforation are serious complications in this group of patients.

Occasionally, children with UC may have a presentation dominated by extraintestinal manifestations, such as growth failure, arthropathy, skin manifestations, or liver disease. This is uncommon in adults and occurs in less than 5% of the pediatric disease.

INDETERMINATE COLITIS

Ten percent to 15% of patients with IBD have a colitis that must be initially designated as indeterminate. In this case, the clinical picture, laboratory data, endoscopic and radiographic information, and the histology do not point to either CD or UC. Ultimately, the distinction between CD and UC allows the selection of the medical and, more importantly, the surgical treatment.

GASTROINTESTINAL COMPLICATIONS

CD and UC are both associated with significant gastrointestinal complications. The major intestinal complications of UC are massive bleeding, toxic megacolon, and carcinoma. In contrast, the major intestinal complications of CD are due to the transmural nature of the disease. This leads to the formation of abscesses, fistulae, strictures, and adhesions, which may also contribute to the development of obstruction or bacterial overgrowth.

The most serious acute complication of UC is toxic megacolon. Although reported to occur in up to 5% of UC patients, it is rare in young patients. Toxic megacolon is a medical and surgical emergency. The colonic dilatation in toxic megacolon results from severe inflammation resulting in disturbed intestinal motility. Disrupted mucosal integrity may allow entry of bacteria into submucosal tissues, leading to necrosis and peritonitis.

Colonic malignancy is a significant complication in both UC and CD patients with pancolitis beginning in childhood. Duration of disease and pancolitis are well recognized as risk factors for the development of malignancy, with the risk of cancer increasing over that of the general population after 10 years of disease. Other risk factors include concomitant sclerosing cholangitis; an excluded, defunctionalized, or bypassed segment; and depressed red blood cell folate levels.

Children who develop UC before 14 years of age have a cumulative colorectal cancer incidence rate of 5% at 20 years and 40% at 35 years. Children who develop the disease between 15 and 39 years of age have a cumulative incidence rate of 5% at 20 years and 30% at 35 years. Therefore, it is estimated that there is an 8% risk of dying from colon cancer 10 to 25 years after diagnosis of colitis if colectomy is not performed for control of disease symptoms. The risk for children with onset of disease in the first decade is unknown, but children who develop colitis before the age of 10 should undergo colonoscopy screening during their adolescence. Epithelial dysplasia generally precedes carcinoma; therefore, yearly surveillance colonoscopies are recommended for these high-risk patients. Because colonoscopies can miss dysplasia, prophylactic colectomy should be considered in any adult who developed UC during childhood. Therefore, adolescent and young adults should be prepared psychologically for the possible need for surgery in the future.

Although the risk of malignancy in CD is not as high as in UC, the risk of adenocarcinoma of the colon for Crohn's colitis is 4 to 20 times that of the general population. Patients with small intestinal disease are 50 to 100 times more likely to develop small intestinal carcinoma. Since small intestinal carcinoma is a rare event in the general population, it is also uncommon in CD.

Fistula and abscess formation is common in CD and due to transmural bowel perforation. Perianal and perirectal fistulization is the most common, with the most common enteroenteric fistula being between the ileum and sigmoid colon. Perianal disease occurs in 15% of pediatric patients with CD. Perianal disease may precede the appearance of the intestinal manifestations of CD by years and is seen most commonly in patients with colitis. When perianal disease does not respond to medical therapy, surgical management is necessary.

EXTRAINTESTINAL MANIFESTATIONS OF PEDIATRIC IBD

The extraintestinal manifestations of IBD in children are summarized in Table 17-1. Twenty-five percent to 35% of patients with IBD have at least one extraintestinal manifestation. These diseases may be diagnosed before, concurrently with, or after the diagnosis of IBD is made. Extraintestinal manifestations can occur even after colectomy for UC. The presence of extraintestinal manifestations may carry prognostic significance. Patients with UC and extraintestinal manifestations have a significantly higher rate of pouchitis following colectomy and ileal pouch-anal anastomosis.

Skin manifestations, which are common in IBD, include erythema nodosum and pyoderma gangrenosum. Erythema nodosum is more common in CD and usually follows the course of the disease. It affects 3% of pediatric patients with CD, which is less frequent than in the adult population. It is estimated that 75% of the patients with erythema nodosum ultimately develop arthritis. The lesions of erythema nodosum are raised, red, tender nodules that appear primarily on the anterior surfaces of the leg. Therapy involves treating the underlying bowel disease. Pyoderma gangrenosum affects less than 1% of patients with UC and even fewer patients with CD. Pyoderma gangrenosum is often an indolent chronic ulcer that may occur even when the disease is in remission. Therefore, medical therapy for the underlying bowel disease is not always successful. Intralesional therapy with steroids is useful, and colectomy results in healing in approximately one-half of cases.

Aphthous ulceration in the mouth is the most common oral manifestation of IBD. This lesion is more common in CD and is commonly associated with skin and joint lesions. Oral lesions appear to parallel intestinal disease in most cases but also may occur before any gastrointestinal symptoms.

For CD and UC, ophthalmologic manifestations occur most frequently when the disease is active. The incidence is reported to be 4% in the adult population but is lower in children and adolescents with UC and CD. The most common ocular findings are episcleritis and anterior uveitis. The uveitis is usually symptomatic, causing pain or decreased vision. Increased intraocular pressure and cataracts may be seen in children receiving corticosteroid therapy. All patients with IBD require ophthalmologic examination at regular intervals.

Arthritis is the most common extraintestinal manifestation in children and adolescents, occurring in 7% to 25% of pediatric patients. The arthritis is usually transient, nondeforming synovitis, asymmetric in distribution and involves the large joints of the lower extremities. In adults, the arthritis occurs when the disease is active, but in children the arthritis may occur years before any gastrointestinal symptoms develop. Ankylosing spondylitis occurs in 2% to 6% of patients and is more common in males. It is associated with HLA-

B27. While not truly an arthritis, clubbing is common in children with CD involving the small intestine.

Hepatobiliary disease is one of the most common extraintestinal manifestations of IBD and its therapies, affecting hepatocytes, the biliary tree, or even the vascular system. Hepatobiliary complications in children may precede the onset of IBD, accompany active disease, or develop after surgical resection of all diseased bowel. Abnormal serum aminotransferases are common during the course of IBD in children. Most aminotransferase elevations are transient and appear to relate to medications or disease activity. Persistent aminotransferase elevations (> 6 months) should be investigated as the likelihood of serious liver disease is increased. Intrahepatic and extrahepatic manifestations of liver disease occur in children with IBD. Intrahepatic manifestations include chronic active hepatitis, granulomatous hepatitis, amyloidosis, fatty liver, and pericholangitis. Extrahepatic manifestations include cholelithiasis and obstruction. Sclerosing cholangitis may severely affect both the intrahepatic and extrahepatic ducts.

Chronic active hepatitis develops in <1% of children with IBD. The colitis may be relatively asymptomatic, although the chronic active hepatitis may proceed to cirrhosis. Granulomatous hepatitis is rare and is identified by noncaseating granulomatous lesions on liver biopsy. Amyloidosis is amyloid deposition in multiple organs including the liver and is secondary to chronic inflammation. Resolution has occurred after complete control of the primary disease. Fatty infiltration of the liver is a macrovesicular, nonprogressive, reversible lesion usually associated with malnutrition or steroid therapy. Pericholangitis may be an early stage of primary sclerosing cholangitis, although few progress to that stage. Sclerosing cholangitis develops in 3.5% of UC pediatric patients and <1% of CD pediatric patients. An inexorably progressive disease in adults, it may remain more dormant in children. It is not related to disease activity and may appear years before any gastrointestinal disease develops or even years after a colectomy for UC. Endoscopic retrograde cholangiopancreatography (ERCP) has significantly improved the ability to diagnose this disease in the pediatric population. Cholelithiasis has been described in both UC and CD, but more frequently in CD, especially after ileal resection. Cholesterol and pigment stones occur in patients with IBD. The urologic manifestations of IBD include nephrolithiasis, hydronephrosis, and enterovesical fistulae.

Nephrolithiasis is a common renal complication in pediatrics and occurs in approximately 5% of the children with IBD. It usually is the result of fat malabsorption that occurs with small bowel CD. Dietary calcium binds to malabsorbed fatty acids in the colonic lumen and free oxalate is absorbed. This results in hyperoxaluria and oxalate stones. In patients with an ileostomy, increased fluid and electrolyte losses may lead to a concentrated, acidic urine and the formation of uric acid stones. External compression of the ureter by an inflammatory mass or abscess may lead to hydronephrosis. Enterovesical fistulae, which are more common in males, may present with recurrent urinary tract infections or pneumaturia.

Thromboembolic disease is an extraintestinal manifestation that occurs in both adults and children with IBD. It is considered to be the result of a hypercoagulable state that parallels disease activity and may be manifested by thrombocytosis, elevated plasma fibrinogen, factor V, factor VIII, and decreased plasma antithrombin III. This may lead to deep vein thrombosis, pulmonary emboli, and neurovascular disease. Vasculitis affecting either the systemic or the cerebral circulation has been described in association with IBD in children.

Other extraintestinal manifestations include pancreatitis, fibrosing alveolitis, interstitial pneumonitis, pericarditis, and peripheral neuropathy. Pancreatitis may result from 5-aminosalicylic acid and 6-mercaptopurine, while peripheral neuropathy may occur with prolonged metronidazole therapy.

DIAGNOSIS OF PEDIATRIC IBD

The initial evaluation of suspected IBD should be performed by the primary physician. The importance of the history cannot be overemphasized. Recent antibiotic intake and family history are important and often overlooked. Abdominal examination is often nonspecific, although a fullness or mass in the right lower quadrant may indicate CD. Rectal examination is important to detect perianal disease fecal blood. A careful assessment of growth and development is an important part of the evaluation of the pediatric patient. Growth abnormalities may be detected by evaluation of several different parameters. These include the measurement of height and weight, the calculation of percent height and weight for age and percent weight for height, measurement of growth velocity, anthropometry to determine body composition, and skeletal bone age to look for delayed bone maturation. The measurement of growth velocity is the most sensitive indicator of growth abnormalities because a decrease in growth velocity may be seen before the crossing of major percentile lines on standard growth curves.

Laboratory data are nonspecific. The complete blood cell count may reveal evidence of hypochromic, microcytic anemia. The sedimentation rate is elevated in 90% of patients with CD. A normal sedimentation rate, however, should not deter further evaluation in a suspicious case. Additional studies should include serum proteins (albumin, transferrin, prealbumin) and micronutrients (folic acid, vitamin B_{12}, serum iron, total iron binding capacity, calcium, magnesium). Anti-*Saccharomyces cerevisiae* antibody (ASCA) is positive in 70% of patients with CD. These antibody tests can, at times, help differentiate between UC and CD colitis. Up to 85% of all patients with CD have evidence of terminal ileal disease, which is confirmed using colonoscopy and ileal biopsy. Colonoscopy with ileoscopy has been used extensively in the management of adults and children with CD. The expanded use of this diagnostic modality was made possible by technological advances in the manufacture of smaller endoscopes and the training of gastroenterologists skilled in pediatric endoscopy.

Consequently, this has led to a reliance on an upper gastrointestinal series with small bowel follow-through (UGI/SBFT) to diagnose small bowel disease, especially terminal ileum (TI) disease. The UGI/SBFT has been found to be highly specific but the sensitivity is low. The terminal ileum in a young child is often nodular but later attains a velvety appearance on direct vision and as seen by contrast radiography in early adulthood. This nodular appearance may be easily misinterpreted as abnormal after SBFT, suggesting the presence of CD. In these instances, the only reliable way of diagnosing IBD is through colonoscopy and terminal ileal biopsy. The presence of granulomata anywhere in the GI tract confirms the diagnosis of CD.

Colonoscopy and ileoscopy have demonstrated an excellent safety profile in centers with trained pediatric gastroenterologists. Most children tolerate the procedure with only minor discomfort under conscious sedation with adequate cardiorespiratory monitoring or general anesthesia. It is estimated that the rate of perforation in pediatric patients is less than 1%.

A pediatric Crohn's disease activity index (PCDAI) was developed in 1990. It included the following parameters:

1. Subjective reporting of the degree of abdominal pain, stool pattern, and general well-being

2. The presence of extraintestinal manifestations, such as fever, arthritis, rash, and uveitis

3. Physical examination findings

4. Weight and height

5. Hematocrit, erythrocyte sedimentation rate, and serum albumin

The PCDAI also includes linear growth and places less emphasis on subjectively reported symptoms when compared to the Crohn's disease activity index (CDAI), but more on laboratory parameters of intestinal inflammation. It is a useful tool to classify patients by disease activity.

TREATMENT OF PEDIATRIC IBD

The general goals of treatment for children with IBD are to achieve the best possible clinical and laboratory control of the inflammatory disease with the least possible side effects from medication, to promote growth through adequate nutrition, and permit the patient to function as normally as possible (ie, school attendance, participation in sports). Not all of these goals are always attainable.

The treatment of pediatric IBD can be divided into four major categories: medical, surgical, nutritional, and psychological.

MEDICAL THERAPY

With the improved understanding of the immune system, many new agents that block specific immune pathways are in clinical trials. It is important to determine the type and location of the IBD in order to utilize these therapies. Although there are many pediatric clinical trials published, none of the medications used in IBD are approved for their use in children. Table 17-2 summarizes the medical therapy for pediatric IBD.

Table 17-2

PHARMACOLOGIC THERAPY FOR IBD IN PEDIATRICS

Mild Disease and Remission

Ulcerative Colitis
- Sulfasalazine 50 to 75 mg/kg/day twice a day (bid) to four times a day (qid) (max 5 g/day)
- Mesalamine (Asacol, Pentasa) 30 to 80 mg/kg/day divided three times a day (tid) to qid (max Asacol 4.8 g/day, Pentasa 4.0 g/day)
- Mesalamine enema (Rowasa [Solvay Pharmaceuticals Inc, West Baudette, Minn]) 4 g every hour (qhs)
- Mesalamine suppository (Canasa [Axcan Scandipharm Inc, Birmingham, Ala]) 500 mg qhs or bid
- Hydrocortisone enema (Cortifoam and Protofoam [Schwarz Pharma Inc, Milwaukee, Wis) every day (qd) to bid
- Budesonide enema (Entocort [AstraZeneca Pharmaceuticals, Canada]) 2 g/100 mL qd

Moderate Disease

Crohn's Disease
- Oral budesonide (Entocort [AstraZeneca Pharmaceuticals, Wilmington, Del) 6 to 9 mg qd
- Metronidazole 10 to 15 mg/kg/day divided bid to tid (max 1 g/day)
- Ciprofloxacin 10 to 15 mg/kg/day divided bid (max 1 g/day)
- Prednisone 1 to 2 mg/kg/day divided qd
- Budesonide (Entocort) 9 mg qd

Refractory Disease

Ulcerative Colitis
- Azathioprine 2.0 to 2.5 mg/kg/day qd (monitor metabolite levels)
- 6-Mercaptopurine 1.0 to 1.5 mg/kg/day qd (monitor metabolite levels)
- Cyclosporine A 4 to 6 mg/kg continuous intravenous (IV) infusion, followed by 4 mg orally divided bid (monitor drug levels)
- IV infusion, then 4 mg/kg po divided bid (monitor drug levels)

Crohn's Colitis
- Methotrexate 0.3 to 0.5 mg/kg/dose sq once a week (max 25 mg), supplement with 1 mg/day of folic acid
- Infliximab (Remicade [Centocor, Malvern, Pa) 5 mg/kg/dose IV

Anti-Inflammatory Drugs

5-AMINOSALICYLATES

The use of sulfasalazine in the pediatric population has declined dramatically because of its effects. Eighty percent to 90% of patients intolerant of or allergic to sulfasalazine will tolerate oral 5-ASA preparations. The new 5-ASA preparations that work within the small intestine have been shown to have a greater rate of maintaining remission in CD than placebo. These preparations include Asacol (Proctor & Gamble Pharmaceuticals, Cincinnati, Ohio), which dissolves in the ileum and cecum, and Pentasa (Roberts Pharmaceutical Co, Eatontown, NJ), which is composed of microspheres that release 5-ASA throughout the small intestine. Symptoms of mild inflammation should remit in 60% to 70% of patients within 3 to 4 weeks. Occasionally, hypersensitivity to 5-ASA compounds can mimic colitic symptoms. Balsalazide (eg, Colazal, Salix Pharmaceuticals, Raleigh, NC) is a new mesalamine prodrug activated by colonic bacteria; therefore, its activity is restricted to the colon. The capsule can be opened and the powder can be dissolved in water, making this formulation easier to administrate in the pediatric IBD population.

Children with CD will benefit from 5-ASA products released in the small intestine. More proximal release is achieved by opening up some of the 5-ASA capsules; this allows an anti-inflammatory effect in the esophagus, stomach, duodenum, and proximal small intestine. Some of the 5-ASA compounds are prepared as enemas or suppositories for symptoms related to distal colitis or pouchitis after surgery.

Corticosteroids

Corticosteroids in children with IBD need to be used with great caution. Side effects like striae, acne, moon facies, posterior cataracts, and hirsutism can have a psychological impact on the adolescent patient. The effects on growth and bone mineralization represent more serious side effects. Several enema and suppository corticosteroid formulations are available to treat distal colitis or pouchitis.

Budesonide, a new steroid preparation formulated for topic small intestinal release, has less side effects than systemic steroids. Budesonide has been shown to be more effective than placebo in maintaining remission in CD. Few studies of this drug in children are available.

Corticosteroids are effective in controlling exacerbations of CD and UC. When used for more than 7 days, a weaning dose schedule is recommended to avoid side effects related to the adrenal-pituitary-hypophysis axis. Low dose alternate-day corticosteroid therapy has been proposed as a strategy to achieve remission in IBD but studies have failed to demonstrate its efficacy.

Immunomodulators

Multiple immunosuppressive agents including 6-mercaptopurine (6-MP), azathioprine, cyclosporine, tacrolimus, thalidomide, and methotrexate have been used in IBD.

Azathioprine and its metabolite, 6-MP, are increasingly used to treat children and adolescents with IBD. These drugs have a delayed clinical response time of 3 to 4 months, but side effects can be evident a few days after starting the medication. The advantage of these drugs is the ability to measure the metabolizing enzyme (thiopurine methyltransferase) and metabolite levels (6-methyl mercaptopurine and 6-thioguanine) on the erythrocytes. Compliance issues, especially in adolescent patients, can be addressed by measuring the metabolite levels.

Methotrexate is another drug that has been adopted for the use of IBD. Few studies on children have been published. One of the advantages of this drug is that is administered by a weekly injection.

Antibiotics, Prebiotics, and Probiotics

Recent studies also have shown the usefulness of antibiotic therapy in the treatment of CD. Metronidazole, as well as the combination of metronidazole and ciprofloxacin, is useful in both the management of perianal, small bowel, and colonic diseases.

Probiotics are living micro-organisms that can affect the host in a beneficial manner. Prebiotics are nondigestible food ingredients that stimulate the growth and activity of probiotic bacteria already established in the colon. Probiotics have been shown to be effective in the treatment of *Clostridium difficile*, as well as in preventing the frequency and severity of infectious acute diarrhea in children. The most successful studies involve the use of *Lactobacillus GG* at a dose of 1x1010 viable organisms per day and the yeast boulardii at a dose of 1 g/day. A probiotic preparation (VSL#3 at 6 g/day) that uses a combination of three species of *Bifidobacterium*, four strains of *Lactobacillus*, and one strain of *Streptococcus* has shown promise in maintaining remission in UC and pouchitis, as well as in preventing the postoperative recurrence of CD.

The mechanism of action of probiotics may include receptor competition, effects on mucin secretion, or probiotic immunomodulation of gut-associated lymphoid tissue.

Biologic Agents

Recently, a novel therapeutic approach has been developed from our improved understanding of the immune system. These therapies consist of either anti-inflammatory cytokines (eg, IL-10, IL-11) or antibodies that diminish the effects of proinflammatory cytokines (eg., anti-TNFµ, anti-IL-12).

Infliximab is an antitumor necrosis factor chimeric monoclonal antibody of the IgG1 type that has been used recently in the treatment of CD. In several multicenter studies infliximab has been shown to significantly improve the PCDAI scores in children with IBD. The use of infliximab (5 mg/kg/dose) has been demonstrated to be safe and effective in pediatric patients with IBD.

A more humanized anti-TNFµ antibody of IgG4 subtype, called CDP 571, is currently under study for the pediatric IBD population.

SURGICAL THERAPY

CD is often more difficult to manage because surgery does not cure the disease. It is only considered for uncontrollable bleeding, stenotic bowel, or fistulas unresponsive to medical therapy. Strictureplasty is helpful to open up stenotic areas without removing large segments of small intestine. Some success in decreasing recurrence rates after surgery with the use of mesalamine or 6-MP has recently been reported. However, until a treatment that prevents recurrence in the majority of cases is developed, reliance on medical and nutritional therapy is necessary for CD.

UC can be "cured" with a total proctocolectomy. Various endorectal pullthrough procedures, similar to those performed to treat Hirschsprung's disease or imperforate anus, have been used to treat UC.

NUTRITIONAL THERAPY

Nutritional therapy is more useful in CD than in UC. Its primary goal is to prevent or correct malnutrition, maintain and promote growth, and correct specific micronutrient deficiencies. It also can be used to induce remission, reverse complications, and prevent relapses. The goal is to provide enough calories for both normal and catch-up growth. Improvement in nutritional status may be accomplished by a variety of methods. Occasionally, with heightened awareness of the nutritional needs, patients will be compliant with oral supplemental alimentation with high-caloric formulas. When oral supplementation fails, other means of providing nutritional support include overnight continuous nasogastric feeding and intravenous parenteral alimentation. Enteral nutrition with an oligopeptide formula has fewer relapses when used over 4 weeks of a 20-week cycle, when compared to patients receiving alternate day prednisone. Also, patients who attained remission with exclusive enteral nutrition had prolonged remission and improved linear growth if nighttime nasogastric feedings were continued with an oligopeptide or amino acid-based formula, when compared to children who discontinued the nighttime feeding.

A dramatic reversal of malnutrition and a change in growth velocity can be expected in all children treated with adequate nutrition in conjunction with medical therapy to control symptoms of IBD. Another potential therapy is omega-3 fatty acids (fish oil). Omega-3 fatty acids are known to reduce the production of leukotriene B4 and thromboxane A2, inhibit synthesis of cytokines, and act as free radical scavengers. For CD patents at risk for relapse, enteric-coated preparations of omega-3 fatty acids (1.8 g EPA plus 0.9 g DHA) reduced relapse rates at 1 year as measured by the CDAI when compared to placebo, 28% versus 69%, respectively.

PSYCHOLOGICAL THERAPY

Emotional support of the patient and family during the diagnosis and early phases of therapy is very important. In general, depression is common in chronic disease. Some studies have shown that children with IBD have a higher incidence of low self-esteem and depression than healthy children or children with other pediatric chronic diseases. Lifetime prevalence of depression is higher in CD than in UC. CD is a potentially disabling condition that may cause disruption of family and school life, produce financial burdens, and lead to social isolation. Children on steroids experience depressive symptoms more frequently than children not taking steroids.

The main goal of the psychosocial intervention is to restore emotional health and improve function. A multidisciplinary approach with the patient and his or her family is needed for treatment.

BIBLIOGRAPHY

Baldassano RN, et al. A multicenter study of infliximab (anti-TNF alpha antibody) in the treatment of children with active Crohn's disease. *Gastroenterology.* 1999;116(4):A665.

Baldassano RN, Han PD, Jeshion WC, et al. Pediatric Crohn's disease: risk factors for postoperative recurrence. *Am J Gastroenterol.* 2001;96(7):2169-2176.

Baldassano RN, Piccoli DA. Inflammatory bowel disease in pediatric and adolescent patients. *Gastroenterol Clin North Am.* 1999;28(2):445-458.

Fox VL. Pediatric endoscopy. *Gastrointest Endosc Clin N Am.* 2000;10(1):175-194, viii.

Gupta P, Andrew H, Kirschner BS, Guandalini S. Is lactobacillus GG helpful in children with Crohn's disease? results of a preliminary, open-label study. *J Pediatr Gastroenterol Nutr.* 2000;31(4):453-457.

Gupta PR, Gokhale D, Kirschner BS. 6-mercaptopurine metabolite levels in children with inflammatory bowel disease. *J Pediatr Gastroenterol Nutr.* 2001;33(4):450-454.

Hyams JS, Ferry GD, Mandel FS, et al. Development and validation of a pediatric Crohn's disease activity index. *J Pediatr Gastroenterol Nutr.* 1991;12(4):439-447.

Ling SC, Griffiths AM. Nutrition in inflammatory bowel disease. *Curr Opin Clin Nutr Metab Care.* 2000;3(5):339-344.

Ogura Y, Inohara N, Benito A, Chen FF, Yamaoka S, Nunez G. Nod2, a Nod1/Apaf-1 family member that is restricted to monocytes and activates NF-kappaB. *J Biol Chem.* 2001;276(7):4812-4818.

Semeao EJ, Jawad AF, Zemel BS, Neiswender KM, Piccoli DA, Stallings VA. Bone mineral density in children and young adults with Crohn's disease. *Inflamm Bowel Dis.* 1999;5(3):161-166.

Sentongo TA, Semeao EJ, Piccoli DA, Stallings VA, Zemel BS. Growth, body composition, and nutritional status in children and adolescents with Crohn's disease. *J Pediatr Gastroenterol Nutr.* 2000;31(1):33-40.

Steinhart AH, Ewe K, Griffiths AM, Modigliani R, Thomsen OO. Corticosteroids for maintaining remission of Crohn's disease (Cochrane Review). *Cochrane Database Syst Rev.* 2001;3:CD000301.

Stephens M, Batres LA, Ng D, Baldassano RN. Growth failure in the child with inflammatory bowel disease. *Semin Gastrointest Dis.* 2001;12(4):253-262.

Vasiliauskas E. Pediatric inflammatory bowel disease. *Curr Treat Options Gastroenterol.* 2000;3(5):403-424.

Zachos M, Tandeur M, Griffiths AM. Enteral nutritional therapy for inducing remission of Crohn's disease (Cochrane review). *Cochrane Database Syst Rev.* 2001;3:CD000542.

chapter 18

Medical Approach to the Patient With Inflammatory Bowel Disease

Peter D. Han, MD and Russell D. Cohen, MD

INTRODUCTION

The successful treatment of patients with inflammatory bowel disease (IBD) requires careful attention to the patient's symptoms, with discrimination of which symptoms are due to IBD and which symptoms are due to separate disease processes. Establishing the cause of symptoms in these patients who are often prone to infections or have had previous bowel surgery may be diagnostically challenging.

Key in the evaluation of patients with IBD is the identification of the location and severity of disease. Treating IBD consists of a two-staged process: *induction* of remission, followed by *maintenance* of that remission. Crohn's disease and ulcerative colitis are invariably life-long diseases, and failure to maintain remission often leads to relapse. As a result, the selection of safe and effective medications for both remission induction and maintenance must be understood. The panoply of medications available to treat Crohn's disease and ulcerative colitis can be fit into a framework of treatment for certain disease types and severities, allowing for a logical approach to each patient's case.

This chapter will review the medical approach to patients with IBD. First, the general principles in the evaluation and management of symptoms suggestive of active IBD will be highlighted. Diarrhea, anorexia, nausea, vomiting, fever, or abdominal pain may in fact be due to other, more common causes that may coexist with active IBD. Next, the management of specific clinical presentations of ulcerative colitis and then Crohn's disease will be reviewed. Finally, a discussion of novel therapies will give the reader insight into potential future treatment approaches. The reader is encouraged to first review the chapters on etiology and pathogenesis of these diseases and pharmacology of IBD drugs to gain a better understanding of the treatment principles.

Principles in the Evaluation and Management of IBD Symptoms

Diarrhea

Patients with IBD frequently complain of *diarrhea*, which may refer to increased stool frequency, altered stool consistency, increased stool volume/ weight, and/or fecal incontinence. A thorough history will help to define the precise nature of the complaint and guide therapy. Diarrhea in patients with IBD may result from a number of etiologies (Table 18-1).

Active IBD is often the cause of diarrhea in these patients. Disease activity can be determined directly through the use of endoscopic or radiographic imaging or by other "indirect" methods. Elevations of serum levels of C-reactive protein (CRP), erythrocyte sedimentation rate (ESR), white blood cell counts (especially with elevated band-forms), and/or platelet counts may all be reflective of an IBD "flare." The presence of fecal leukocytes is indicative of an inflammatory bowel process but not a reliable gauge of disease activity.

Diet is a frequent concern of patients with IBD. Patients may notice that certain foods tend to exacerbate their diarrhea or other bowel symptoms. Avoidance of these foods while taking care to maintain adequate nutritional status may help to control symptoms. It should be stressed that there are no particular foods that increase disease activity in IBD. Rather particular foods in certain individuals may exacerbate diarrhea or other bowel symptoms resulting from IBD. Patients are often advised to adhere to a "low residue diet," avoiding high fiber grains; raw produce; and difficult-to-digest foods, such as nuts, seeds, corn, and popcorn. The exception may be patients with solely distal ulcerative colitis or proctitis and constipation in which fiber may be needed for relief of symptoms.

Lactase deficiency may occur in patients with IBD. Suspected lactase-deficiency should be confirmed by a lactose breath test to avoid inappropriate avoidance of all dairy products, an important source of calcium for patients at possible increased risk of osteoporosis. A lactose-free diet or the use of lactase enzyme supplements may help to control symptoms.

Enteric infections may cause diarrhea. Patients with IBD are prone to develop infections with pathogenic strains of *Clostridium difficile* even without

Table 18-1

ETIOLOGIES FOR DIARRHEA IN PATIENTS WITH IBD

Etiology	Diagnostic Test	Treatment
Diet	Empiric avoidance of certain foods (highly patient-specific)	Avoidance of inciting foods while ensuring adequate nutritional intake
Lactase deficiency	Lactose breath test or empiric trial of lactose-free diet	Lactose-free diet
Enteric infection	Stool culture, *Clostridium difficile* toxin, ova, and parasites (other stool studies as situation warrants)	Antibiotic/antiparasitic therapy
Bacterial over-therapy	Hydrogen breath test or empiric trial of antibiotics	Antibiotic therapy
Enteroenteral fistula	Computed tomography scan Barium study (UGI, SBFT, BE)	Treat if symptomatic (surgery, medical therapy)
Bile salt diarrhea	Response to empiric therapy with bile acid binding resins	Oral bile acid sequestrants
Steatorrhea	Fecal fat determination	Bile salt supplementation, medium-chain triglycerides, pancreatic enzymes
Medications	Use of laxatives or magnesium-containing medications	Discontinue offending agent
Ischemic bowel disease	Clinical exam, radiologic studies, and/or endoscopy	Optimize enteric circulation, surgical consultation

continued on next page

Table 18-1 (Continued)

ETIOLOGIES FOR DIARRHEA IN PATIENTS WITH IBD

Etiology	Diagnostic Test	Treatment
Bowel obstruction	History, physical, and radiologic studies	Nasogastric decompression, surgical consultation
Irritable bowel syndrome/ functional bowel disorder	History and physical, and exclusion of other causes	Antispasmodics, antidiarrheals, antidepressants
Factitious diarrhea	Laxative screen, history	Counseling
Active IBD	Clinical, laboratory, imaging evaluation	Treatment of IBD

UGI = upper gastrointestinal barium study, SBFT = small bowel follow-through barium study, BE = barium enema

---

antecedent use of antibiotics. Infections with enteric pathogens such as *Salmonella, Shigella, Campylobacter,* enterohemorrhagic *E. coli, Giardia lamblia, Entamoeba histolytica,* and cytomegalovirus (CMV) may cause increased bowel symptoms. Patients with IBD and diarrhea should have stool samples sent for *C. difficile* toxin, stool culture, and ova and parasites at their initial presentation and also for diarrheal attacks that differ from typical IBD flares or are refractory to IBD therapies. In addition, CMV may need to be excluded in patients on immunosuppressive agents.

Bacterial overgrowth in the small intestine may result in diarrhea due to malabsorption caused by bacterial degradation of carbohydrates, fatty acids, and bile salts. Predisposing factors in patients with IBD include intestinal stasis, bowel obstruction, resection of the ileocecal valve, and intestinal resection or fistulous disease resulting in blind loops. A small bowel series or enteroclysis may help to define anatomic abnormalities that can lead to bacterial overgrowth. Although culture of jejunal aspirates is the gold standard diagnostic test, [14C]-D-xylose or hydrogen breath testing may also be used to establish the diagnosis. Treatment regimens should consist of alternating regimens of antibiotics effective against anaerobic and aerobic enteric bacteria. Although presumptive treatment of overgrowth without prior testing is discouraged due to the risk of unnecessary antibiotic-related complications, the efficacy of antibiotics in some patients with IBD leads some physicians to "treat and see" if patients improve.

Bile salt malabsorption may cause diarrhea in patients with terminal ileal involvement or resection. In mild cases of ileal impairment, increased hepatic synthesis of bile salts is adequate to allow micelle formation, and normal fat absorption occurs. The increased delivery of bile acids to the colon leads to diarrhea due to impaired electrolyte and water absorption as well as chloride ion secretion caused by bile acids in the colon. Treatment with cholestyramine or colestipol (typically before meals) is often immediately effective in these patients; failure to notice an impact suggests that the diarrhea is from a different etiology. In more severe cases of ileal impairment (ie, less than 100 inches of healthy small bowel remaining), hepatic synthesis is not able to provide enough bile acids for adequate fat absorption and steatorrhea results. Testing the stool for fecal fat may confirm the presence of steatorrhea, which may require supplementation of bile acids and reduction in dietary intake of long-chain fatty acids.

Medications may also result in diarrhea. Medication history should be closely examined for use of prescribed or over-the-counter laxatives or other magnesium-containing products. Antibiotic use may predispose to *C. difficile* colitis. Many IBD physicians suggest avoiding nonsteroidal anti-inflammatory drugs (NSAIDs) (and perhaps COX-II inhibitors) due to the risk of inducing flares of disease. Even some of the medications typically used to treat IBD, especially olsalazine but also mesalamine, sulfasalazine, and the immunomodulators, may cause diarrhea in certain individuals. Holding a few doses will often determine whether these are indeed the culprits.

Bowel ischemia may result in inflammatory diarrhea. The diarrhea may contain significant amounts of blood, and abdominal pain may be present. Diagnosis involves radiologic imaging and endoscopy. Mesenteric ischemia (ie, ischemia involving the distribution of the superior mesenteric artery and sometimes the celiac artery) may present with postprandial pain, bloating, weight loss, and diarrhea. Diagnosis is often made by a mesenteric doppler ultrasound, followed by an aortogram. Ischemic colitis (ie, colitis involving the distribution of the inferior mesenteric and sometimes the superior mesenteric arteries) more commonly presents with bloody diarrhea. Diagnosis can be made on colonoscopy with biopsy, although the endoscopic appearance may be confused with infectious or inflammatory colitis. Typically, the rectum is spared due to the dual systemic and portal blood supplies.

Bowel obstruction due to adhesions, herniations, or stricture formation may cause diarrhea due to flow of liquid stool around the obstruction or due to bacterial overgrowth in the proximal, dilated segments of bowel. Evaluation consists of clinical and radiologic examinations.

ANOREXIA, NAUSEA, AND VOMITING

Anorexia, nausea, and vomiting are not uncommon in IBD patients and may result in poor nutrition. A common cause is obstruction of the bowel, either directly due to IBD or due to adhesions or hernias from previous abdominal surgeries. Patients with Crohn's disease may form partial (or rarely, complete) small or large bowel obstructions at the site of small intestinal or colonic strictures. Small bowel disease or adhesions may serve as the lead point of an intussusception. Due to the mucosal nature of the disease, stricture formation is less common in ulcerative colitis and should prompt an evaluation for colonic malignancy when present.

Anorexia may result from the elevation of inflammatory cytokines that occurs with active inflammation. In addition, unabsorbed fat and carbohydrate in the terminal ileum can slow the transit of food through the jejunum and delay gastric emptying through a hormonally mediated mechanism. This gastric stasis can also contribute to nausea and vomiting. Alternatively, direct disease involvement of the upper GI tract in Crohn's disease may lead to these symptoms.

Drug side effects are a common cause of anorexia, nausea, and vomiting in IBD patients. Ten percent to 20% of patients treated with sulfasalazine develop nausea and vomiting—likely due to the sulfa-moiety. However, 5-aminosalicylate (5-ASA) compounds can also cause nausea and vomiting. Nausea and hypogeusia are also common during treatment with metronidazole. Trace metal deficiencies, particularly zinc, may lead to anorexia due to hypogeusia and hyposmia. Nausea and vomiting may also occur in association with pancreatitis, which may be caused by 6-mercaptopurine (6-MP) or azathioprine.

The clinical approach to these symptoms should focus on maintaining an adequate nutritional status. Unnecessary medications should be eliminated. If the patient is on sulfasalazine, a mesalamine compound may be substituted (Table 18-2). Upper endoscopy may be helpful in establishing the presence of gastroduodenal Crohn's disease, requiring adjustments to therapy. A gastric emptying study may indicate gastric stasis requiring treatment with prokinetic agents, although these are discouraged in patients with bowel obstruction. Diet can also be adjusted to consist of soft and easily digestible foods while maintaining adequate nutritional intake.

FEVER

In many patients, fever is due to active IBD. Inflammation of the bowel, active perianal disease, or the presence of an inflammatory phlegmon or abscess may result in fevers. The release of pyrogenic cytokines may cause fevers in IBD patients with no other localized sources. If warranted by clinical circumstances, evaluation for active disease consisting of laboratory, radiologic, and endoscopic evaluation should be undertaken. Some patients may have an increased susceptibility to infection due to immunosuppressive medications. Evaluation of potential infectious etiologies based on the clinical scenario should be undertaken. Fever can also occur as a hypersensitivity reaction to medications used in the treatment of IBD.

ABDOMINAL PAIN

Abdominal pain is one of the most common symptoms among IBD patients, with several potential etiologies.

Intestinal obstruction due to strictures or adhesions can lead to abdominal pain through stretching of the bowel wall. In patients with IBD who have

Table 18-2

AMINOSALICYLATE FORMULATIONS

Medication	Site of Delivery	Dosage	Formulation
Oral Agents			
Sulfasalazine (eg, Azulfidine [Pharmacia & Upjohn, Peapack, NJ])	Colon	Start at 500 mg bid Titrate up to 3 to 6 g/day as tolerated	Sulfa moiety linked to 5-ASA bond cleaved by colonic bacteria
Olsalazine (eg, Dipentum [Pharmacia & Upjohn, Peapack, NJ])	Colon	1 to 3 g/day bid	Two 5-ASA molecule-linked bonds cleaved by colonic bacteria
Balsalazide (eg, Colazal [Salix Pharmaceuticals Inc, Raleigh, NC])	Colon	6.75 g/day tid	Aminobenzoyl-alanine (inert) linked to 5-ASA; bond cleaved in colon
Mesalamine (eg, Asacol)	Distal ileum/ colon	2.4 to 4.8 g/day bid to tid	5-ASA in eudragit S resin (releases drug at pH 7)
Mesalamine (eg, Pentasa)	Stomach to colon	3 to 4 g/day bid to qid	5-ASA in ethylcellulose granules (sustained release)
Rectal Agents			
Mesalamine suppository (eg, Canasa)	Rectum	500 mg suppository bid to tid	5-ASA suppository
Mesalamine enema (eg, Rowasa)	Rectum to splenic flexure	4 g enema qhs	5-ASA enema

strictures or adhesions, a low-residue diet is advised to help prevent intestinal obstruction. Patients should be counseled to thoroughly chew their food and avoid "anything that cannot be converted to liquid mush in their mouth," such as raw vegetables or other high fiber foods.

Active inflammation can lead to abdominal pain if the inflammation is transmural and affects the serosa. Typically, superficial ulcerations do not lead to significant abdominal pain. Rectal inflammation can sensitize the walls of the bowel to distension, leading to the sensation of tenesmus.

Abdominal pain may represent perforation of the bowel with generalized or localized peritonitis. It is not unusual for a Crohn's patient to seal over a microperforation, and develop a tender inflammatory mass on examination. Abdominal x-rays and a CT scan may help to evaluate for free air and abscess formation.

Abdominal pain, nausea, and vomiting may be due to pancreatitis, particularly in patients taking purine analogues (6-MP, azathioprine), and less commonly with mesalamine. IBD patients are at higher risk for gallstones and kidney stones, which may also result in abdominal pain. The same etiologies of abdominal pain that are often considered in a non-IBD setting, such as appendicitis, diverticulitis, incarcerated hernias, or gynecological pain, also need to be excluded in IBD patients.

An overlapping functional bowel disorder may contribute to abdominal pain in a number of patients with IBD. This is thought to be related to increased irritability of the intestine due to active inflammation and increased sensitivity to stretching of the bowel wall. Abdominal pain, bloating, and cramping out of proportion to the established degree of bowel inflammation may suggest a functional component. Treatment with antispasmodic agents (dicyclomine 20 to 40 mg four times a day [qid], hyoscyamine 0.125 to 0.25 mg qid) or antidepressants (such as nortriptyline or amitriptyline 10 to 50 mg/day or selective serotonin reuptake inhibitors) may be helpful. Care should be taken to avoid any anticholinergic medications in severe disease to avoid precipitating toxic megacolon.

THERAPY OF SPECIFIC CLINICAL PRESENTATIONS

ULCERATIVE COLITIS

A thorough clinical history and comprehensive review of the patient's laboratory, endoscopic, radiologic, and histologic examinations are essential to formulate an effective treatment plan. Knowing what parts of the colon are inflamed allows one to tailor the available therapies to the particular patient. Although the diagnosis can be made initially on flexible sigmoidoscopy with biopsy, it is often helpful to perform a full colonoscopy to establish the extent and severity of the disease. Biopsies should be taken separately from endoscopically normal and abnormal areas and placed in separate, labeled jars to allow for an accurate assessment of microscopic extent of disease, and thus appropriate colorectal cancer risk stratification. In patients with symptoms of diarrhea and abdominal pain, it is also important to rule out intestinal infections through examination of stool for culture, ova and parasites, and *C. difficile*. *C. difficile* infection in patients with IBD may develop in the absence of prior antibiotic use. The clinical approach to patients with ulcerative colitis classified by extent and severity of disease is detailed below.

Ulcerative Proctitis

Ulcerative colitis with inflammation limited to the rectum is termed *ulcerative proctitis*. Symptoms often include rectal bleeding, tenesmus, multiple frequent small bowel movements, and a sensation of incomplete evacuation. Patients may even complain of constipation due to decreased motility of the proximal unaffected colon, with bowel movements often consisting of only blood and pus.

In patients with active disease, topical aminosalicylate therapy is the most effective initial approach to induce remission. Mesalamine can be administered topically as 500 mg suppositories every morning (qam) and every hour (qhs) (Canasa [Axcan Scandipharm, Birmingham, Ala]) or 4 g enemas qhs (Rowasa [Solvay, Brussels, Belgium]). In patients with difficulty retaining mesalamine enemas, corticosteroid enemas (Cortenema 100 mg qhs) are often easier to hold initially. The patient can gradually be transitioned to mesalamine as symptoms improve. Corticosteroids may also be administered as suppositories or foam (Cortifoam), which are easier to tolerate and often all that is needed for proctitis. Several weeks may be required to achieve the full effect of these preparations. It is important to remember that systemic absorption of these steroid preparations may eventually lead to side effects, and thus long-term therapy is discouraged.

Patients often prefer the use of oral medications, but they are rarely effective alone. 5-ASA formulations that release in the colon (see Table 18-2) can be tried, but the large doses needed are difficult to justify, given the efficacy of the rectal formulations. Systemic corticosteroids are often ineffective for the treatment of ulcerative proctitis, and their side-effects are prohibitive.

Failure of a patient with ulcerative proctitis to respond to topical therapies prompts re-evaluation of the case. Compliance to the prescribed therapeutic regimen should be verified. Stool studies should be re-examined for enteric infection. Sigmoidoscopy with biopsies is useful to confirm the diagnosis and determine the proximal extent of disease. As many as 30% of patients initially diagnosed with ulcerative proctitis experience proximal extension of their disease, and therapies may need to be adjusted. In some cases, it may be necessary to exclude sexually transmitted diseases due to anal intercourse (which can mimic ulcerative proctitis).

Once a patient has achieved clinical remission, the focus shifts to prevention of relapse. Continuation of the type of mesalamine therapy that was successful in inducing remission is the advised course. Some patients treated with topical mesalamine preparations may be gradually tapered to decreasing frequencies of administration, but relapses should be treated immediately with re-establishment of the active therapy dosage. Patients initially treated with topical corticosteroid preparations should be transitioned to topical mesalamine and gradually tapered off of the steroid preparation.

Left-Sided Colitis

Ulcerative colitis extending up to but not beyond the splenic flexure (or 60 cm from the anal verge) is termed left-sided ulcerative colitis. Topical therapy with mesalamine enemas 4 g qhs (eg, Rowasa) is first-line therapy for patients with left-sided ulcerative colitis. Radioscintographic data have shown that enemas administered with the patient in left lateral decubitus position reach up to the splenic flexure. The addition of mesalamine suppositories in the morning and afternoon may be necessary in some patients. Those who prefer oral agents may be given a mesalamine formulation that releases in the colon (see Table 18-2). However, it is important to note that oral agents are often slower to work and less effective than topical therapies in these patients, perhaps due to proximal colonic stasis leading to decreased distal delivery of medication. There is a direct relationship between oral mesalamine dose and efficacy, and doses at the upper limits shown in Table 18-2 may be needed. Combination therapy with topical and oral mesalamine is superior to oral mesalamine in the induction and maintenance of remission.

Patients intolerant to or with inadequate response to mesalamine may need corticosteroids, preferably as an enema formulation (Cortenema 100 mg qhs), or oral prednisone. Failure to improve or to wean off of corticosteroids despite optimal dosing of oral and rectal mesalamine suggests that the patient needs therapies for refractory colitis (see below).

Maintenance therapy to prevent relapse should be instituted once patients achieve clinical remission. Continuation of the mesalamine therapy successful in inducing remission is the advised course, often at the dose required to induce remission. If patients decrease the dose or discontinue the topical therapies and subsequently relapse, reinstitution of the previously successful regimen is advised. Patients who achieved remission with steroid preparations should be transitioned to topical and/or maximal dose oral mesalamine, and the steroid agents should be tapered. Corticosteroids should not be used in an attempt to maintain remission.

Extensive Colitis/Pancolitis

Ulcerative colitis extending beyond the splenic flexure is termed extensive colitis; when it reaches the cecum, it is referred to as pancolitis. Patients with extensive colitis or pancolitis and only mild to moderate symptoms can be treated as outpatients. Because the disease extends beyond the reach of topical preparations, oral aminosalicylates are the initial medications of choice. These medications should be used in appropriate doses to induce remission as outlined in Table 18-2 (3 to 4 g/d of sulfasalazine or 2.4 to 4.8 g/d of mesalamine). Topical aminosalicylates or steroids may be used for additional symptom relief if patients complain of left-sided symptoms such as tenesmus or fecal urgency. In patients with mild symptoms, antispasmodic or antidiarrheal medications (such as hyoscyamine, dicyclomine, or loperamide) may also be used for additional symptom relief. Oral aminosalicylates should be continued at maintenance doses once clinical remission has been achieved.

Systemic corticosteroid therapy may need to be initiated in patients who do not achieve clinical remission with maximal doses of oral and topical aminosalicylates. The initial dose of corticosteroids (typically 20 to 40 mg of prednisone daily) should be maintained until remission is achieved and then slowly tapered (one may choose to decrease the dose by 5 mg/d (daily) every week until 20 mg/d is reached, then decrease by 2.5 to 5 mg/d every 1 to 2 weeks, if tolerated without relapse). Maximal oral and topical mesalamine should be continued in most cases. Patients who have recurrent symptoms during the steroid taper may need to have an initial dose escalation followed by a slower taper. The management of patients with steroid dependent or refractory disease is discussed in the section on refractory disease.

Severe Disease

Patients with severe flares of ulcerative colitis should be managed in the inpatient setting. Indications for admission include failure of outpatient medical management, fever, hypotension, dehydration, >10 stools per day, severe rectal bleeding, and/or abdominal tenderness/distension. Treatment should be initiated with intravenous steroids in divided doses or as a continuous infusion (prednisolone 40 to 60 mg/d, methylprednisolone 32 to 48 mg/d, or hydrocortisone 300 to 400 mg/d). Higher doses of steroids often provide little additional benefit at the cost of a higher incidence of side effects. Oral 5-ASA compounds are often held and anticholinergics, antidiarrheals, and narcotic analgesics avoided as they can precipitate toxic megacolon. Supportive care should include correction of fluid and electrolyte imbalances and transfusions to correct anemia. Patients with severe symptoms should initially be kept on a nothing-by-mouth diet (NPO) with intravenous (IV) fluid supplementation, but as symptoms begin to resolve, they may be maintained on a low-residue diet. Patients who are malnourished or who do not quickly improve and restart eating should receive parenteral nutrition support. Hydrocortisone enemas (100 mg qhs) may provide additional symptomatic relief to patients who have prominent rectal symptoms such as tenesmus or fecal urgency.

Intravenous steroids should be continued at the initial dosage until patients are in remission (having a reasonable number of formed stools without blood, pain, or urgency and can take adequate oral nutrition). Subsequently, oral steroids can be substituted for intravenous steroids at an initial dosage of 40 mg/d of prednisone in divided doses. Therapy with aminosalicylates may be resumed at this point. Any recrudescence of disease activity should be aggressively treated with reinitiation of IV corticosteroids as well as re-examination of stools for new enteric infection. Patients who remain in remission after switching to oral steroids may be tapered slowly (decrease by 5 mg/d every week until 20 mg/d is reached, then decrease by 2.5 to 5 mg/d every 1 to 2 weeks). Recurrence of disease activity during this taper should be treated promptly with resumption of previous steroid dose and a slower steroid taper once recurrent symptoms are controlled.

If patients do not improve during the first week of intravenous steroid therapy, the likelihood of future improvement is small. These patients should be considered for cyclosporine therapy or surgery (proctocolectomy). The use of cyclosporine should be limited to centers with access to same or next day cyclosporine levels, with expertise in treating IBD, and in which appropriate surgical back-up is available. Cyclosporine is administered as a continuous infusion at a dose of 4 mg/kg body weight every 24 hours. The dose should be adjusted to achieve a target level of 350 to 550 ng/mL (radio-immuno-assay [RIA]). Intravenous steroids are typically continued along with hydrocortisone enemas (100 mg every day). Patients receiving cyclosporine should begin to respond within the first 3 to 5 days. If no response is seen within the first week of therapy or if the patient's condition worsens, they should have an immediate colectomy.

The following criteria should all be met prior to switching from IV to oral cyclosporine therapy: a reasonable number of formed bowel movements with no pain, minimal blood per rectum, and tolerance of a reasonable oral diet. Failure to achieve these criteria should result in a colectomy. Patients who enter remission are then switched to oral cyclosporine dosed bid at a total daily dose twice that of the final IV dose. Oral cyclosporine is dosed to maintain drug levels of 200 to 350 ng/mL (RIA). Azathioprine or 6-MP should be started or optimized, and corticosteroids switched to oral dosing. Prophylaxis against Pneumocystis carinii pneumonia is advised. Over the subsequent 2 to 3 months, cyclosporine and corticosteroids are tapered off.

Cyclosporine is only intended for short-term use, with long-term maintenance of response via therapy with azathioprine or 6-MP. Patient intolerance of or refusal to take long-term immunosuppressive therapy precludes the use of cyclosporine. There are multiple serious potential side effects and contraindications to cyclosporine use, and dose-reduction is needed in patients with low serum cholesterol levels. Prior to using cyclosporine, providers are strongly encouraged to read the "user's guide" to cyclosporine.

Toxic Megacolon/Fulminant Colitis

Patients with fulminant colitis present with high fever, abdominal tenderness, abdominal distention, and anemia due to colonic blood loss. Rapid extension of inflammation through the bowel wall into the serosa may result in toxic megacolon manifested by colonic dilation and increasing signs of systemic toxicity. In patients with severe colitis, toxic megacolon may be precipitated by the use of narcotics, antidiarrheals, or anticholinergics; electrolyte abnormalities (particularly hypokalemia); or coexisting infection (*C. difficile* or cytomegalovirus). Colonoscopy or barium enema in patients with fulminant colitis may also precipitate toxic megacolon.

Patients with fulminant colitis/toxic megacolon should be referred immediately for colectomy. Patients should receive IV corticosteroids at a dose of 40 to 60 mg/d, and broad-spectrum antibiotic coverage should be started. Electrolytes and a complete blood cell count (CBC) should be followed at least daily and more frequently if circumstances warrant. Serial abdominal films should be obtained in patients with fulminant colitis to evaluate for colonic dilation or perforation. Hematocrit should be maintained with transfusion and coagulation abnormalities corrected. Patients should be maintained NPO with adequate supplementation of IV fluids. Frequent repositioning of the patient from supine to decubitus to prone positions (ie, "rolling technique") may help decompress the dilated colon through successful passage of trapped colonic gas.

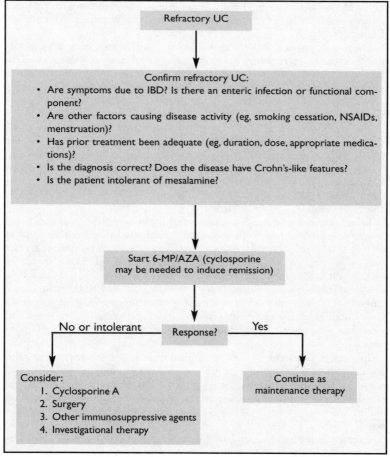

Figure 18-1. Algorithm for treatment of refractory ulcerative colitis.

Refractory Disease

Failure of medical therapy in ulcerative colitis may be classified as failure to either induce or maintain remission. Patients who respond to corticosteroids but are unable to discontinue them are termed steroid dependent, while those who remain active despite high-dose steroids are steroid refractory. Figure 18-1 presents an algorithm for treatment of refractory ulcerative colitis. First, the presence of active IBD should be reconfirmed by objective means. It is often helpful to perform a flexible sigmoidoscopy with biopsies to rule out other etiologies of colitis. For example, the presence of colonic pseudomembranes can suggest concomitant *C. difficile* infection. Abdominal cramping and diarrhea out of proportion to the level of observed inflammation may indicate a functional bowel disorder, which may be responsive to antispasmodics or antidiarrheals.

Once the presence of active UC has been established, prior attempts at therapy should be scrutinized to ensure that optimal doses of medication have been used for sufficient lengths of time to ensure an appropriate attempt at inducing and maintaining remission. Potential patient nonadherence with prescribed regimens (and the reasons) should be investigated. The appropriate duration for a therapeutic trial of a medication to induce remission of active disease varies depending on the clinical circumstance. Some cases of distal ulcerative colitis may take months to resolve on adequate therapy. On the other hand, in severe disease treated as an inpatient with IV corticosteroid therapy, remission should be expected in 7 to 10 days. In some cases in which mesalamine is used, an uncommon intolerance reaction occurs. If this is suspected, then a trial off of all 5-ASA compounds or a change to a different 5-ASA compound may be attempted.

Other factors that may affect disease activity in women include menstruation or pregnancy. Those with menstrual cycle related flares may respond to hormonal manipulation with oral contraceptive pills or disruption of menses with progesterone or leuprolide. In all patients, the use of NSAIDs should be discouraged as they may lead to increased disease activity. In ulcerative colitis, abrupt discontinuation or reduction of smoking can lead to flares in disease activity, which may respond to treatment with nicotine-containing agents. In some instances, short-term resumption of smoking may lead to remission and allow time for slower acting immunomodulators to become effective as maintenance therapy.

In cases of persistent disease, the clinical history of disease as well as prior evaluation should be carefully scrutinized for any signs indicating Crohn's disease. Careful review of family history for individuals with Crohn's disease, re-examination of pathology specimens, repeat physical exam with emphasis on findings of fistulous or small bowel disease, or ANCA and ASCA serologies may be useful in this regard.

Patients with steroid-dependent disease are often treated with 6-MP or azathioprine (6MP/AZA). Two strategies to dosing are start low and work up or start high. In strategy 1, patients are typically started at 50 to 100 mg of either agent and then slowly increased in dose (typically in 25 mg increments) over the course of the ensuing weeks to months while monitoring for evidence of hematologic or hepatic toxicity. Maximum dose is achieved when either the patients white blood cell count dips into the low-normal range, ANC approaches 2000, or at a "target" dose of 1.5 to 2.0 mg of 6-MP/kg body or 2.5 to 3.0 mg azathioprine/kg body weight. Benefits of this approach include safety and accurate assessment of side-effects, as many of the serious side effects and intolerances are dose-related. Drawbacks are the delay in time to reach "therapeutic" doses, prolonging exposure to corticosteroids, and the failure of many clinicians to appropriately increase the dose.

Strategy 2 requires initial testing of TPMT levels (available commercially) to exclude patients who are deficient for this enzyme and will develop profound pancytopenia. Then, 6-MP or AZA is started at the target levels as stated above. The benefits and drawbacks of this approach are the converse of those stated above for strategy 1.

In an attempt to further refine the dosing of these agents, metabolite levels of these drugs are now commercially available (most commonly through Prometheus Laboratories, San Diego, Calif). Recent studies in IBD patients suggest that levels of the 6-thioguanine (6-TGN) metabolite may correlate with efficacy, with a goal 6-TGN level of >235. However, not all studies agree. Until appropriate prospective analyses are completed in IBD patients, clinicians should be cautious in interpreting these levels. The 6-methylmercaptopurine (6-MMP) metabolite seems to correlate with hepatotoxicity, with a level of >5600 indicating the need for caution. Investigational studies of the therapeutic use of 6-TGN as a treatment for IBD, bypassing the 6-MMP metabolite and thus the idiosyncratic pancreatitis that some patients develop, are ongoing.

After initiating 6-MP or AZA, a steroid taper should be initiated after a few weeks, if the patient's disease allows. The speed and success of the taper may vary based on individual disease characteristics. A steroid taper should not be initiated if the patient is still flaring. The dose of 6-MP/AZA may be optimized over the next few weeks to months while the steroids are being tapered. Patients should not be considered "failures" of therapy with 6MP/AZA until they have been on adequate doses of these agents for at least 6 months.

Patients who are allergic, intolerant, or unresponsive to 6MP/AZA are often relegated to surgery, although referral to a specialized IBD center for consideration of more "investigational therapies" may be an option. Agents such as mycophenolate mofetil, tacrolimus, methotrexate, and infliximab have been tried with varying success, and novel agents may be available in the setting of controlled clinical trials.

Pouchitis

Modern surgical approaches to patients with ulcerative colitis have resulted in the construction of ileoanal pouches in many patients who have undergone proctocolectomy for refractory disease or the development of dysplasia or cancer, precluding the need for a permanent ileostomy. These ileal pouches, often referred to as a J, W, or S pouch, depending upon the anatomy utilized, are prone to developing inflammation or pouchitis. While mild cases occur in as many as 50% of patients with pouches, 5% to 10% of patients may develop chronic pouchitis.

Pouchitis is diagnosed by endoscopy with biopsy. It is often easiest to scope the pouch using an upper endoscope to allow comfortable passage through the surgically-constructed narrow ileal pouch-anal anastomosis. The use of a Fleets enema preparation allows for better visualization. The ileal pouch and the afferent ileal limb should be inspected and biopsied (in separate containers). The endoscopic appearance of pouchitis may be similar to that of Crohn's or ulcerative colitis, with erythema, edema, and ulcerations; however, true pouchitis should not extend into the proximal ileal limb. Disease proximal to the pouch is suggestive of Crohn's, as is the formation of perianal or anovaginal fistulas.

Stool samples should be sent for the usual pathogens (especially *C. difficile*). Pouchitis is usually responsive to a 2- to 4-week course of ciprofloxacin 500 mg po bid or metronidazole 250 to 500 mg po tid. Refractory cases may respond to combination therapy with the antibiotics or with agents such as topical mesalamine or corticosteroids (similar to the approach used in ulcerative proctitis). Other agents such as systemic corticosteroids, AZA, 6-MP, cyclosporine, tacrolimus, and infliximab have been used in some instances. Surgical removal of the pouch with permanent ileostomy is a last resort.

Successfully treated pouchitis may require "maintenance" therapy with these same agents in patients who are prone to relapse. Maintenance of "remission" has also been successfully shown with the probiotic formulation VSL#3, and other probiotic agents are currently undergoing investigation.

CROHN'S DISEASE

A thorough clinical history and review of the patient's laboratory, endoscopic, radiologic, and histologic examinations is important to formulate an appropriate treatment plan for the patient with Crohn's disease. Focus should be on defining the location of disease, severity of disease, intestinal complications (such as stricture, fistula, or abscess), extra-intestinal manifestations (skin, joints, eye, liver), and nutritional status.

The clinical approach to patients with various presentations of Crohn's disease is detailed below.

Ileocolitis/Colitis (Figure 18-2)

First line therapy for patients with Crohn's colitis is identical for that of ulcerative colitis, and the reader is referred to the previous section for details. Patients with ileocolitis are preferentially treated with a mesalamine-based agent that releases in both small and large bowel, typically Pentasa (Shire US, Newport, Ky), although Asacol (Proctor and Gamble, Cincinnati, Ohio) may also be effective in certain individuals. Topical therapies may be effective in patients with distal colonic and rectal Crohn's. The dose of the aminosalicylates required for the induction and maintenance of remission are typically higher in Crohn's than in UC patients.

Antibiotics are thought to be effective alternative first-line therapies in some Crohn's patients. If patients do not improve on aminosalicylate therapy, metronidazole (10 to 20 mg/kg/d po) or ciprofloxacin (500 mg po bid) may be added. If patients improve within 2 to 4 weeks on the antibiotic, the dose may be tapered over the ensuing weeks to months, although some patients may require long-term use of antibiotics for their disease.

If patients do not improve on the first-line therapies, corticosteroids are typically added at an initial dose of 20 to 40 mg/d. Patients who respond should be tapered off of steroids over 2 to 3 months as described in the previous section on ulcerative colitis. The Entocort EC budesonide formulation recently released in the United States has been shown to be effective in Crohn's disease affecting the ileum and right colon and is preferable to conventional corticosteroids due to a reduced side-effect profile. Budesonide is initially start-

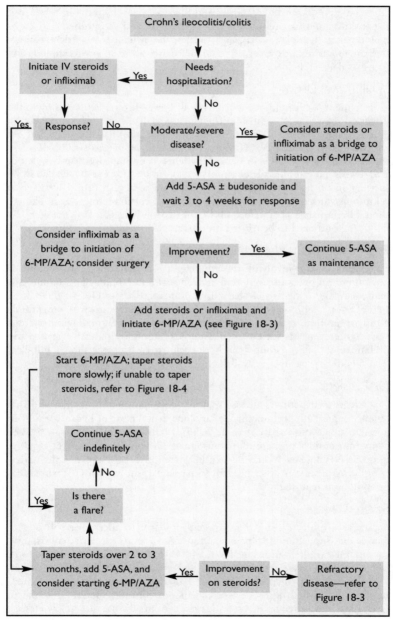

Figure 18-2. Algorithm for treatment of Crohn's ileocolitis/colitis.

ed at 9 mg po qd for 8 to 10 weeks and then decreased by 3 mg intervals over the ensuing months. Steroids are often ineffective and inappropriate to use as maintenance therapies, so patients need to be switched to other therapies. Infliximab has recently emerged as an alternative agent to corticosteroids and its use is detailed below.

Small Bowel Disease.

In patients with mild to moderate small bowel disease, Pentasa is often the preferred mesalamine agent due to its guaranteed release in the small bowel. Asacol releases at a pH of 7 and is thought to be appropriate for some, but not all, patients with distal ileal Crohn's. Mesalamine often needs to be dosed in the 3.0 to 4.8 g/day range in Crohn's patients. If no improvement is noted in 2 to 4 weeks, metronidazole or ciprofloxacin can be added as detailed above in the section on ileocolitis/colitis. If no response is seen in 2 to 4 weeks or if symptoms worsen, then budesonide, traditional corticosteroids, or infliximab should be initiated as described above for ileocolitis/colitis. Patients who still fail to respond need to be treated for refractory disease.

Esophagogastroduodenal Disease

Crohn's disease involving the esophagus, stomach, and/or duodenum is uncommon. A previously reported incidence of only 5% may be an underestimate, as many patients may have asymptomatic disease. Due to their distal sites of release, aminosalicylates are not helpful. Monotherapy with omeprazole 40 mg/d has been reported to be helpful in inducing and maintaining remission. Systemic agents such as corticosteroids, immunosuppressive agents, and infliximab are often required and have been used with some success but clear data on efficacy are not yet available.

Oral Lesions

Patients with Crohn's disease may develop aphthous stomatitis and oral lesions. Topical application of triamcinolone dental paste or hydrocortisone in a pectin or gelatin carrier may be helpful. If the disease persists, a 1-week course of steroids (20 mg/d of prednisone or a Medrol [Pharmacia & Upjohn, Peapack, NJ] dose pack) may be helpful. Systemic therapy aimed at the underlying bowel disease is often needed. In particular, success with infliximab has recently been reported.

Severe Disease

Severe Crohn's disease may present similarly to ulcerative colitis with bloody diarrhea, abdominal pain, and fever. As in severe ulcerative colitis, indications for hospitalization are fever >40°C, hypotension, dehydration, >10 stools per day, severe rectal bleeding, and abdominal tenderness/distension. Once infection is ruled out, IV steroid therapy such as 40 mg/d of prednisolone in divided doses or as a continuous infusion should be initiated. Cyclosporine is infrequently used in severe Crohn's disease due to low efficacy rates, safety concerns, and the availability of infliximab.

Infliximab therapy may be effective once infection (abscess, enteric infection) is ruled out. At a dose of 5 mg/kg of body weight, median response and remission times of 1 to 2 weeks have been reported. Given the mean 2- to 3-month duration of response and remission, most patients need reinfusions of the agent. Concerns over the formation of antibodies to the chimeric agent with subsequent loss of efficacy has convinced many specialists to infuse infliximab at 0, 2, and 6 weeks, and then at 8-week intervals. Dose escalation to 10 mg/kg may be needed in occasional patients who lose efficacy with the 5 mg/kg dose. Practice guidelines with this novel agent may change over time, and the reader is encouraged to update this information frequently.

Refractory Disease (Figure 18-3)

The evaluation and treatment of refractory Crohn's patients is similar to that for ulcerative colitis (see previous section), with a few notable exceptions. The first is the influence of cigarette smoking. Most studies have shown a relationship between cigarette smoking and refractory or recurrent Crohn's disease (the same probably holds true for smoking other tobacco products, and perhaps for chewing tobacco). All Crohn's disease patients should be strongly encouraged to stop smoking.

There are also a few differences in the therapeutic approach to the patient with refractory Crohn's disease (Table 18-3) compared to the approach to refractory ulcerative colitis. While AZA or 6-MP is typically used for steroid-dependent or steroid-refractory disease, Crohn's patients who are intolerant, allergic, or unresponsive to these agents may be switched from the purine analogues to treatment with methotrexate (MTX). MTX is initially dosed at 25 mg intramuscularly or subcutaneously (sc) every week and is effective at inducing and maintaining remission in Crohn's patients. Frequent monitoring of hepatic function tests and complete blood and platelet counts (monthly at first, then every 3 months) and daily supplementation with folic acid (1 mg orally) is advised. Side effects such as nausea, headache, and fatigue are often transient and responsive to 25% to 50% dose reductions.

MTX's onset of action is typically 1 to 3 months, and steroids should be tapered slowly over this time period. If remission and steroid withdrawal are successful with MTX, it is continued as a maintenance therapy at a dose of 15 to 25 mg/week. Due to the extremely rare incidence of liver pathology, liver biopsies after each 1.5 g cumulative dose are no longer routinely required but need to be checked if there is suspicion for potential hepatotoxicity. Patients at risk for liver fibrosis, such as diabetics, obese patients, those being treated with other potentially hepatotoxic medications, or those with underlying liver disease, should not be treated with MTX.

Infliximab is a chimeric monoclonal antibody to TNF-a that has been shown to be effective in the treatment of refractory Crohn's disease through multiple randomized, placebo-controlled trials. In cases of refractory disease, infliximab is used in patients whose disease has not responded to optimal doses of immunomodulatory agents such as 6-MP/AZA after an appropriate duration of therapy. In patients with moderate to severe symptoms who cannot comfortably wait several months to achieve remission, infliximab has been advocated as a bridge to the ini-

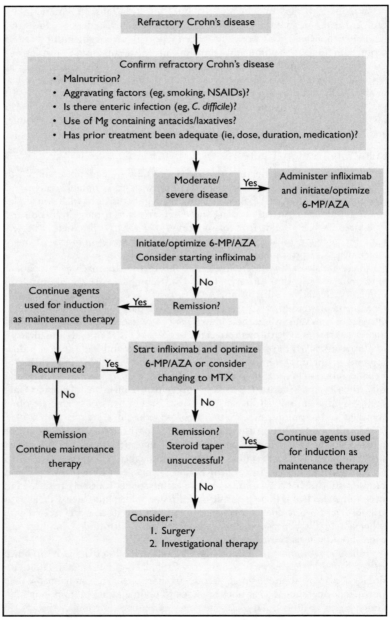

Figure 18-3. Treatment algorithm for refractory Crohn's disease.

Table 18-3

MEDICAL THERAPY FOR
REFRACTORY CROHN'S DISEASE

Medication	Dose	Typical Response Time	Side Effects
6-MP/AZA	Low: 50 mg/d titrate upward High: 1.5 to 2.0 mg/kg/d 6-MP or 2.0 to 2.5 mg/kg/d AZA	2 to 6 months	Uncommon: leukopenia, nausea, pancreatitis, fevers, arthralgias, hepatitis
Methotrexate	25 mg im/sc every week	2 to 4 months	Common: nausea, diarrhea, stomatitis, leukopenia, hair loss Rare: hypersensitivity pneumonitis, transaminase elevations, hepatic fibrosis
Infliximab	5 mg/kg IV every 8 weeks or as needed	1 to 2 weeks	Uncommon: headache, nausea, upper respiratory tract infection, hypersensitivity reactions

tiation of slower acting immunomodulatory agents. However, the realization that many of these patients require repeat infliximab infusions and that prolonging the time between the infusions increases the risk of the development of antibodies to the agent and intolerance and/or diminished response to subsequent infusions have resulted in the gradual adoption of an initial series of one to three infusions of 5 mg/kg IV at 0, 2, and 6 weeks and then repeat infusions every 8 weeks (6 to 12 weeks) afterward in many patients.

If the patient continues to have active disease despite therapy with immunomodulatory agents and infliximab, surgical therapy should be considered. This is covered in detail in other chapters in this book. As Crohn's disease typically recurs after surgery, postoperative prophylaxis is advised in many patients, as detailed below. Alternatively, there are a number of experimental therapies that are undergoing investigation.

Postoperative Prophylaxis

Given enough time, Crohn's disease inevitably recurs after surgical resection, typically at the proximal side of the surgical anastomosis. There are a few notable exceptions; most (but not all) patients with Crohn's colitis do not experience disease recurrence following a total proctocolectomy with end-ileostomy. Some Crohn's perianal fistulas never recur after corrective surgery, and occasionally some other Crohn's patients appear to be long-term surgical cures. Cigarette smoking again arises as a very strong risk factor for early postoperative recurrence of disease.

The decision to treat a Crohn's patient prophylactically following surgery should be based on the location of disease, previous severity of disease, disease type (penetrating or fistulizing disease seems particularly likely to recur sooner), previous bowel resections, amount of remaining healthy small bowel, and the efficacy (and risks) of the medications.

The most benign postoperative prophylactic therapy is mesalamine. High-dose mesalamine (3 g or more daily) has been shown to be effective in delaying symptomatic postoperative recurrence in patients with ileal Crohn's disease, although the effect is modest (at best) and the number of pills (up to 16 daily) difficult to justify in many cases.

Low dose 6-MP (50 mg daily) has been shown to be superior to mesalamine and placebo in preventing symptomatic, endoscopic, and radiographic postoperative recurrence in ileal Crohn's disease. Higher doses of 6-MP or AZA may be more effective, as may infliximab, MTX, and other immunomodulatory agents, but these have yet to be formally studied. Metronidazole given at 20 mg/kg for the first 3 months following ileal resection also showed a trend toward delayed postoperative recurrence of disease, but its limited efficacy and high rate of side effects have shifted attention toward other antibiotics (such as ornidazol) and probiotics.

Fistulous/Perianal Disease

The formation of fistulas in IBD is unique to Crohn's patients and may lead to the reclassification of a previous "ulcerative colitis" diagnosis. Up to one third of Crohn's patients may develop fistulas. It is helpful to consider two main subtypes of fistulas when evaluating and treating these patients: perianal and internal fistulas. In all instances, involvement of an experienced surgeon in the evaluation of the refractory fistula patient is advised.

Perianal fistulas typically start at the anorectal junction at the dentate line. They often exit in the perianal, perineal, or gluteal region but may also involve the nearby scrotum or vaginal vestibule. Fistulas may drain mucus, pus, blood, stool, or simply air and often close intermittently. Fistulas that fail to exit may result in perianal abscesses. Careful examination (often under anesthesia) to exclude an abscess should be considered in patients with initial presentation or worsening of their perianal disease.

The treatment of fistulas is detailed in Table 18-4 and Figure 18-4. First-line therapies include ciprofloxacin 500 mg po bid or metronidazole 250 to 500 mg po tid to qid, with the addition of the second antibiotic if the first proves ineffective. Successful fistula closures may allow for gradual tapering of these agents, although many patients require chronic antibiotic therapy. Patients with fistulas that fail to close or stay closed are often treated with AZA or 6-MP, as detailed in previous sections. Infliximab infusions (5 mg/kg) at 0, 2, and 6 weeks are effective in closing most fistulas, although repeat infusions (every 8 weeks or sooner if needed) are often necessary and increasingly being given as a maintenance strategy. Other agents that have been used with success include cyclosporine (limited by toxicity and failure to maintain fistula closure), tacrolimus, and MTX. Maintenance therapy with the agent utilized to close the fistulas is advised. Experimental therapies with other immunomodulatory agents and approaches such as hyperbaric oxygen have had mixed success. There are no data supporting the efficacy of aminosalicylates or corticosteroids in the treatment of fistulizing Crohn's disease, although select patients seem to benefit from rectally applied mesalamine or steroid preparations. Some clinical trials have shown a trend toward worse outcomes with systemic corticosteroid therapy, which also may adversely impact postsurgical healing.

Internal fistulas often start at a diseased section of bowel just proximal to a Crohn's stricture and may connect to a variety of locations, most commonly another section of bowel, another internal organ such as the bladder, or the skin, often along a previous scar tract. If the fistula cannot drain into another organ or drain exteriorly, an abscess may result. There are little data on pharmacological therapy of internal fistulas other than for enterocutaneous fistulas, which may be treated similarly to perianal fistulas. However, patients with internal fistulas often are already surgical candidates due to severe Crohn's strictures. Serious consideration should be given to proceeding directly to surgical resection and closure of the fistulous tract.

EXPERIMENTAL AGENTS

Due to the chronic, relapsing nature of IBD, the unacceptable side-effect profile of long-term corticosteroids, and the realization that certain individuals do not have an adequate response to the medications previously discussed in this chapter, new agents are constantly being sought. Some represent adaptations of currently available drugs used in other disease states, while others are novel, experimental therapies.

Existing Immunomodulatory Agents

The use of agents such as mycophenolate mofetil, tacrolimus, and thioguanine has already been discussed. Thalidomide, leflunomide, cyclophosphamide, penicillamine, pentoxifylline, and hydroxychloroquine have also been utilized in some instances. Although initially touted as a possible alterna-

Table 18-4

MEDICAL THERAPY OF FISTULIZING CROHN'S DISEASE

Medication	Dose*	Typical Response Time	Side Effects
Metronidazole	10 to 20 mg/kg/d in divided doses	2 to 8 weeks	Common: peripheral neuropathy/ paresthesias, dyspepsia, metallic taste, disulfiram-like effect
Ciprofloxacin	1 g/d dosed bid	2 to 8 weeks	Rare: seizures, photosensitivity, tendon rupture
6-MP/AZA	Low: 50 mg/d, titrate upward High: 1.5 to 2.0 mg/kg/d 6-MP or 2.0 to 2.5 mg/kg/d AZA	2 to 6 months	Uncommon: leukopenia, nausea, pancreatitis, fevers, arthralgias, hepatitis
Cyclosporine	4 mg/kg IV as a continuous infusion converted to 4 mg/kg po bid	3 to 14 days	Common: hypertension, nephrotoxicity Uncommon: seizures, leukopenia, infections
Infliximab	5 mg/kg IV at weeks 0, 2, 6 and then as needed	3 to 14 days	Uncommon: headache, nausea, upper respiratory tract infection, hypersensitivity reactions

*See text for dosing details and warnings.

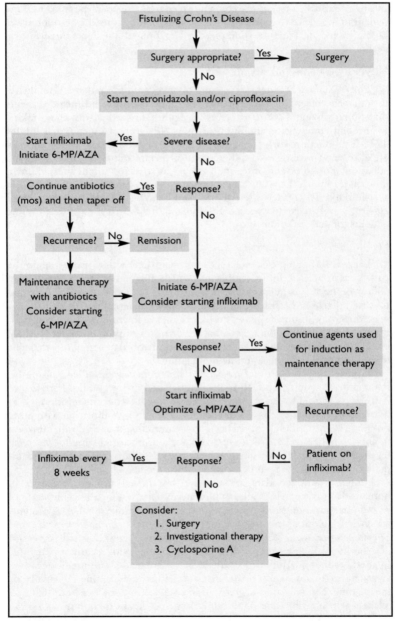

Figure 18-4. Algorithm for treatment of fistulizing Crohn's disease.

tive to infliximab, a recent placebo-controlled trial of etanercept failed to show benefit in moderate-to-severe Crohn's patients, highlighting the need for placebo-controlled data before widespread adaptation of these potentially toxic agents.

Novel Investigational Agents

There seems to be a constant stream of novel agents as potential candidates for effective therapy in IBD patients. The most recent trend includes agents directly targeted at TNF-α, either as antibodies directed against the cytokine or through competitive inhibition of the TNF receptor. Agents that inhibit TNF-α production, such as pentoxifylline or thalidomide (and its conjugates), are also being investigated. Other types of therapies include those targeting adhesion molecules and integrins such as interferons, interleukins, human growth hormone, heparins, nicotine-containing agents, and novel steroid preparations. The reader is referred to the Crohn's and Colitis Foundation of America's web page (www.ccfa.org) for a current listing of sites enrolling patients for various studies.

Probiotics

There is intriguing evidence that intestinal bacteria may play a role in the pathogenesis of IBD. In susceptible individuals, inflammation may result from failure of normal regulatory constraints to the mucosal immune response toward indigenous enteric bacteria. Most current therapies for IBD act to suppress the host immune response. Probiotics are live micro-organisms that modify the intestinal microflora. Potential mechanisms of probiotic effect include competitive interactions, production of antimicrobial metabolites, dialogue with the epithelium, and immune modulation.

Bacterial species such as *Lactobacillus* and *Bifidobacterium* have no proinflammatory capacity and thus are often used as probiotics. Strains of *Escherichia coli* and *Enterococcus*, as well as nonbacterial organisms such as *Saccharomyces boulardii*, have also been used, often in combination with other probiotic agents. Probiotics are effective in controlling intestinal inflammation in animal models of IBD such as IL-10 knockout mice and lymphocyte transfer models. Probiotics may also diminish the rate of progression from inflammation to dysplasia to colon cancer in animal models.

Limited controlled data are available on the efficacy of probiotics in humans. In two separate studies in ulcerative colitis, a nonpathogenic strain of *E. coli* was found to exhibit efficacy similar to that of mesalamine. A probiotic cocktail containing strains of *Lactobacillus*, *Bifidobacterium*, and *Streptococcus salivarus thermophilus* (VSL#3) showed significant efficacy versus placebo in the maintenance of remission in patients with recurrent pouchitis. In another randomized trial, 32 patients with Crohn's disease in remission were allocated to maintenance treatment with either mesalamine 3 g daily or mesalamine 2 g daily plus a preparation of *Saccharomyces boulardii*. Clinical relapses at 6 months were significantly less frequent in the group taking the probiotic agent. Despite these favorable results, it is unlikely that a single probiotic agent will be effective in all individuals with IBD as different bacteria may contribute to the persistence of intestinal inflammation in different patients. Commercially available probiotic agents abound, but the lack of regulation on these products makes it difficult to rely on claims that these products contain the exact organisms, in the specific concentrations advertised, and that the contents are still viable. More rigorous controlled studies on the efficacy of probiotics are needed to determine the efficacy of different preparations on different populations of patients.

CONCLUSION

Due to its idiopathic nature and varied presentations, the approach to the treatment of IBD may be challenging and perhaps daunting. Identification of the location and severity of the disease process, exclusion of symptoms that may in fact be due to coexistent infections or other noninflammatory etiologies, and then subsequent application of medical therapies appropriate for each patient's condition will hopefully lead to successful induction and maintenance of disease remission. The methodological approach discussed in this chapter will aid the physician in utilizing the safest, effective agents in each case. While the armamentarium of treatment options will likely continue to grow in the future, the majority of patients should expect to do well with the currently available therapies and lead productive, comfortable lives.

BIBLIOGRAPHY

Bitton A, Peppercorn MA. Medical management of specific clinical presentations. *Gastroenterol Clin North Am.* 1995;24(3):541-558.

Chung PY, Cohen RD. Evolving medical therapies for ulcerative colitis. *Curr Gastroenterol Rep.* 2001;3(6):464-470.

Cohen RD, Stein R, Hanauer SB. Intravenous cyclosporine in ulcerative colitis: a five-year experience. *Am J Gastroenterol.* 1999;94(6):1587-1592.

Cohen RD, Woseth DM, Thisted RA, Hanauer SB. A meta-analysis and overview of the literature on treatment options for left-sided ulcerative colitis and ulcerative proctitis. *Am J Gastroenterol.* 2000;95(5):1263-1276.

Cuffari C, Hunt S, Bayless T. Utilization of erythrocyte 6-thioguanine metabolite levels to optimize azathioprine therapy in patients with inflammatory bowel disease. *Gut.* 2001;48(5):642-646.

Dubinsky MC, Lamothe S, Yang HY, et al. Pharmacogenomics and metabolite measurement for 6-mercaptopurine therapy in inflammatory bowel disease. *Gastroenterology.* 2000;118(4):705-713.

Ehrenpreis ED, Kane SV, Cohen LB, Cohen RD, Hanauer SB. Thalidomide therapy for patients with refractory Crohn's disease: an open-label trial. *Gastroenterology.* 1999;117(6):1271-1277.

Feagan BG, Fedorak RN, Irvine EJ, et al. A comparison of methotrexate with placebo for the maintenance of remission in Crohn's disease. North American Crohn's Study Group Investigators. *N Engl J Med.* 2000;342(22):1627-1632.

Feagan BG, Rochon J, Fedorak RN, et al. Methotrexate for the treatment of Crohn's disease. The North American Crohn's Study Group Investigators. *N Engl J Med.* 1995;332(5):292-297.

Greenberg GR, Feagan BG, Martin F, et al. Oral budesonide for active Crohn's disease. Canadian Inflammatory Bowel Disease Study Group. *N Engl J Med.* 1994;331(13):836-841.

Hanauer SB. Inflammatory bowel disease. *N Engl J Med.* 1996;334(13):841-848.

Hanauer SB, Dassopoulos T. Evolving treatment strategies for inflammatory bowel disease. *Annu Rev Med.* 2001;52:299-318.

Hanauer SB, Feagan BG, Lichtenstein GR, et al. Maintenance infliximab for Crohn's disease: the ACCENT I randomized trial. *Lancet.* 2002;359(9317):1541-1549.

Kornbluth A, Present DH, Lichtiger S, Hanauer S. Cyclosporine for severe ulcerative colitis: a user's guide. *Am J Gastroenterol.* 1997;92(9):1424-1428.

Lichtenstein GR. Treatment of fistulizing Crohn's disease. *Gastroenterology.* 2000;119(4):1132-1147.

Lichtenstein GR. Approach to corticosteroid-dependent and corticosteroid-refractory Crohn's disease. *Inflamm Bowel Dis.* 2001;7 (Suppl 1):S23-S29.

Lichtiger S, Present DH, Kornbluth A, et al. Cyclosporine in severe ulcerative colitis refractory to steroid therapy. *N Engl J Med.* 1994;330:1841-1845.

Mahadevan U, Sandborn WJ. Evolving medical therapies for Crohn's disease. *Curr Gastroenterol Rep.* 2001;3(6):471-476.

Prakash A, Markham A. Oral delayed-release mesalazine: a review of its use in ulcerative colitis and Crohn's disease. *Drugs.* 1999;57(3):383-408.

Present DH, Korelitz BI, Wisch N, Glass JL, Sachar DB, Pasternack BS. Treatment of Crohn's disease with 6-mercaptopurine: a long-term, randomized, double-blind study. *N Engl J Med.* 1980;302(18):981-987.

Present DH, Rutgeerts P, Targan S, et al. Infliximab for the treatment of fistulas in patients with Crohn's disease. *N Engl J Med.* 1999;340(18):1398-1405.

Sandborn WJ, Hanauer SB. Antitumor necrosis factor therapy for inflammatory bowel disease: a review of agents, pharmacology, clinical results, and safety. *Inflamm Bowel Dis.* 1999;5(2):119-133.

Sands BE. Therapy of inflammatory bowel disease. *Gastroenterology.* 2000;118(2 Suppl 1):S68-S82.

Schwartz DA, Pemberton JH, Sandborn WJ. Diagnosis and treatment of perianal fistulas in Crohn disease. *Ann Intern Med.* 2001;135(10):906-918.

Targan SR, Hanauer SB, van Deventer SJ, et al. A short-term study of chimeric monoclonal antibody cA2 to tumor necrosis factor alpha for Crohn's disease. Crohn's Disease cA2 Study Group. *N Engl J Med.* 1997;337(15):1029-1035.

INDEX

Build Your Library

Along with this title, we publish numerous products on a variety of topics. We are sure that you will find the title below to be an essential addition to your library. Order your copies today or contact us for a copy of our latest catalog for additional product information.

THE CLINICIAN'S GUIDE TO INFLAMMATORY BOWEL DISEASE

Gary R. Lichtenstein, MD

400 pp., Soft Cover, 2003, ISBN 1-55642-554-6, Order #75546, $45.00

Inside this state-of-the-art guide, you will find line drawings and photos, tables, algorithms, and bulleted text with key facts. Some topics that are covered inside this essential learning tool are Epidemiology, Disease Modifiers, Extraintestinal Manifestations, Nutrition, Pregnancy & Fertility, Surgical & Medical Therapy, as well as Considerations for the Pediatric and Adolescent patients.

Contact us at

SLACK Incorporated, Professional Book Division
6900 Grove Road, Thorofare, NJ 08086
1-800-257-8290/1-856-848-1000, Fax: 1-856-853-5991
E-Mail: orders@slackinc.com or www.slackbooks.com

ORDER FORM

QUANTITY	TITLE	ORDER #	PRIC
	The Clinician's Guide to Inflammatory Bowel Disease	75546	$45.
		Subtotal	$
		Applicable state and local tax will be added to your purchase	$
		Handling	$4.5
		Total	$

Name _____

Address: _____

City: _____ State:_____ Zip: _____

Phone:_____ Fax_____

Email: _____

•

• Check enclosed (Payable to SLACK Incorporated)_____

• Charge my: ___ [American Express] ___ [VISA] ___ [MasterCard]

Account #: _____

Exp. date: _____ Signature _____

NOTE: Prices are subject to chang without notice.
Shipping charges will apply.
Shipping and handling charges are Non-Returnable.

CODE: 328